Antihypertensives

ACE inhibitors	Fetal renal failure teratogenic (3% risk)	Avoid nifedipine	Methyldopa	Captopril safe
Methyldopa	Nil known	Best 1st line	N/A	Safe
β-Blockers	Possible IUGR if early	Caution, 3rd line	Methyldopa	Safe
Ca antagonists	Nil known	Best 2nd line (e.g. nifedipine)	N/A	Safe
Thiazide diuretics	Maternal hypovolaemia. Fetal thrombocytopenia.	Avoid	Methyldopa	Safe

Fundamentals: severe hypertension in pregnancy is common and life threatening and requires treatment. Avoid ACE inhibitors prenatally

Endocrine/ hormone treatments

Thyroid hormone	Replacement therapy	Use if indicated	N/A	Safe
Propylthiouracil	Fetal hypothyroidism (rare).	Use, minimum dose	N/A	Monitor thyroid
Carbimazole	Fetal hypothyroidism (rare), aplasia cutis	Use, minimum dose	Propylthiouracil	Monitor thyroid
Insulin	Replacement therapy, maternal hypoglycaemia	Use with usual precautions	N/A	Safe
Metformin	probably safe, little data	Caution.	Insulin	safe

Fundamentals: treatment of underlying disease greatly reduces maternal and fetal risks.

Immunosuppresants

Ciclosporin	Nil known	Continue, monitor levels	N/A	Probably safe
Azathioprine	Minimal	Continue if indicated	N/A	Safe
Prednisolone	No fetal effects	Use minimum dose	N/A	Safe
	Maternal gestational diabetes, hypertension			

Fundamentals: treatment of underlying disease (e.g. transplant) imperative and reduces maternal and, therefore, fetal risks.

Oxford Handbook of
Obstetrics and Gynaecology

Third Edition WITHDRAWN

Edited by

Sally Collins

Specialist Registrar in Obstetrics and Gynaecology,
The John Radcliffe Hospital,
Oxford, UK

Sabaratnam Arulkumaran

Professor of Obstetrics and Gynaecology,
St George's Hospital Medical School,
University of London, UK

Kevin Hayes

Senior Lecturer/Honorary Consultant in Obstetrics
and Gynaecology, and Medical Education,
St George's Hospital Medical School,
University of London, UK

Simon Jackson

Consultant Gynaecologist,
The John Radcliffe Hospital,
Oxford, UK

Lawrence Impey

Consultant in Obstetrics and Fetal Medicine,
The John Radcliffe Hospital,
Oxford, UK

OXFORD
UNIVERSITY PRESS

OXFORD
UNIVERSITY PRESS

Great Clarendon Street, Oxford, OX2 6DP,
United Kingdom

Oxford University Press is a department of the University of Oxford.
It furthers the University's objective of excellence in research, scholarship,
and education by publishing worldwide. Oxford is a registered trade mark of
Oxford University Press in the UK and in certain other countries

First edition published 2005
Second edition published 2008
Third edition published 2013

Impression: 10

Reprinted 2013 ,2014 ,2015 ,2016 ,2017 ,2018 ,2019 ,2020

British Library Cataloguing in Publication Data
Data available

ISBN 978–0–19–969840–0

Printed in China by
C&C Offset Printing Co. Ltd.

Contents

Preface

Welcome to the third edition of this Oxford Handbook. In obstetrics and gynaecology, as in all fields of medicine, the available evidence, technology and guidelines can move forward at a rapid pace and often prove difficult to keep up with. As the majority of junior doctors are well aware, the gaps in our knowledge often become apparent at the most inopportune moments; this book seeks to fill those gaps rapidly and effectively. It uses the well-known Oxford Handbook format to facilitate easy navigation around concise, clinically relevant, evidence-based information. It can be quickly dipped into for specific answers between seeing patients in clinic or on delivery suite, as well as providing a solid, general grounding for those just beginning in the specialty. It also has sufficient depth and detail to provide a good starting point in the preparation for postgraduate exams. To ensure the most up-to-date information is always available, emphasis has been placed on providing relevant web addresses, especially for guidelines and useful organizations. Text boxes have also been employed to help highlight some of the more important pieces of information.

Although this handbook is most likely to be used by trainees within the specialty, we envisage it will be useful for all those involved in women's health, including GPs, midwives, and medical students. We hope you find it a helpful resource and that it proves to be a valuable companion and guide in your everyday practice of obstetrics and gynaecology.

Acknowledgements

We would like to thank all our second edition authors, especially the trainees at the John Radcliffe and St George's hospitals. Additionally, we are very grateful to those who have gone the extra mile to ensure that our third edition chapters are up to date, especially Charlotte Bennett, Lucy MacKillop, and Jo Morrison who reviewed the highly specialized areas of neonatology, maternal medicine, and oncology to ensure that they contained the best available evidence. We would also like to thank the doctors of all grades who anonymously reviewed some of the text, providing valuable feedback and further fine-tuning the finished manuscript. To conform to the Oxford Handbook style and to avoid overlap and repetition, some contributions have been considerably edited and we thank all our authors for their understanding. We are most grateful to Prof. Basky Thilaganathan for providing many of the ultrasound images and Ms Penny Trotter for the colposcopy pictures. Last, but definitely not least, we would like to thank our partners and families who continue to remain so patient and supportive throughout this project, especially Berni O'Connor 'for doing all the real work on the home front' and David Reynard 'for putting up with all this'.

Sally Collins, Sabaratnam Arulkumaran,
Kevin Hayes, Simon Jackson, and Lawrence Impey
London and Oxford, October 2012

Abbreviations

1°	primary
2°	secondary
+ve	positive
−ve	negative
A&E	Accident and Emergency
AA	Alcoholics Anonymous
AAT	aspartate aminotransferase
ABC	airway, breathing, and circulation
ABG	arterial blood gases
AC	abdominal circumference
ACE	angiotensin converting enzyme
ACEI	angiotensin-converting enzyme inhibitor
ACL	anticardiolipin
ACTH	adrenocorticotrophic hormone
ADH	antidiuretic hormone
AEDF	absent end diastolic flow
AF	atrial fibrillation
AFE	amniotic fluid embolism
AFI	amniotic fluid index
AFLP	acute fatty liver of pregnancy
AFP	alpha-fetoprotein
AIN	peri-anal intraepithelial neoplasia
AIS	androgen insensitivity syndrome
AJCC	American Joint Committee on Cancer
ALP	alkaline phosphatase
ALT	alanine transaminase
AMH	antimüllerian hormone
AN	antenatal
ANA	antinuclear antibody
APH	antepartum haemorrhage

APR	Antiretroviral Pregnancy Registry
APS	antiphospholipid syndrome
APTT	activated partial thromboplastin time
ARDS	adult respiratory distress syndrome
AREDF	absent/reversed end diastolic flow
ARM	artificial rupture of membranes
ART	assisted reproductive technologies
ASD	atrial septal defect
ASIS	anterior superior iliac spines
AST	aspartate amniotransferase
AVM	arteriovenous malformation
AWE	aceto-white epithelium
AXR	abdominal X-ray
BCE	Bacillus Calmette–Guerin
bd	twice daily
BEP	bleomycin, etoposide, and cisplatin
BFHI	Baby-Friendly Hospital Initiative
BM	blood sugar monitoring
BMD	bone mineral density
BMI	body mass index
BOTS	Borderline Ovarian Tumour Study
BP	blood pressure
BPD	biparietal diameter
BRCA	breast cancer gene
BSO	bilateral salpingo-oophrectomy
BV	bacterial vaginosis
CA125	cancer antigen 125
CAH	congenital adrenal hyperplasia
CAIS	complete androgen insensitivity syndrome
cART	combination antiretroviral therapy
CBAVD	congenital bilateral absence of the vas deferens
CBT	cognitive-behavioural therapy
CCAM	congenital cystic adenomatoid malformation
CCT	controlled cord traction

CEA	carcinoembryonic antigen
CEMACH	Confidential Enquiry into Maternal and Child Health
CEMD	Confidential Enquiry into Maternal Deaths
CESDI	Confidential Enquiry into Stillbirths and Deaths in Infancy
CF	cystic fibrosis
CFTR	cystic fibrosis transmembrane conductance regulation
cGIN	cervical glandular intraepithelial neoplasia
CHD	congenital heart disease
CIN	cervical intraepithelial neoplasia
CL	corpus luteum
CMACE	Centre for Maternal and Child Enquiries
CMV	cytomegalovirus
CNS	central nervous sytem
CNST	Clinical Negligence Scheme for Trusts
COCP	combined oral contraceptive pill
CP	cerebral palsy
CPP	chronic pelvic pain
CPR	cardiopulmonary resuscitation
CrHD	coronary heart disease
CRL	crown–rump length
CRP	C-reactive protein
CS	Caesarean section
CSE	combined spinal epidural
CSF	cerebrospinal fluid
CT	computed tomography
CTG	cardiotocography
CV	cyclophosphamide and vincristine
CVA	cerebrovascular accident
CVD	cardiovascular disease
CVP	central venous pressure
CVS	chorionic villus sampling
CXR	chest X-ray
DCDA	dichorionic, diamniotic
DES	diethylstilbestrol

DH	Department of Health
DHEAS	dehydroepiand osterone sulphate
DIC	disseminated intravascular coagulation
DO	detrusor overactivity
DOA	direct occipito-anterior
DOL	direct occipito-lateral
dRVVT	Dilute Russell Viper Venom Test
DSD	disorders of sex development
DUB	dysfunctional uterine bleeding
DVT	deep vein thrombosis
EAS	external anal sphincter
EBRT	external beam radiotherapy
EBV	Epstein–Barr virus
EC	emergency contraception
ECG	electrocardiograph
ECOG	Eastern Cooperative Oncology Group
ECT	electroconvulsive therapy
ECV	external cephalic version
ED	erectile dysfunction
EDD	expected date of delivery
EFM	electronic fetal monitoring
EFW	estimated fetal weight
EGFR	epidermal growth factor receptor
EIA	enzyme immunoassay
EL	elevated liver enzymes
EMA	etoposide, methotrexate, and dactinomycin
EOC	epithelial ovarian cancer
EP	ectopic pregnancy
EPAU	early pregnancy assessment unit
EPDS	Edinburgh Postnatal Depression Scale
EPU	early pregnancy unit
ERCP	endoscopic reterograde cholangio-pancreatography
ERPC	evacuation of retained products of conception

ESR	erythrocyte sedimentation rate
ET	endometrial thickness
ETT	endotracheal tube
EUA	examination under anaesthetic
FBC	full blood count
FDA	Food and Drug Administration
FDP	fibrin degradation product
FETO	fetoscopic tracheal occlusion
FEV_1	forced expiratory volume in 1s
FFN	fetal fibronectin
FFP	fresh frozen plasma
FGM	female genital mutilation
FH	fetal heart
FHR	fetal heart rate
FIGO	International Federation of Gynaecology and Obstetrics
FISH	fluorescent in situ hybridization
FL	femur length
FM	fetal movement
FPR	false positive rate
FSD	female sexual dysfunction
FSE	fetal scalp electrode
FSH	follicle-stimulating hormone
FU	5-Fluorouracil
FVS	fetal varicella syndrome
GA	general anaesthesia
GAS	group A streptococcus
GBS	group B streptococcus
GCSF	granulocyte colony-stimulating factor
GDM	gestational diabetes mellitus
GFR	glomerular filtration rate
GI	gastrointestinal
GMC	General Medical Council
GnRH	gonadotrophin-releasing hormone

GT	γ-glutamyltranferase
GTD	gestational trophoblastic disease
GTT	glucose tolerance test
GUM	genitourinary medicine
H	haemolysis
HAART	highly active antiretroviral therapy
Hb	haemoglobin
HBeAg	hepatitis B E antigen
HBsAg	hepatitis B surface antigen
HBV	hepatitis B virus
HC	head circumference
hCG	human chorionic gonadotrophin
hct	haematocrit
HCV	hepatitis C virus
HDL	high density lipoprotein
HDU	high dependency unit
HELLP	haemolysis, elevated liver enzymes, and low platelets
HFEA	Human Fertilization and Embryology Authority
HH	hypogonadotrophic hypogonadism
HIV	human immune deficiency virus
HLA	human leucocyte antigen
HNIG	human normal immunoglobulin
HNPCC	hereditary non-polyposis colorectal cancer
HOCM	hypertrophic obstructive cardiomyopathy
HP	hypothalamo-pituitary
hPL	human placental lactogen
HPO	hypothalamus-pituitary-ovary
HPU	Health Protection Unit
HPV	human papillomavirus
HRT	hormone replacement therapy
HSDD	hypoactive sexual desire disorder
HSG	hysterosalpingography
HSV	herpes simplex virus

5-HT	5-hydroxytryptamine
HTLV	human lymphotropic virus
HVS	high vaginal swab
HyCoSy	hysterosalpingo-contrast-sonography
IA	intermittent auscultation
IAS	internal anal sphincter
IBD	inflammatory bowel disease
IBS	irritable bowel syndrome
IC	interstitial cystitis
ICS	International Continence Society
ICSI	intracytoplasmic sperm injection
ICU	intensive care unit
IDS	interval debulking surgery
IgG	immunoglobulin G
IgM	immunoglobulin M
IGT	impaired glucose tolerance
IL	interleukin
IM	intramuscular
IMB	intermenstrual bleeding
INR	international normalized ratio
IOL	induction of labour
Ip	intraperitoneal
ITP	idiopathic thrombocytopaenic purpura
IUCD	intrauterine contraceptive device
IUD	intrauterine death (of the fetus)
IUGR	intrauterine growth restriction
IUI	intrauterine insemination
IUP	intrauterine pregnancy
IUS	intrauterine system
IV	intravenous
IVF	*in vitro* fertilization
IVU	intravenous urogram
JVP	jugular venous pressure

LA	local anaesthetic
LARC	long-acting reversible contraceptive
LATS	long-acting thyroid stimulator
LAVH	laparoscopic-assisted vaginal hysterectomy
LDH	lactate dehydrogenase
LDL	low density lipoprotein
LE	lupus-erythematosus
LFT	liver function test
LH	luteinizing hormone
LLETZ	large loop excision of the transformation zone
LMP	last menstrual period
LMWH	low-molecular-weight heparin
LN	lymph node
LNG	levonorgestrel
LNMP	last normal menstrual period
LP	low platelets
LR	likelihood ratio
LSCS	lower segment Caesarean section
LSD	lysergic acid diethylamide
LUNA	laparoscopic uterine nerve ablation
LVEF	left ventricular ejection fraction
LVS	low vaginal swab
MA	mentoanterior
MAIS	mild androgen insensitivity syndrome
MAS	meconium aspiration syndrome
MCA	middle cerebral artery
MCDA	monochorionic, diamniotic
MCHC	mean corpuscular haemoglobin concentration
MCMA	monochorionic, monoamniotic
MCV	mean corpuscular volume
MDMA	3, 4-methylenedioxy-N-methylamphetamine
MDT	multidisciplinary team
MEA	microwave endometrial ablation

MEOW	modified early obstetric warning system
MI	myocardial infarction
MMMT	mixed mesodermal Müllerian tumour
MMP	matrix metalloproteinase
MMR	mumps, measles, and rubella
MMtR	maternal mortality ratio
MoM	multiples of median
MP	mentoposterior
MPA	medroxyprogesterone acetate
MRKH	Mayer–Rokitansky–Küster–Hauser
MRI	magnetic resonance imaging
MROP	manual removal of placenta
MS	multiple sclerosis
MSAF	meconium-stained amniotic fluid
MSU	midstream urine (sample)
MTCT	mother-to-child transmission
MTHFR	methylenetetrahydrofolate reductase
MWS	Million Women Study
NAAT	nucleic acid amplification test
NBM	nil by mouth
NCSP	National Chlamydia Screening Programme
NEC	necrotizing enterocolitis
NHSCSP	National Health Service Cervical Screening Programme
NHSLA	National Health Service Litigation Authority
NK	natural killer
NNM	neonatal mortality
NNRTI	Non-nucleoside analogue reverse transcriptase
NPSA	National Patient Safety Agency
NPV	negative predictive value
NSAID	non-steroidal anti-inflammatory drug
NSC	National Screening Committee
NT	nuchal translucency
NTD	neural tube defect

NYHA	New York Heart Association
OA	occipito-anterior
OAB	overactive bladder
OATS	oligoasthenoteratozoospermia
od	once daily
OGTT	oral glucose tolerance test
OHSS	ovarian hyperstimulation syndrome
OL	occipito-lateral
OP	occipito-posterior
OTIS	Organization of Teratology Information Specialists
PAIS	partial androgen insensitivity syndrome
PAPP-A	pregnancy-associated plasma protein-A
PCA	patient-controlled analgesia
PCB	postcoital bleeding
PCI	percutaneous coronary intervention
PCO_2	partial pressure of carbon dioxide
PCOS	polycystic ovary syndrome
PCP	primary pneumocystis pneumonia
PCR	polymerase chain reaction
PDA	patent ductus arteriosus
PDS	polydioxanone suture
PE	pulmonary embolism
PEFR	peak expiratory flow rate
PEP	post-exposure prophylaxis
PET	pre-eclamptic toxaemia
PFME	pelvic floor muscle exercises
PG	prostaglandin
PGD	preimplantation genetic diagnosis
PGS	preimplantation genetic screening
PI	protease inhibitor
PID	pelvic inflammatory disease
PlGF	placental growth factor
PIH	pregnancy-induced hypertension

PLCO	Prostate, Lung, Colorectal, and Ovarian
PMB	postmenopausal bleeding
PMS	premenstrual syndrome
PO	per oral (by mouth)
POCT	point of care test
POF	premature ovarian failure
POP	progesterone-only pill
PP	placenta praevia
PPH	post-partum haemorrhage
PPROM	preterm prelabour rupture of membranes
PPV	positive predictive value
PR	progesterone
PROM	prelabour rupture of membranes
PS	performance status
PSV	peak systolic velocity
PT	prothrombin time
PTT	partial thromboplastin time
PTU	propylthiouracil
PUL	pregnancy of unknown location
PV	per vaginam
Q	ventilation
qds	four times daily
QOL	quality of life
RCOG	Royal College of Obstetricians and Gynaecologists
RCT	randomized controlled trial
RECIST	response evaluation criteria in solid tumours
REDF	reversed end diastolic flow
Rh	rhesus
RMI	risk of malignancy index
ROM	rupture of membrane
RPR	rapid plasma reagin
RR	relative risk
RUQ	right upper quadrant (of abdomen)

SADS	sudden adult/arrhythmic death syndrome
SAH	subarachnoid haemorrhage
SARC	Sexual Assault Referral Centre
SB	stillbirth
SC	subcutaneous
SCBU	special care baby unit
SERM	selective oestrogen reuptake modulator
SFH	symphysis fundal height
SFLt-1	soluble-like tyrosine kinase
SGA	small for gestational age
SHBG	sex hormone-binding globulin
SHO	senior house officer
SIDS	sudden infant death syndrome
SLE	systemic lupus erythematosus
SNRI	serotonin and norepinephrine reuptake inhibitor
SOL	space-occupying lesion
SPD	symphysis pubis dysfunction
SpR	specialist registrar
SROM	spontaneous rupture of membranes
SSRI	selective serotonin reuptake inhibitor
STAN	ST waveform analysis
STI	sexually transmitted infection
SUI	stress urinary incontinence
SVT	supraventricular tachycardia
$t_{1/2}$	half-life
T_3	triiodothryonine
T_4	thyroxine
TAH	total abdominal hysterectomy
TAS	transabdominal scan
TB	tuberculosis
TBG	thyroid-binding globulin
TBI	total body irradiation
tds	three times daily

TENS	transcutaneous electrical nerve stimulation
TFT	thyroid function test
TIBC	total iron-binding capacity
TNF	tumour necrosis factor
TOP	termination of pregnancy
TORCH	toxoplasmosis, rubella, cytomegalovirus, herpes simplex, and HIV
TOT	transobturator tape
TRAP	twin reversed arterial perfusion
TSH	thyroid-stimulating hormone
TTP	thrombotic thrombocytopaenic purpura
TTTS	twin-to-twin transfusion syndrome
TVS	transvaginal scan
TVT	tension-free vaginal tape
TVUSS	transvaginal ultrasound scan
TZ	transformation zone
U&E	urea and electrolytes
UC	ulcerative colitis
UKFOCCS	UK Collaborative Trial of Ovarian Cancer Screening
UFH	unfractionated heparin
UPSI	unprotected sexual intercourse
USI	urodynamic stress incontinence
USS	ultrasound scan
UTI	urinary tract infections
VAIN	vaginal intraepithelial neoplasia
VBAC	vaginal birth after Caesarean
VBP	vinblastin, bleomycin, and cisplatin
VDRL	Venereal Disease Research Laboratory
VE	vaginal examination
VEGF	vascular endothelial growth factor
VIN	vulval intraepithelial neoplasia
VL	viral load
VMA	vanillylmandelic acid
V/Q scan	ventilation/perfusion scan

VSD	ventricular septal defect
VTE	venous thromboembolism
vWF	von Willebrand's factor
VZIG	varicella-zoster immunoglobulin
VZV	varicella zoster virus
WCC	white cell count
WHI	Women's Health Initiative
WHO	World Health Organization
ZDV	zidovudine

Contributors

Editors

Miss Sally Collins
John Radcliffe Hospital, Oxford, UK

Professor Sabaratnam Arulkumaran
St George's Hospital, London, UK

Mr Kevin Hayes
St George's Hospital, London, UK

Mr Simon Jackson
John Radcliffe Hospital, Oxford, UK

Mr Lawrence Impey
John Radcliffe Hospital, Oxford, UK

Contributors

Miss Karolina Afors
St George's Hospital, London, UK

Dr Christian Becker
John Radcliffe Hospital, Oxford, UK

Dr Amy Bennett
Dept of Genitourinary Medicine, Oxford University Hospitals NHS Trust, Oxford, UK

Mrs Rebecca Black
John Radcliffe Hospital, Oxford, UK

Dr Shabana Bora
St George's Hospital, London, UK

Dr Brian Brady
John Radcliffe Hospital, Oxford, UK

Mr Paul Bulmer
St George's Hospital, London, UK

Mr Edwin Chandraharan
St George's Hospital, London, UK

Dr Noan-Minh Chau
Specialist Registrar rotation in Medical Oncology, London Deanery, UK

Dr Mellisa Damodaram
Queen Charlotte's and Chelsea Hospital, London, UK

Miss Claudine Domoney
Chelsea and Westminster Hospital, London, UK

Dr Stergios K. Doumouchtsis
St George's Hospital, London, UK

Dr Suzy Elniel
Chelsea and Westminster Hospital, London, UK

Dr Cleave W. J. Gass
St George's Hospital, London, UK

Dr Ingrid Granne
John Radcliffe Hospital, Oxford, UK

Miss Catherine Greenwood
John Radcliffe Hospital, Oxford, UK

Mr Manish Gupta
John Radcliffe Hospital, Oxford, UK

Miss Pauline Hurley
John Radcliffe Hospital, Oxford, UK

Dr Nia Jones
Queens Medical Centre, Nottingham, UK

Miss Brenda Kelly
John Radcliffe Hospital, Oxford, UK

Dr Nigel Kennea
St George's Hospital, London, UK

Dr Andy Kent
St George's Hospital, London, UK

Dr Su-Yen Khong
John Radcliffe Hospital, Oxford, UK

Dr Emma Kirk
St George's Hospital, London, UK

Dr Samatha Low
Royal Berkshire Hospital,
Reading, UK

Dr Jo Morrison
Musgrove Park Hospital,
Taunton, UK

**Dr Neelanjana
Mukhopadhaya**
St George's Hospital,
London, UK

Dr Faizah Mukri
Specialist Registrar rotation,
London Deanery, UK

Dr Santosh Pattnayak
St George's Hospital,
London, UK

Dr Natalia Price
John Radcliffe Hospital,
Oxford, UK

Dr Aysha Qureshi
Royal United Hospital, Bath, UK

Dr Devanna Rajeswari
St George's Hospital, London, UK

Dr Gowri Ramanathan
St George's Hospital, London, UK

Dr Margaret Rees
John Radcliffe Hospital, Oxford, UK

Dr Jackie Sherrard
Dept of Genitourinary Medicine,
Oxford University Hospitals NHS
Trust, Oxford, UK

Dr Lisa Story
John Radcliffe Hospital, Oxford, UK

Ms Louise Strawbridge
University College London,
London, UK

Mr Alex Swanton
Royal Berkshire Hospital,
Reading, UK

Dr Linda Tan
St George's Hospital, London, UK

Dr Katy Vincent
John Radcliffe Hospital, Oxford, UK

Miss Cara Williams
Clinical Fellow in Paediatric and
Adolescent Gynaecology,
University College London
Hospital, UK

Dr Niraj Yanamandra
St Peter's Hospital, Chertsey, UK

Chapter 1

Normal pregnancy

Obstetric history: current pregnancy

Obstetric history taking has many features in common with most other sections of medicine, along with certain areas specific to the specialty. The basic framework can be easily learned; however, competence requires good clinical knowledge and a lot of practice. As obstetrics often requires intimate examination and discussion of sensitive information, it is important to ensure privacy, and to demonstrate respect and confidentiality. It is important to offer a health professional as a chaperone. Translation may be required and it is best to have an official translator. The family, especially the husband, translating may not divulge or may distort certain information. It is also important to ask about domestic violence when the mother is alone and offer help if appropriate.

A carefully obtained history taken in a logical sequence avoids inadvertent omission of important details, and guides the examination to follow.

Current pregnancy

Much of this information will be contained in the patient's 'hand-held' notes:
- Name.
- Age.
- Occupation.
- Relationship status.
- Gravidity (i.e. number of pregnancies, including the current one).
- Parity (i.e. number of births beyond 24wks gestation).

The expected date of delivery (EDD) can be calculated from the last menstrual period (LMP) using Naegele's rule (add 1yr and 7 days to the LMP and subtract 3mths), most often done with an obstetric calendar ('wheel'). Enquire about details that may affect the validity of the patient's EDD as calculated from her LMP including:
- Long cycles.
- Irregular periods.
- Recent use of the combined oral contraceptive pill (COCP).

▶ Dating scans between 8 and 13wks are more reliable than LMP and should be used to provide an EDD where possible.

Enquire about the current pregnancy, including:
- General health (tiredness, malaise, and other non-specific symptoms).
- If >20wks, enquire about fetal movements.
- General details of pregnancy to date (previous admissions and current problems).
- Results of all antenatal (AN) blood tests—routine and specific.
- Results of anomaly and other scans (details of results can be cross-checked with the notes).
- If she is postnatal:
  - labour and delivery
  - history of the postnatal period.

An obstetric history

Should include:
- Current pregnancy details.
- Past obstetric history.
- Past gynaecological history.
- Past medical and surgical history.
- Drug history and allergies.
- Social history, including:
  - recreational drug use
  - domestic violence
  - psychiatric illness especially in the postnatal period.
- Family history especially with regard to:
  - multiple pregnancy
  - diabetes
  - hypertension
  - chromosomal or congenital malformations.

Gravidity and parity explained

The terminology used is gravida **x**, para **a + b**:
- x is the total number of pregnancies (including this one).
- a is the number of births beyond 24wks gestation.
- b is the number of miscarriages or termination of pregnancies before 24wks gestation.

Example

A woman who is pregnant for the 4th time with 1 normal delivery at term, 1 termination at 9wks, and 1 miscarriage at 16wks would be gravida 4, para 1+2.

Obstetric history: other relevant features

▶ History often repeats itself, so previous AN, intrapartum, or postpartum complications should influence the management of this pregnancy.

Past obstetric history includes:
- Details of all previous pregnancies (including miscarriages and terminations).
- Length of gestation.
- Date and place of delivery.
- Onset of labour (including details of induction of labour).
- Mode of delivery.
- Sex and birth weight.
- Fetal and neonatal life.

Clear details of any complications or adverse outcomes (such as shoulder dystocia, postpartum haemorrhage, or stillbirth).

Past gynaecological/medical/surgical history
- Method of contraception before conception.
- Previous gynaecological procedures.
- Cervical smear history.
- Medical conditions, such as hypertension, epilepsy, or diabetes.
- Details of any consultations with other physicians (neurologist or endocrinologist, psychiatrists).
- Involvement of multidisciplinary teams (MDT).
- Details of any previous surgery.

Drug and allergy history
- Current medications.
- Medications taken at any time during the pregnancy.
- Any allergies and their severity (anaphylaxis or a rash?).

Family history
Any history of hereditary illnesses or congenital defects is important and is required to ensure adequate counselling and screening is offered.
- Familial disorders such as thrombophilias.
- Previously affected pregnancies with any chromosomal or genetic disorders, hypertensive disorders, early pregnancy loss, or preterm delivery.
- Consanguinity.

Social history
- Smoking.
- History of drug or alcohol abuse.
- Plans for breast-feeding.
- Social aspects, such as plans for childcare arrangements.
- Domestic violence screening.

Obstetric physical examination

At initial visit, a complete physical examination should be undertaken.

Abdominal examination: inspection

- Note the apparent size of the abdominal distension.
- Note any asymmetry.
- Fetal movements.
- Cutaneous signs of pregnancy:
  - linea nigra (dark pigmented line stretching from the xiphi sternum through the umbilicus to the suprapubic area)
  - striae gravidarum (recent stretch marks are purplish in colour)
  - striae albicans (old stretch marks are silvery-white)
  - flattening/eversion of umbilicus (due to ↑ intra-abdominal pressure).
- Superficial veins (alternative paths of venous drainage due to pressure on the inferior vena cava by a gravid uterus).
- Surgical scars (a low Pfannenstiel incision may be obscured by pubic hair, and laparoscopy scars hidden within the umbilicus).

Abdominal examination: palpation

- *Symphysis fundal height* (SFH):
  - palpated <20wks
  - measured in centimetres >20wks.
- Estimation of number of fetuses: ?multiple fetal poles.
- *Fetal lie* (relationship of longitudinal axis of fetus to that of the uterus):
  - *longitudinal*—fetal head or breech palpable over pelvic inlet
  - *oblique*—the head or breech is palpable in the iliac fossa and nothing felt in the lower uterus
  - *transverse*—fetal poles felt in flanks and nothing above the brim.
- *Presentation* (part of the fetus overlying the pelvic brim):
  - cephalic (this could be vertex, face, or brow presentations determined vaginally)
  - breech
  - other (shoulder, compound).
- *Amniotic fluid volume*:
  - ↑ tense abdomen with fetal parts not easily palpated
  - ↓ compact abdomen with fetal parts easily palpable.

Auscultation of the fetal heart

The fetal heart (FH) is best heard at the anterior shoulder of the fetus:

- A Doppler ultrasound device (Sonicaid) from about 12wks.
- A fetal stethoscope (Pinard) from about 24wks gestation.
- In a breech presentation it is often heard at, or above, the level of the maternal umbilicus.
- Rate and the rhythm of the FH should be determined over 1min.
- The recent NICE guidelines raise the need for routine fetal heart rate (FHR) auscultation in the presence of fetal movement (FM); but mothers enjoy listening to the fetal heart.

General examination

- Body mass index (BMI) calculated [weight (kg)/height (m)^2].
  ⚠ Pregnancy complications are increased with a BMI <18.5 and >25.
- Blood pressure (BP) measured in the semi-recumbent position (45° tilt).
  ⚠ Use an appropriate size cuff; too small a cuff gives a falsely high BP.
- *Auscultation of the heart and lungs:*
  - flow murmurs are common in pregnancy and are not significant
  - cardiac murmurs may be detected for the first time in pregnancy.
- Thyroid gland (exclude a goitre).
- Breasts (exclude any lumps).
- Varicose veins and skeletal abnormalities (kyphosis or scoliosis):
  normal pregnancy is associated with an increase in lumbar lordosis,
  which can lead to lower backache.

Normal uterine size

- The uterus normally becomes palpable at 12wks gestation.
- It reaches the level of the umbilicus at 20wks gestation.
- It is at the xiphi sternum at 36wks gestation.

Symphysis fundal height

▶ The SFH detects approximately 40–60% of small-for-gestational age
fetuses, but its predictive value in detecting large-for-dates fetuses is
considerably less.

The uterine size is objectively measured with a tape measure from
the highest point of the fundus to the upper margin of the symphysis
pubis (see Fig. 1.1).

Appropriate growth is usually estimated to be the number of weeks
gestation in centimetres (at 30wks the SFH should be 30 ± 2cm):

- ± 2cm from 20 until 36wks gestation.
- ± 3cm between 36 and 40wks.
- ± 4cm at 40wks.

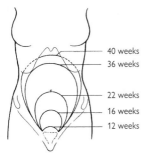

40 weeks
36 weeks

22 weeks
16 weeks
12 weeks

Fig. 1.1 Typical fundal heights at various stages of pregnancy. Reproduced from
Wyatt JP, Illingworth RN, Graham CA, *et al.* (eds) (2006). *Oxford Handbook of
Emergency Medicine.* Oxford: OUP. By permission of Oxford University Press.

Engagement of the fetal head

Conventionally, engagement or the passage of the maximal diameter of the presenting part beyond the pelvic inlet is estimated using the palm width of the five fingers of the hand (Fig. 1.2). If five fingers are needed to cover the head above the pelvic brim, it is five-fifths palpable, and if no head is palpable, it is zero-fifths palpable.

- Normally, the fetus engages in an attitude of flexion in the larger transverse diameter of the pelvic inlet, unless the pelvis is very roomy where it may engage in any diameter (see Fig. 1.3).
- In nulliparous women, engagement usually (not in all) occurs beyond 37wks, but in multiparous women it may not occur until the onset of labour.
- Rare causes of non-engagement should always be considered and investigated with an ultrasound scan (USS) (including placenta praevia and fetal abnormality).
- In women of Afro-Caribbean origin, engagement may only occur at the onset or during the course of labour, even in nulliparous women due to the shape of the pelvic inlet.

Paulik's grip

This is a one-handed technique that uses a cupped right hand to grasp and assess the lower pole of the uterus (usually the fetal head).

▶ This can be very uncomfortable and is not necessary if the head can be palpated using two hands.

Engagement

- A head that is only two-fifths palpable is usually considered to be engaged (and therefore fixed in the pelvis; see Fig. 1.2).
- Put simply, an easily palpable head is not engaged, whereas a head more difficult to palpate is more likely to be deeply engaged.

⚠ Care must be taken, as a breech presentation can sometimes be mistaken for a deeply engaged head.

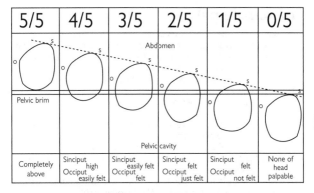

5/5	4/5	3/5	2/5	1/5	0/5
Completely above	Sinciput high Occiput easily felt	Sinciput easily felt Occiput felt	Sinciput felt Occiput just felt	Sinciput felt Occiput not felt	None of head palpable

Fig. 1.2 Clinical estimation of descent of the fetal head and engagement. Reproduced from Arulkumaran S, Symonds IM, Fowlie A. (2004). *Oxford Handbook of Obstetrics and Gynaecology.* Oxford: OUP. By permission of Oxford University Press.

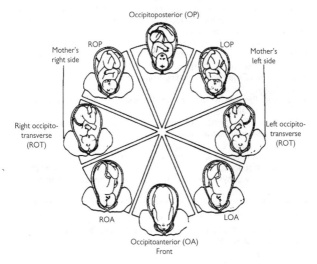

Fig. 1.3 Fetal position. Reproduced from Collier J, Longmore M, *et al.* (2008). *Oxford Handbook of Clinical Specialties*, 8th edn. Oxford: OUP. By permission of Oxford University Press.

The female pelvis

The bony ring of the pelvis is made up of two symmetrical innominate bones and the sacrum. Each innominate bone is made up of the ilium, ischium, and the pubis, which are joined anteriorly at the symphysis pubis and posteriorly to the sacrum at the sacroiliac joints.

The female pelvis has evolved for giving birth, and differs from the male pelvis in the following ways:
- The female pelvis is broader, and the bones more slender than those of the male.
- The male pelvic brim is heart-shaped and widest towards the back, whereas the female pelvic brim is oval-shaped transversely and widest further forwards; the sacral promontory is less prominent.
- The female pelvic cavity is more spacious and has a wider outlet than the male pelvis.
- The subpubic angle is rounded in a female pelvis (like a Roman arch) and more acute in the male pelvis (like a Gothic arch).

Pelvic muscles and ligaments

The pelvis gains its strength and stability through numerous muscles and ligaments. The inner aspect of the pelvic bones is covered by muscles. Above the pelvic brim are the iliacus and psoas muscles; the obturator internus and its fascia occupies the side walls; the posterior wall is covered by the pyriformis; and the levator ani and coccygeus, with their opposite counterparts, constitute the pelvic floor.

Pelvic ring stability is provided by the following ligaments:
- *Sacrospinous ligament:* extending from the lateral margin of the sacrum and coccyx to the ischial spine.
- *Sacrotuberous ligament:* extending from the sacrum to the ischial tuberosity.
- *Iliolumbar ligament:* extending from the spine to the iliac crest at the back of the pelvis.
- *Dorsal sacroiliac ligament:* a heavy band passing from the ilium to the sacrum posterior to the sacroiliac joint.
- *Ventral sacroiliac ligament:* bridging the sacroiliac joint anteriorly, and is an important stabilizing structure of the joint.
- *Inferior and superior pubic ligament:* a band across the lower and upper part of the symphysis respectively, providing further strength to the joint.
- *Inguinal ligament:* running from the anterior superior iliac spine of the ilium to the pubic tubercle of the pubic bone.

The remaining ligaments that surround the pelvis are ligaments that do not provide stabilization of the pelvis.

Pelvic boundaries
The pelvis is divided by an oblique plane passing through the prominence of the sacrum, the arcuate, and pectineal lines, and the upper margin of the symphysis pubis, into the greater and the lesser pelvis. The circumference of this plane is termed the pelvic brim. This pelvic brim separates the false pelvis above from the true pelvis below. The plane of the pelvis is at an angle of 55° to the horizontal.

Pelvic shapes
There are four basic shapes of the female pelvis, as illustrated in Fig. 1.4.
- *Gynaecoid*: the classical female pelvis with the inlet transversely oval and a roomier pelvic cavity.
- *Anthropoid*: a long, narrow and oval-shaped pelvis due to the assimilation of the sacral body to the fifth lumbar vertebra.
- *Android*: the inlet is heart-shaped and the cavity is funnel-shaped with a contracted outlet.
- *Platypolloid*: a wide pelvis flattened at the brim with the sacral promontory pushed forward.

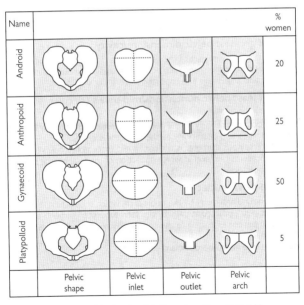

Fig. 1.4 Basic shapes of the female pelvis. Reproduced from Abitbol M, Chervenak F, Ledger WJ. (1996). *Birth and human evolution: anatomical and obstetrical mechanics in primates.* New York: Bergin & Garvey.

Diameters of the female pelvis

The female bony pelvis is not distensible, and only very minor degrees of movement are possible at the symphysis pubis and the sacroiliac joints. Its dimensions are, hence, critical for normal childbirth.

▶ The diameters of the female pelvis vary at different parts of the pelvis:
- The true pelvis is bound anteriorly by the symphysis pubis (3.5cm long) and posteriorly by the sacrum (12cm long).
- The superior circumference of the true pelvis is the pelvic inlet and the inferior circumference is the outlet (Fig. 1.5).

The true pelvis has four planes.

Plane of pelvic inlet

- This is bound anteriorly by the upper border of the pubis, laterally by the iliopectineal line, and posteriorly by the sacral promontory.
- The average transverse diameter is 13.5cm and the average anteroposterior diameter is 11cm (obstetric conjugate diameter) (transversely oblong).
- It is not possible to measure these diameters clinically, and the only diameter at the pelvic inlet amenable to clinical assessment is the distance from the inferior margin of the pubic symphysis to the midpoint of the sacral promontory (the diagonal conjugate), which is ~1.5cm greater than the obstetric conjugate diameter.

Plane of greatest pelvic dimensions/cavity

- This is the roomiest part of the pelvis and has little clinical significance.
- It is almost round in shape with an average transverse diameter of 13.5cm and an average anteroposterior diameter of 12.5cm.

Plane of least pelvic dimensions/mid-pelvis (circular in shape)

- This is bound anteriorly by the apex of the pubic arch, laterally by the ischial spines, and posteriorly by the tip of the sacrum.
- The interspinous diameter is the narrowest space in the pelvis (10cm) and represents the level at which impaction of the fetal head is most likely to occur.

Plane of pelvic outlet

- This is bound anteriorly by the pubic arch, which should have a desired angle of >90°, posterolaterally by the sacrotuberous ligaments and ischial tuberosities leading to the coccyx posteriorly (anteroposteriorly oblong).
- The average intertuberous diameter is 11cm.

Assessment of 'pelvic adequacy'

Examination of the pelvis before labour does not accurately discriminate between those who will achieve vaginal birth and those who will not. Even computed tomography (CT) or magnetic resonance imaging (MRI) scanning, together with ultrasound of the fetal head, is not helpful, unless there is a gross abnormality, which will be evident from the history or gait. This is because of the dynamic nature of labour, when the head 'moulds' (reducing the head circumference by a few centimetres) and the joints of the pelvis can move, increasing the pelvic dimensions slightly.

The ideal female pelvis has the following features:

- Oval brim.
- Shallow cavity.
- Non-prominent ischial spines.
- Curved sacrum with large sciatic notches (>90∞).
- Sacrospinous ligament >3.5cm long.
- Rounded subpubic arch >90∞.
- Intertuberous distance of at least 10cm.

Diagonal conjugate diameter of at least 12cm.

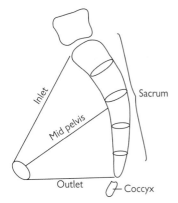

Fig. 1.5 Median sagittal section of the female pelvis showing the pelvic inlet and outlet. Reproduced from Collier J, Longmore M, *et al.* (2008). *Oxford Handbook of Clinical Specialties*, 8th edn. Oxford: OUP. By permission of Oxford University Press.

Fetal head

Anatomy of the fetal skull

The fetal cranium is made up of five main bones, two parietal bones, two frontal bones, and the occipital bone. These are held together by membranous areas called *sutures*, which permit movement during birth (Fig. 1.6).

• The *coronal suture* separates the frontal bones from the parietal bones.
• The *sagittal suture* separates the two parietal bones.
• The *lambdoid suture* separates the occipital bone from the parietal bones.
• The *frontal suture* separates the two frontal bones.

When two or more sutures meet, there is an irregular membranous area between them called a *fontanelle* (Fig 1.6).

• The *anterior fontanelle* or *bregma* is a diamond-shaped space at the junction of the coronal and sagittal sutures; this measures about 3cm in anteroposterior and transverse diameters, and usually ossifies at ~18mths after birth.
• The *posterior fontanelle* or the *lambda* is a smaller triangular area that lies at the junction of the sagittal and lambdoid sutures.

⚠ The positions of the sutures and fontanelles play a very important role in identifying the position of the fetal head in labour.

Regions of the fetal head

The fetal head has different regions assigned to help in the description of the presenting part felt during vaginal examination in labour.

• The *occiput* is the bony prominence that lies behind the posterior fontanelle.
• The *vertex* is the diamond-shaped area between the anterior and posterior fontanelles, and between the parietal eminences.
• The *bregma* is the area around the anterior fontanelle.
• The *sinciput* is the area in front of the anterior fontanelle, which is divided into the brow (between the bregma and the root of the nose) and the face (lying below the root of the nose and the supraorbital ridges).

Caput and moulding of the fetal head

During labour, the dilating cervix may press firmly on the fetal scalp preventing venous blood and lymphatic fluid from flowing normally. This may result in a tissue swelling beneath the skin called *caput succedaneum*. It is soft and boggy to touch and usually disappears within 24h of birth.

There is usually some alteration in the shape of the fetal head and a reduction in the head circumference in labour by a process of overlapping of the cranial bones (a reduction of up to 4cm is possible). This moulding is physiological and disappears a few hours after birth. The frontal bones can slip under the parietal bones and, in addition, one parietal bone can override the other and in turn slip under the occipital bone.

The degree of moulding can be assessed vaginally:
- *No moulding*: when the suture lines are separate.
- *1+ moulding*: when the suture lines meet.
- *2+ moulding*: when the bones overlap but can be reduced with gentle digital pressure.
- *3+ moulding*: when the bones overlap and are irreducible with gentle digital pressure.

▶ The presence of caput and moulding can play an important part in diagnosing obstructed labour.

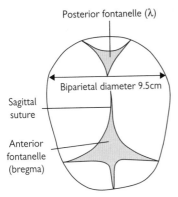

Fig. 1.6 Fontanelles, sagittal suture, and biparietal diameter. Reproduced from Collier J, Longmore M, et al. (2008). *Oxford Handbook of Clinical Specialties*, 8th edn. Oxford: OUP. By permission of Oxford University Press.

Diameters and presenting parts of the fetal head

The region that presents in labour depends on the degree of flexion or deflexion of the fetal head on presentation to the maternal pelvis. The important diameters of the fetal head as well as the presenting parts are as described below (Fig. 1.7):

- *Suboccipitobregmatic diameter (9.5cm):* presentation of a well-flexed vertex. Diameter extends from the middle of the bregma to the undersurface of the occipital bone where it joins the neck. Fetal head circumference is smallest at this plane and measures 32cm.
- *Suboccipitofrontal diameter (10.5cm):* partially flexed vertex, with diameter extending from the prominent point of the mid-frontal bone to the undersurface of occipital bone where it joins the neck.
- *Occipitofrontal diameter (11.5cm):* presentation of a deflexed head. Diameter extends from the prominent point of the mid-frontal bone to the most prominent point on the occipital bone. Fetal head circumference at this plane measures 34.5cm.
- *Mentovertical diameter (13cm):* brow presentation, with the diameter extending from the chin to the most prominent point of the midvertex. Presents with the largest anteroposterior diameter.
- *Submentobregmatic diameter (9.5cm):* face presentation, with diameter extending from just behind chin to the middle of the bregma.

Other noteworthy diameters of the fetal head include:

- *Biparietal diameter (BPD, 9.5cm):* greatest transverse diameter of the head, extending from one parietal eminence to the other.
- *Bitemporal diameter (8cm):* greatest distance between two temporal eminences.
- *Bimastoid diameter (7.5cm):* distance between the tips of the two mastoid processes.

See 📖 Malpresentations in labour: overview, p. 316.

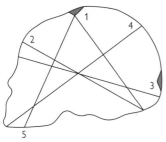

1 Suboccipitobregmatic 9.5cm
  flexed vertex presentation
2 Suboccipitofrontal 10.5cm
  partially deflexed vertex
3 Occipipitofrontal 11.5cm
  deflexed vertex
4 Mentovertical 13cm brow
5 Submentobregmatic 9.5cm face

Fig. 1.7 Different presenting diameters of the fetal head. Reproduced from Collier J, Longmore M, Turmezei T, et al. (2008) *Oxford Handbook of Clinical Specialties*, 8th edn. Oxford: OUP. By permission of Oxford University Press.

Useful definitions when discussing the presenting part

- *Presentation* is the lowermost part of the fetus presenting to the pelvis. In more than 95% of cases the vertex is the presenting part and is called normal presentation. Any other presentation (e.g. face, brow, breech, and shoulder) is called malpresentation.
- *Denominator* is the most definable peripheral landmark of the presenting part, i.e. occiput for the vertex, mentum for the face, and sacrum for the breech presentation.
- *Position of the presenting part* is the relationship of the denominator to the fixed points of the maternal pelvis, i.e. sacrum posteriorly, pubic symphysis anteriorly, sacro-iliac joints posterolaterally, and ileo-pectineal eminences anterolaterally.
- *Station* is the relationship of the most prominent leading part of the presenting part to the ischial spines expressed as ± 1,2,3cm.

▶ In the vertex presentation more than 90% present in the occipito-anterior position, i.e. the occiput is in the anterior half of the pelvis and is called the normal position. If the occiput is pointing laterally or is in the posterior half of the pelvis, it is called malposition and is associated with deflexed head presenting a larger anteroposterior diameter of the vertex (11.5cm) and, hence, difficulties with progress of labour (Fig. 1.3).

Placenta: early development

The placenta is the organ responsible for providing endocrine secretions and selective transfer of substances to and from the fetus. It serves as an interface between the mother and developing fetus. Understanding the development of the placenta is important, as it is the placental trophoblasts that are critical for a successful pregnancy.

Embryological development

- After fertilization, the zygote enters the uterus in 3–5 days and continues to divide to become the blastocyst.
- Implantation of the blastocyst starts on day 7 and is finished by day 11:
  - the inner cell mass of the blastocyst forms the embryo, yolk sac, and amniotic cavity
  - the trophoblast forms the future placenta, chorion, and extraembryonic mesoderm.
- When the blastocyst embeds into the decidua, trophoblastic cells differentiate and the embryo becomes surrounded by two layers of trophoblasts:
  - the inner mononuclear cytotrophoblast
  - the outer multinucleated syncytiotrophoblast.
- The invading trophoblast penetrates endometrial blood vessels forming intertrophoblastic maternal blood-filled sinuses (lacunar spaces).
- Trophoblastic cells advance as early or primitive villi, each consisting of cytotrophoblast surrounded by the syncytium.
- These villi mature into 2° and 3° villi, and the mesodermal core develops to form fetal blood vessels (completed by day 21).
- On days 16–17, the surface of the blastocyst is covered by branching villi which are best developed at the embryonic pole: the chorion here is known as chorionic frondosum; the future placenta develops from this area.
- Simultaneously, the lacunar spaces become confluent with one another and, by weeks 3–4, form a multilocular receptacle lined by syncytium and filled with maternal blood: this becomes the future intervillous space.
- With further growth of the embryo the decidua capsularis becomes thinner, and both villi and the lacunar spaces in the decidua are obliterated, converting the chorion into chorionic levae.
- The villi in the chorionic frondosum show exuberant division and subdivision, and with the accompanying proliferation of the decidua basalis, the future placenta is formed.
- This process starts at 6wks and the definitive numbers of stem villi are established by 12wks.

Placenta: later development

Placental growth continues to term.
- Until week 16, the placenta grows both in thickness and circumference due to growth of the chorionic villi with accompanying expansion of the intervillous space.
- After 16wks growth occurs mainly circumferentially.

Placental villi
- Functional units of the placenta.
- There are ~60 stem villi in human placenta with each cotyledon containing 3–4 major stem villi.
- Despite their close proximity (0.025mm), there is no mixing of maternal and fetal blood.
- Placental barrier is made of outer syncytiotrophoblast, which is in direct contact with maternal blood, the cytotrophoblast layer, basement membrane, stroma containing mesenchymal cells, and the endothelium and basement membrane of fetal blood vessels

---

The placenta at term
- Circular, diameter 15–20cm, thickness ~2.5cm at the centre.
- Weight ~500g (ratio of fetal:placental weight at term is about 6:1).
- Occupies ~30% of the uterine wall at term and has two surfaces.

Fetal surface
- Covered by a smooth, glistening amnion with the umbilical cord usually attached at or near its centre.
- Branches of the umbilical blood vessels are visible beneath amnion as they radiate from the insertion of the cord.
- Amnion can be peeled off from underlying chorion, except at insertion of cord.

Maternal surface
- Rough and spongy appearance, divided into several velvety bumps called cotyledons (15–20) by septa arising from the maternal tissues.
- Each cotyledon may be supplied by its own spiral artery.
- Numerous small greyish spots may be visible on the maternal surface representing calcium deposition in degenerated areas.

Umbilical cord
- Vascular cable that connects the fetus to the placenta.
- Varies from 30 to 90cm long, covered by amniotic epithelium.
- Contains two umbilical arteries and one umbilical vein embedded into the Wharton's jelly.
- Arteries carry deoxygenated blood from fetus to placenta and the oxygenated blood returns to fetus via the umbilical vein.
- In a full-term fetus, blood flow in the cord is ~350mL/min.

Placenta: circulation

The placental circulation consists of two distinctly different systems—the uteroplacental circulation and the fetoplacental circulation.

Uteroplacental circulation

- Uteroplacental circulation is the maternal blood circulating through the intervillous space (Table 1.1).
- Intervillous blood flow at term is estimated to be 500–600mL/min, and blood in the intervillous space is replaced 3–4 times/min.
- Pressure and concentration gradients between fetal capillaries and intervillous space favours placental transfer of oxygen and other nutrients to the fetus.

Arterial system

- Spiral arteries respond to the ↑ demand of blood supply to the placental bed by becoming low-pressure, high-flow vessels.
- They become tortuous, dilated, and less elastic by trophoblastic invasion, which starts early in pregnancy and occurs in two stages:
  - in first trimester, the decidual segments of the spiral arterioles are structurally modified
  - in second trimester, second wave of trophoblastic invasion occurs, resulting in invasion of myometrial segments of spiral arteries.

▶ Failure of this physiological change, particularly second wave of trophoblastic invasion, is implicated in development of pre-eclampsia and intrauterine growth restriction.

Venous system

- Blood entering the intervillous space from the spiral artery becomes dispersed to reach the chorionic plate and gradually the basal plate, being facilitated by mild movements of villi and uterine contractions.
- From basal plate, uterine veins drain the deoxygenated blood.
- Venous drainage only occurs during uterine relaxation.
- Spiral arteries are perpendicular and veins are parallel to uterine wall, making large volumes of blood available for exchange at the intervillous space even though the rate of flow is decreased during contraction, i.e. the veins are blocked for a longer time to allow pooling of blood in the retroplacental area.

Fetoplacental circulation (see Table 1.2)

- Two umbilical arteries carry deoxygenated blood from the fetus and enter the chorionic plate underneath the amnion.
- Arteries divide into small branches and enter the stem of the chorionic villi, where further division to arterioles and capillaries occurs.
- The blood then flows to the corresponding venous channel and subsequently to the umbilical vein.
- Maternal and fetal bloodstreams flow side by side, in opposite directions, facilitating exchange between mother and fetus.

Table 1.1 Haemodynamics of uteroplacental circulation

Volume of blood in the intervillous space	150mL
Blood flow in the intervillous space	500–600mL/min
Pressure changes in the intervillous space	
Height of uterine contraction	30–50mmHg
Uterine relaxation	10–15mmHg
Pressure in the spiral artery	70–80mmHg
Pressure in the uterine veins	8–10mmHg

Table 1.2 Haemodynamics in the fetoplacental circulation

Fetal blood flow through placenta	400mL/min
Pressure	
In the umbilical artery	60–70mmHg
In the umbilical vein	10mmHg
Oxygen saturation and partial pressure of oxygen	
In the umbilical artery	60%; 20–25mmHg
In the umbilical vein	70–80%; 30–40mmHg

Placenta: essential functions

The placenta is directly responsible for mediating and/or modulating the maternal environment necessary for normal fetal development.

> **Principal functions of the placenta**
> - To anchor the fetus and establish the fetoplacental unit.
> - To act as an organ for gaseous exchange.
> - Endocrine organ to bring the needed changes in pregnancy.
> - Transfer of substances to and from the fetus.
> - Barrier against infection.

The placenta as an endocrine organ

As an active endocrine organ, the placenta produces a number of hormones, growth factors, and cytokines. The production of human chorionic gonadotrophin (hCG), oestrogens, and progesterone by the placenta is vital for the maintenance of pregnancy.

hCG

- Primarily produced by syncytiotrophoblasts.
- Detected from 6 days after fertilization; forms basis of modern pregnancy testing.
- Concentrations reach a peak at 10–12wks gestation, then plateau for remainder of the pregnancy.

The placenta as a barrier

The placenta acts as a barrier for the fetus against pathogens and the maternal immune system.

Infection

The placenta forms an effective barrier against most maternal blood-borne bacterial infections. However, some important organisms, such as syphilis, parvovirus, hepatitis B and C, rubella, human immune deficiency virus (HIV), and cytomegalovirus (CMV) are able to cross it and infect the fetus during pregnancy.

Drugs

Many drugs administered to the mother will pass across the placenta into the fetus; exceptions include low-molecular-weight heparin (LMWH).

Some drugs may have little effect on the fetus and be considered 'safe' (e.g. paracetamol), but others (e.g. warfarin) may significantly affect development, structure, and function of the fetus—a process known as *teratogenesis*.

Before prescribing any drug to a pregnant woman it is the prescriber's obligation to ensure it is considered safe for stage of pregnancy.

See ▢ Drugs in pregnancy, p. 261.

Placental transfer

Although the placenta acts as a barrier to most substances, it allows exchange of gases, transfer of fetal nutrition, and removal of waste products in a highly effective manner. Speed of exchange and concentration of substance exchanged depends upon:

- Concentration of the substance on each side of the placenta.
- Molecular size.
- Lipid solubility.
- Ionization.
- Placental surface area.
- Maternofetal blood flow.

A low-molecular-weight lipid-soluble substance with a high concentration gradient across the placenta, for example, will be transferred quickly to the fetus. Actual transfer occurs by simple diffusion, facilitated diffusion, active transport, and/or endocytosis (Table 1.3).

Table 1.3 Transfer mechanisms across the placenta for common anabolites and catabolites

Substance	Transfer mechanism(s)	Direction of transfer
Oxygen	Simple diffusion	To fetus
Carbon dioxide	Simple diffusion	From fetus
Glucose	Simple and facilitated diffusion	To fetus
Amino acids	Facilitated diffusion	To fetus
Iron	Endocytosis	To fetus
Fatty acids	Facilitated diffusion	To fetus
Water	Simple diffusion	To and from fetus
Electrolytes	Counter-transport mechanism	To and from fetus
Urea and creatinine	Simple diffusion	From fetus

Physiology of pregnancy: endocrine

Physiological and anatomical changes occur during the course of pregnancy to provide a suitable environment for the growth and development of the fetus. Early changes are due, in part, to metabolic demands brought on by the fetus, placenta, and uterus, and, in part, to increasing levels of pregnancy hormones, particularly those of progesterone and oestrogen. Later changes are more anatomical in nature and are caused by mechanical pressure from the expanding uterus.

Endocrine changes

Progesterone ↑ throughout pregnancy
- Synthesized by the corpus luteum until 35 days and by the placenta thereafter.
- Progesterone promotes smooth muscle relaxation (gut, ureters, uterus) and raises body temperature.
- It is the principal hormone that prevents preterm labour and is now increasingly administered to prevent preterm labour.

Oestrogens, mainly oestradiol (90%)
- ↑ Breast and nipple growth, and pigmentation of the areola.
- Promote uterine blood flow, myometrial growth, cervical softening.
- ↑ Sensitivity and expression of myometrial oxytocin receptors.
- ↑ Water retention and protein synthesis.

Human placental lactogen (hPL)
- Has a structure and function similar to growth hormone.
- Modifies maternal metabolism to ↑ the energy supply to the fetus.
- ↑ Insulin secretion, but ↓ insulin's peripheral effect (liberating maternal fatty acids and sparing glucose enabling it to be diverted to the fetus).

The pituitary gland in pregnancy
- Enlarges mainly due to changes in the anterior lobe.
- Prolactin levels increase substantially, probably due to oestrogen stimulation of the lactotrophes.
- Gonadotrophin secretion is inhibited, whilst plasma adrenocorticotrophic hormone (ACTH) levels ↑.
- Maternal plasma cortisone output ↑, but the unbound levels remain constant.

The posterior pituitary releases oxytocin principally during the first stage of labour and during suckling.

Effect of pregnancy on the thyroid

- The maternal thyroid gland enlarges due to ↑ demand in pregnancy.
- ↑ Renal clearance of iodine results in a relative iodide deficiency.
- The thyroid responds by tripling its iodide uptake from the blood, which results in follicular enlargement.
- Thyroid-binding globulin (TBG) is doubled by the end of the first trimester due to high oestrogen levels.
- As a result, total T_3 (triiodothryonine) and T_4 (thyroxine) levels rise early in pregnancy, then fall to remain within normal non-pregnant range.
- Thyroid-stimulating hormone (TSH) may decrease slightly in early pregnancy, but tends to remain within the normal range.
- T_3 and T_4 cross the placental barrier in very small amounts.

⚠ Iodine, antithyroid drugs, and long-acting thyroid stimulator (LATS) or antibodies associated with Graves' disease can cross the placenta and affect the fetal thyroid function, which starts as early as 12wks.

Physiology of pregnancy: haemodynamics

Plasma volume
- ↑ By 10–15% at 6–12wks of gestation.
- Expands rapidly until 30–34wks.
- Total gain at term ~1100–1600mL (total plasma volume of 4700–5200mL, a 30–50% ↑ from the non-pregnant state).
- Acute excessive weight gain is commonly due to oedema.

Red cell volume (or red cell mass)
- Rises from 1400 to 1640mL at term (↑ 18%).
- With iron and folate supplements, an ↑ of 30% has been reported.

▶ The discrepancy between the rate of ↑ of plasma volume and that of red cell mass results in a relative haemodilution or 'physiological anae-mia' with the haemoglobin (Hb) concentration, haematocrit, and red cell counts all ↓ (particularly in the second trimester).

▶ Mean corpuscular Hb concentration remains constant.

Total white cell count
- ↑ Mainly due to the ↑ in neutrophil polymorphonuclear leucocytes, which peaks at 32wks.
- A further massive neutrophilia occurs during labour.
- Eosinophils, basophils, and monocytes remain relatively constant, but there is a profound ↓ in eosinophils during labour, being virtually absent at delivery.
- Although lymphocyte count and the number of B and T cells remain constant, lymphocyte function and cell-mediated immunity are profoundly depressed, giving rise to lowered resistance to viral infections.

Platelets
- ↓ Slightly during pregnancy.
- Platelet function is unchanged.

Clotting factors
- Pregnancy is a hypercoagulable state.
- Most clotting factors ↑, especially fibrinogen.

▶ Erythrocyte sedimentation rate (ESR) levels can also be elevated up to 4-fold in pregnancy.

Physiology of pregnancy: cardio-respiratory

Cardiovascular changes

Major changes occur in the cardiovascular system in pregnancy; the most significant of these changes occur within the first 12wks.

- Cardiac output ↑ from 5 to 6.5L/min by ↑ stroke volume (10%) and pulse rate (~15 beats/min).
- During labour, contractions may ↑ cardiac output by 2L/min, probably due to injection of blood from the distended intervillous space.
- With progressive enlargement of the uterus, the heart and diaphragm are displaced upwards.
- The heart enlarges and ↑ in volume by 70–80mL due to ↑ diastolic filling and muscle hypertrophy.

▶ Pregnancy may proceed normally even when the mother has an artificial cardiac pacemaker, compensation occurring mainly from increased stroke volume.

Blood pressure in pregnancy

- Peripheral resistance ↓ by nearly 50% (probably due to the ↑ production of vasodilator prostaglandins).
- BP (most noticeably diastolic) ↓ mid-pregnancy by 10–20mmHg and ↑ to non-pregnant levels by term.
- Profound ↓ can occur late in pregnancy when lying supine, due to compression of the inferior vena cava leading to ↓ venous return and ↓ cardiac output (supine hypotension syndrome).
- Aortic compression may also occur causing a conspicuous difference between brachial and femoral pressures giving a pressure difference of 10–15% from the supine to the lateral position.
- The balance of vasoconstrictor and vasodilator factors regulating peripheral resistance may be the basis of BP regulation in pregnancy and implicated in development of pregnancy-induced hypertension.
- Vasodilatation and hypotension also stimulate renin–angiotensin release, which plays a part in BP regulation.

Respiratory system changes

- The level of the diaphragm rises in pregnancy and the intercostal angle ↑ from 68° in early pregnancy to 103° in late pregnancy: breathing becomes more diaphragmatic than costal.
- Tidal volume ↑ ~40% (500–700mL) due to effect of progesterone.
- Inspiratory capacity (tidal volume plus inspiratory reserve volume) ↑ progressively in late pregnancy.
- Respiratory rate changes slightly, hence the resting pregnant woman ↑ ventilation by breathing more deeply and not more frequently.
- Breathlessness is common in pregnancy as maternal partial pressure of carbon dioxide (pCO_2) is set lower to allow the fetus to offload CO_2.

Physiology of pregnancy: genital tract and breast

Uterus

- Undergoes a 10-fold ↑ in weight to 1000g at term.
- Muscle hypertrophy occurs up to 20wks, after which stretching of the muscle fibres occurs.
- Uterine blood flow has been shown to ↑ from ~50mL/min at 10wks to 500–700mL/min at term.
- The uterine and ovarian arteries and branches of the superior vesical arteries undergo massive hypertrophy.

> *The uterus is divided functionally and morphologically into three sections:*
> - Cervix.
> - Isthmus (which later develops into the lower segment).
> - Body of the uterus (corpus uteri).

Cervix

- Reduction in cervical collagen towards term enables its dilatation.
- Hypertrophy of cervical glands leads to the production of profuse cervical mucus, and the formation of a thick mucus plug or operculum that acts as a barrier to infection.
- Vaginal discharge ↑ due to cervical ectopy (proliferation of columnar epithelium into vaginal portion of the cervix) and cell desquamation.

Uterine body

- ↑ In size, shape, position, and consistency.
- Uterine cavity expands from 4 to 4000mL.

Vagina

- A rich venous vascular network in connective tissue surrounds vaginal walls with blood and gives rise to slightly bluish appearance.
- High oestrogen levels stimulate glycogen synthesis and deposition:
  - action of lactobacilli on glycogen in vaginal cells produces lactic acid
  - lactic acid lowers the vaginal pH to keep the vagina relatively free from any bacterial pathogens.

Breast

- The lactiferous ducts and alveoli develop and grow under the stimulus of oestrogen, progesterone, and prolactin.
- From 3–4mths, colostrum (thick, glossy, protein-rich fluid) can be expressed from the breast.
- Prolactin stimulates the cells of the alveoli to secrete milk:
  - effect is blocked during pregnancy by the peripheral action of oestrogen and progesterone
  - shortly after delivery the sudden ↓ in these hormones enables prolactin to act uninhibited on the breast, and lactation begins.
- Suckling further stimulates prolactin and oxytocin release: oxytocin stimulates contraction of the myoepithelial cells to cause ejection of milk.

Physiology of pregnancy: other changes

Urinary tract

Various anatomical and physiological changes occur in pregnancy:

- Kidney size ↑ by about 1cm in length.
- Marked dilatation of the calyces, renal pelvis, and ureter from first trimester.
- Vesicoureteric reflux occurs sporadically: a combination of reflux and ureteric dilatation leads to urinary stasis and ↑ infection.
- Although bladder muscle relaxes in pregnancy, residual urine is not normally present after micturition.
- Uric acid clearance increases from 12 to 20mmol/mL, causing reduction in plasma uric acid levels: as pregnancy progresses, the filtered load of uric acid ↑, while the excretion remains constant, resulting in plasma levels returning to non-pregnant values.
- Renal blood flow ↑ by 30–50% in the first trimester, in line with the ↑ in cardiac output that occurs, and remains elevated:
  - results in ↑ glomerular filtration rate (GFR) and effective renal plasma flow, causing a ↓ in plasma levels of urea and creatinine
  - plays an important role in the variable glycosuria (due to exceeding the tubular maximum of absorption caused by more volume filtered) and urinary frequency that occurs in pregnancy.

⚠ Creatinine within the normal range for non-pregnant women may indicate renal impairment in pregnancy.

Alimentary system

- ↓ Tone of oesophageal sphincter and displacement through the diaphragm due to ↑ abdominal pressure causes reflux oesophagitis (heartburn).
- Gastric mobility is low and gastric secretion is reduced, resulting in delayed gastric emptying.
- Gut motility is generally ↓, and with possible ↑ sodium and water absorption in the large bowel, there is a tendency to constipation.

Skin

- Pigmentation in linear nigra, nipple, and areola or chloasma (brown patches of pigmentation seen especially on the face).
- Palmar erythema and spider naevi are also common.
- Incidence of striae varies in different populations:
  - represents the effect of disruption of collagen fibres in the subcuticular zone
  - probably related to the effect of ↑ production of adrenocortical hormones, as well as to the actual stress in the skin associated with relatively rapid expansion of the abdomen.

Preparing for pregnancy

A woman's body undergoes significant changes in pregnancy, with the developing fetus making increasing demands. Preparation for pregnancy should begin before conception, as fetal development begins from the third week after the last menstrual period. Damaging effects (e.g. exposure to drugs) may occur before the woman is even aware she is pregnant. Being as fit and healthy as possible before conception maximizes chances of a healthy pregnancy, but not all poor obstetric outcomes can be avoided. Pre-pregnancy counselling by a specialist team is recommended where specific risks and diseases are identified.

Specific risks for older mothers

- Advanced maternal age is a risk factor for adverse outcome.
- A woman >35yrs old has a reduced chance of conceiving. This rate of decline drops very quickly by 40yrs.
- Age also carries an increased risk of chromosomal abnormalities in the baby (most common abnormality being Down's syndrome).
- Older mothers are more likely to develop complications in pregnancy, e.g. pre-eclampsia and diabetes mellitus.

Exercise and stress

- Moderate exercise should be encouraged, as it improves a woman's cardiovascular and muscular fitness.
- Women should be reassured that beginning or continuing a moderate course of exercise during pregnancy is not associated with adverse outcome. Best exercises are low-impact aerobics, swimming, brisk walking, and jogging.
- Contact and high-impact and vigorous racquet sports that may involve the risk of abdominal trauma should be avoided.
- Exercise is also associated with higher self-esteem and confidence.
- Relaxation and avoiding stress should be encouraged when planning for pregnancy.

⚠ Scuba diving may result in fetal birth defects and fetal decompression disease and, therefore, is not recommended.

Stopping contraception

- There is no delay in return to fertility after stopping the pill or having the coil removed.
- Women using contraceptive injection may experience a delay of several months.
- Often recommended that women wait 3mths after stopping the pill before trying to conceive.

Supplements and lifestyle advice

Folic acid and other vitamins

Folic acid is the only vitamin supplement that is recommended for use before pregnancy and up to 12wks gestation for women who are otherwise eating a healthy balanced diet.

> **Recommended doses of folic acid**
> - 400micrograms/day folic acid has been shown to reduce the occurrence of neural tube defects.
> - For women at higher risk (e.g. previous affected child, women with epilepsy, diabetes, and obesity), a dose of 5mg/day is recommended.

Iron
- Routine supplementation is not necessary and should be only prescribed when medically indicated. However, it may be considered routine in areas where incidence of iron-deficiency anaemia is high.
- The amount of elemental iron in an adult female is 5g. She will need 1mg/day before menstrual age, 2mg/day during reproductive age, and 3mg/day during pregnancy.

Calcium
Supplementation may be necessary if intake of calcium is low; however, the ideal is increased calcium by dietary intake.

Iodine
Deficiency is endemic in some parts of the world, and can cause cretinism and neonatal hypothyroidism. Supplementation with iodinized salt or oil should be considered.

Zinc
Low serum levels have been associated with an increased risk of preterm labour and growth restriction, but increased intake from dietary sources, such as milk and dairy products, should be sufficient.

⚠ Vitamin A supplementation (intake >700micrograms/day) might be teratogenic and should be avoided, as should consumption of products high in vitamin A, such as liver and pate.

Alcohol, smoking, and recreational drugs

Excessive alcohol intake has been conclusively shown to cause fetal malformations. The exact threshold of alcohol that will cause malformation in the fetus has not been established.

⚠ Avoid alcohol or limit consumption to one standard unit per day.

Smoking during pregnancy has an adverse effect on the developing fetus (e.g. preterm labour, low birth weight). Women should be encouraged to stop and supported through smoking cessation. If they cannot stop, reduction should be promoted.

▶ Stopping smoking at any stage has a beneficial effect.

⚠ Recreational and illegal drugs cause significant problems including miscarriage, preterm birth, poor fetal development, and intrauterine death. Help and support for dealing with any addiction should be sought from the appropriate agencies.

Weight and diet

- Fertility may be reduced in women who are significantly overweight (BMI >30) or underweight (BMI <18.5).
- Obesity is the most common nutritional disorder in the industrialized world, with increased risks including gestational diabetes and hypertension; also, monitoring and assessment may be difficult during pregnancy and labour (see 📖 Obesity in pregnancy: maternal risks, p. 258).
- Obesity has been recognized by the Confidential Enquiry into Maternal Deaths (CEMD) as carrying a greater risk of maternal death (see 📖 The Confidential Enquiry into Maternal Deaths, p. 408).
- Malnutrition, on the other hand, is a major life hazard in the developing world and is a cause of other problems such as anaemia that has its own inherent risk for both mother and fetus.
- Poor nutrition in pregnant women is associated with the delivery of low birth weight (<2500g) babies, and improving the nutritional status and maternal weight can have a positive effect on the birth outcome.
- Weight gain should be around 11–16kg during pregnancy, and women should consume an additional 350kcal (1500kJ) a day.
- A nutritious, well-balanced diet includes foods rich in protein, dairy foods (which supply calcium), starchy foods, and plenty of fruit and vegetables that supply vitamins and fibre.
- It is best to avoid a lot of sugary, salty, or fatty foods.
- Food delicacies such as undercooked meats and eggs, pates, soft cheeses, shellfish and raw fish, and underpasteurized milk should be avoided as they are potential sources of *Listeria* and *Salmonella* that could lead to adverse perinatal outcome.

⚠ Listeriosis in pregnancy is a known but rare cause of poor obstetric outcome and fetal death.

General health check

Planning a pregnancy provides a good opportunity for a general health check by the GP and may identify any potential obstetric risk factors well in advance.

Pre-pregnancy general health check

May include:
- A general examination including BP, heart, and lungs.
- Family history of inherited disorders or congenital abnormalities.
- Urine dipstick.
- Blood tests such as thalassaemia and sickle cell disease may be offered if at risk.
- Rubella (and hepatitis) status should be ascertained and vaccination given if not immune (women should be advised to avoid pregnancy for 3mths after immunization).
- HIV screening if at risk.
- Dental examination.

Pre-existing medical disorders

Pregnancy can have an adverse effect on pre-existing medical disorders (see 📖 Medical disorders in pregnancy, p. 185).
- The effect may be transient, returning to normal after delivery (e.g. diabetes mellitus), or it may be permanent and progressive, leading to maternal mortality (e.g. severe renal impairment or severe cardiac disease).
- For a woman with a pre-existing disorder contemplating pregnancy, the advice of a specialist should be sought early. If the risk is very high, pregnancy may be discouraged altogether (e.g. Eisenmengher's complex—ventricular septal defects (VSD) with pulmonary hypertension).
- Optimal control of certain diseases before conception may be very important to avoid the risk of fetal malformation or adverse outcome (e.g. diabetes mellitus).
- Some medications may be changed before conception to reduce the risk of teratogenesis (e.g. antiepileptics).
- Pregnancy undertaken when the illness is in remission, stable, or cured will ensure a better outcome.

Medication

In general, both prescription drugs and over-the-counter medication should be used as little as possible. Most drugs carry warnings about use in pregnancy. However, the benefit may outweigh the risks, even in pregnancy, so a doctor should be consulted before stopping or starting any medication in pregnancy or before conception.

Working during pregnancy

- Women should be reassured that it is safe to continue working before and during pregnancy.
- Some workplaces are more likely to present hazards (e.g. chemical factories, operating theatres, X-ray departments); hence, precautions may be necessary—specific advice should be sought from the employer's occupational health department.
- Women should be reassured that use of computers and video display units has not been proven to be linked with any adverse outcome.
- See 📖 Vaccination and travel, p. 183.

Diagnosis of pregnancy

The most obvious symptom of pregnancy is cessation of periods, i.e. a period of amenorrhoea in a woman having regular menstruation.

Other common symptoms of early pregnancy

Nausea and vomiting (morning sickness)
- Common in the 1st trimester.
- May occur at any time of the day.
- May sometimes persist throughout pregnancy.

Frequency of micturition
- ↑ Plasma volume and ↑ urine production.
- Pressure effect of the uterus on the bladder.
- Make sure the frequency is not associated with dysuria, which may denote possible infection.

Excessive lassitude or fatigue
- Common in early pregnancy.
- Tends to disappear after 12wks gestation.

Breast tenderness or 'heaviness'
Often seen early in pregnancy, particularly in the month after the first period is missed.

Fetal movements or quickening
- ~20wks gestation in the nullipara.
- 18wks in the multipara.
- Many women may experience fetal movements earlier than this and some may not perceive movements until term.

Occasionally a pregnant woman may experience an abnormal desire to eat something not normally regarded as nutritive (such as dirt). This is known as **pica**.

Clinical examination
- The vagina and cervix have a bluish tinge due to blood congestion.
- The size of the uterus may be estimated by bimanual examination (reasonably accurate in early pregnancy).
- After 12wks the uterus is palpable abdominally and the fetal heart may be heard using a hand-held Doppler.

The pregnancy test
- The hormone hCG is secreted by trophoblastic tissue:
  - ↑ exponentially from ~8 days after ovulation (doubles every second day in an ongoing pregnancy)
  - peaks at 8–12wks gestation.
- hCG levels can be measured in blood or urine.
- Test kits are available commercially (home pregnancy tests):
  - can show a positive result with urinary hCG levels >50IU/L.
  - some 'early' pregnancy test kits will detect levels of >25IU/L.
- These tests can confirm pregnancy within 1 week of a missed period.

Dating of pregnancy

Menstrual history

- The first day of the LMP may be used to calculate the gestational age and the EDD (Obstetric history: current pregnancy, p. 2), but this may be inaccurate as:
  - many women may not be certain of their LMP
  - ovulation does not always occur on day 14 and the proliferative phase may vary considerably in shorter or longer menstrual cycles.
- The EDD can be calculated using Naegele's formula (Obstetric history: current pregnancy, p. 2).
- About 40% of women will deliver within 5 days of the EDD and about 2/3 within 10 days.

⚠ 11–42% of gestational age estimates from LMP may be inaccurate.

▶ Pregnancies resulting from *in vitro* fertilization (IVF) can be dated using the day of embryo transfer.

Dating ultrasound scan

- Between 8 and 13wks USS provides the most accurate measure of gestational age and, where possible, should be used to calculate EDD.
- Before 8wks it is unreliable due to the small size of the gestation sac and fetal pole.
- After 13wks other factors may affect fetal growth; therefore, although an estimate can be made using BPD and femur length (FL), it may be unreliable.

Crown–rump length

Crown–rump length (CRL; Fig. 1.8) is used to calculate gestation between 8 and 13wks. It is measured from one fetal pole to the other along its longitudinal axis in a straight line.

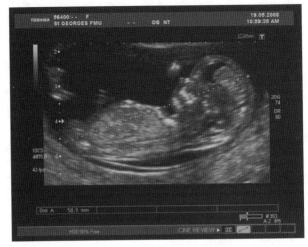

Fig. 1.8 Ultrasound image of a 12wk fetus measuring the CRL.

Ultrasound assessment of fetal growth

Any clinical suspicion that the fetus may be small or large for gestational age should be followed by a formal ultrasound assessment of fetal growth and amount of amniotic fluid (liquor volume).

The measurements used are (Fig. 1.9):

Biparietal diameter and head circumference

- The anatomical landmarks used to ensure the accuracy and reproducibility of the measurement are a midline falx, the thalami symmetrically positioned on either side of the falx, the visualization of the cavum septum pellucidum at one-third the fronto-occipital distance, and the lateral ventricles with their anterior and posterior horns identifiable.
- The calipers are placed between the leading edge of the proximal and distal skull bones (BPD) and circumferentially around the head (HC).

Abdominal circumference

- The abdominal circumference (AC) is the single most important measurement in assessing fetal size and growth.
- It is measured where the image of the stomach and the portal vein is visualized in a tangential section.

Femur length

By convention, measurement of the FL is considered accurate only when the image shows two blunted ends.

⚠ FL can be underestimated if the correct plane is not obtained.

See 📖 Intrauterine growth restriction: overview, p. 142.

Uterus measurement anomalies

The uterus may measure small for dates because of:
- Wrong dates.
- Oligohydramnios.
- Intrauterine growth restriction.
- Presenting part deep in the pelvis.
- Abnormal lie of the fetus.

The uterus may measure large for dates because of:
- Wrong dates.
- Macrosomia.
- Polyhydramnios.
- Multiple pregnancy.
- Presence of fibroids.

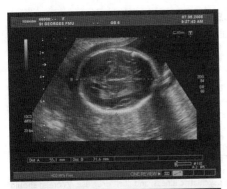

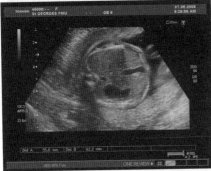

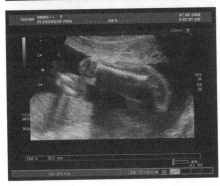

Fig. 1.9 Ultrasound measurement of biparietal diameter, abdominal circumference, and femur length.

Booking visit

The needs of each pregnant woman should be assessed at the first appointment and a plan of care made for her pregnancy. This should be reassessed at each appointment as new problems can arise at any time. Many women in the UK have 'shared obstetric care' whereby the woman's GP and community midwife undertake most of the obstetric care, with a limited number of visits to the hospital.

Routine involvement of an obstetrician in the care of women with uncomplicated pregnancy does not appear to improve perinatal outcomes compared with involving obstetricians when complications arise.

There should be continuity of care throughout the AN period and this should be provided by a small group of carers with whom the woman feels comfortable. The environment in which AN appointments take place should enable women to discuss sensitive issues, such as domestic violence, sexual abuse, psychiatric illness, and illicit drug use. Women should be given the information needed to choose between giving birth at home, in a midwifery-led unit, or in hospital.

Booking should ideally be early in pregnancy (before 12wks) in order to take full advantage of AN care. However, many women are seen for the first time in the second trimester.

⚠ Children born to very late bookers or unbooked women have a higher risk of perinatal mortality (4–5-fold) and morbidity, with an attendant increase in maternal morbidity and mortality.

Booking visit: history

A comprehensive history should be elicited (see 📖 Obstetric history: current pregnancy, p. 2) and a full physical examination undertaken (see 📖 Obstetric physical examination, p. 6).

- Risk factors from past history should be highlighted.
- It is essential to obtain past obstetric notes if it is thought that this information may change the management.
- History of inheritable diseases in close relatives should be sought, and history of migration and travel may identify risk for diseases such as haemoglobinopathies, some forms of hepatitis, and HIV infection.
- Histories of alcohol abuse, smoking, and addictive drug use are useful behavioural markers of potential risks (e.g. fetal abnormalities, impaired fetal growth, preterm labour, and neonatal drug withdrawal problems).
- It is important to identify women at risk of postnatal depressive illness:
  - women should be asked about previous and family history of psychiatric disorders, and social problems including domestic violence and previous self-harm
  - women at risk should have full psychiatric care and social support.
- Advice and support should be given on healthy lifestyles (including diet and exercise), pregnancy care services available, maternity benefits, and sufficient information to enable informed decision-making following screening tests.

First contact with healthcare professionals

Ensure the woman is given information on:
- Folic acid supplementation.
- Lifestyle advice.
- Antenatal screening.
- Booking appointment.

Booking appointment

- Identify high risk women who need additional care.
- Calculate BMI.
- Measure BP.
- Dipstick test urine (protein, glucose, blood, etc.).
- Ultrasound for gestational age and gross structural anomalies.
- Take blood tests for:
  - haemoglobinopathies
  - rubella
  - Venereal Disease Research Laboratory test (VDRL)
  - HIV
  - hepatitis B virus
  - red cell allo-antibodies
  - Hb for anaemia.
- Give information on:
  - AN classes
  - pregnancy care pathway
  - nutrition, diet, and vitamin supplementation
  - maternity benefits
  - how baby develops.

Antenatal care: planning

The basic aims of AN care are:
- To provide evidence-based information and support to women and their partners, to enable them to make informed decisions regarding their care.
- To advise on minor problems and symptoms of pregnancy.
- To assess maternal and fetal risk factors at the onset of pregnancy.
- To facilitate provision of prenatal screening and subsequent management of any abnormalities detected.
- To monitor fetal and maternal well-being throughout pregnancy and screen for commonly occurring complications (most notably BP and urine check at every visit to detect signs of developing pre-eclampsia and diabetes).
- To determine timing and mode of delivery when complications arise or if pregnancy continues after the EDD.

▶ The needs of each pregnant woman should be assessed at each appointment as new problems can arise at any stage in pregnancy.

⚠ Urine should be dipstick tested and BP measured at every AN visit.

Screening for chromosomal and structural abnormalities

Ideally, screening should be offered to all women at the time of booking. Detailed, unbiased, written information should be provided about the conditions being screened for, types of test available, and the implications of the results.

⚠ It is important for a woman to understand that a negative result in any screening test does not guarantee that her baby does not have that or another abnormality.

For full details on current UK screening see 📖 Prenatal diagnosis: overview, p. 108.

Antenatal appointment schedule

A schedule of AN appointments and what needs to be done at each visit has been described in the recent NICE Antenatal Care Guidelines and is summarized below.

Second trimester

- *16wks:*
  - discuss screening results
  - investigate if Hb level <11g
  - offer information and arrange anomaly scan (18–20wks).
- *25wks*—nulliparaous women only: BP, urine dip, plot symphysis SFH.
- *28wks:*
  - screening for anaemia and atypical red cell allo-antibodies
  - anti D prophylaxis to rhesus (Rh) –ve women
  - BP, urine dip, plot SFH.

Third trimester

- *31wks*—nulliparaous women only: BP, proteinuria, and plot SFH.
- *34wks:*
  - discuss labour and birth (including pain relief and birth plan)
  - give anti-D if rhesus –ve
  - BP, proteinuria, plot SFH.
- *36wks*—discuss:
  - breast-feeding
  - vitamin K prophylaxis
  - postnatal self-care
  - awareness of baby blues and postnatal depression
  - BP, proteinuria, plot SFH.
- *38wks:* BP, proteinuria, plot SFH.
- *40wks:*
  - BP, proteinuria, plot SFH
  - give information about prolonged pregnancy.

Membrane sweep at 41wks and induction of labour at 42wks.

Further reading

NICE. (2008). *Antenatal care: routine care for the healthy pregnant woman.* Antenatal care CG62.
℥ www.nice.org.uk/CG62

Antenatal care: routine blood tests

Antenatal care starts once the pregnancy is confirmed, and a referral is made by the GP to the community midwife for booking.

Routine blood tests

Full blood count (FBC)
- Physiological anaemia means lower limit for a 'normal' Hb is 10.5g/dL in pregnancy.
- Commonest cause of anaemia is iron deficiency. Investigate by assessment of haematinic indices, such as ferritin and total iron-binding capacity (TIBC) in microcytic hypochromic anaemia, serum and red cell folate, and serum B12 levels in macrocytic anaemia.

Blood grouping and antibody screen
Determining the blood group makes it possible to identify rhesus −ve women who are at risk of rhesus isoimmunization and to detect abnormal antibodies such as Kell and Duff (see 📖 Rhesus isoimmunization (immune hydrops), p. 135).

Rubella screen
Around 2% of nulliparous and 1% of multiparous women are not immune to rubella. It is recommended that these women receive post-partum rubella vaccination.

Syphilis screen
- Although incidence of syphilis in the UK is low, outbreaks do occur.
- Early treatment can prevent congenital syphilis in the neonate and screening and treatment is cost effective.

Hepatitis B screen
- Screening for hepatitis B is performed on all women in pregnancy at booking so that effective postnatal intervention can be offered.
- In adults, the virus is cleared within 6mths in 90% of those infected.
- In neonates, 90% become chronic carriers with risk of post-infective hepatic cirrhosis and hepatocellular carcinoma—hence the need to screen and prevent.
- Active immunization with hepatitis vaccine may be adequate for those neonates where mother was surface (s) antigen +ve, but passive and active immunization is recommended for those who are core (e) antigen +ve.

HIV screen
- The recommendation for all maternity units in the UK is for universal screening for HIV at the booking visit ('opt out' policy).
  - vertical transmission from mother to fetus can be significantly reduced (by two-thirds) by treatment of mother with antiretrovirals in pregnancy and labour, and infant for 6wks postnatally
  - risk of transmission is reduced by Caesarean section (CS) and avoidance of breast-feeding (see 📖 HIV and pregnancy, p. 176).

Antenatal care: specific blood tests

Haemoglobin electrophoresis
This should be routinely performed in women of minority ethnic or racial origins with high incidence of haemoglobinopathies.

Some ethnic origins at high risk of thalassaemia
- Cyprus.
- Eastern Mediterranean.
- Middle Eastern.
- Indian subcontinent.
- South-east Asia.

▶ Women of African or Afro-Caribbean origin are at risk of sickle cell disease or trait.

▶ If a woman is affected, testing her partner's status would enable appropriate counselling and further prenatal testing.

⚠ Persistent anaemia, of undiagnosed cause, may be an indication for Hb electrophoresis in any woman, regardless of racial origin.

Miscellaneous tests
A variety of other blood tests may be indicated on an individual basis. For example, thyroid function tests (TFTs, history of thyroid disease), HbA1c (to assess long-term control of diabetes), or baseline urea and creatinine (in chronic hypertensives with renal complications).

Screening for gestational diabetes
🖝 There is little consensus as to who, when, how, or even whether to screen for gestational diabetes mellitus (GDM). At present there is insufficient evidence to support routine screening for GDM. The timing of any screening is equally controversial as the later the test is performed, the higher the detection rate since glucose tolerance progressively deteriorates. On the other hand, the earlier in pregnancy GDM is diagnosed and hyperglycaemia treated, the greater the likelihood of positively influencing the outcome. Most units currently use targeted screening based on known risk factors.

Risk factors for gestational diabetes
- Previous GDM.
- Family history of diabetes (first-degree relative with diabetes).
- Previous macrosomic baby.
- Previous unexplained stillbirth.
- Obesity (BMI>30).
- Glycosuria on more than one occasion.
- Polyhydramnios.
- Large for gestational age fetus in current pregnancy.

Antenatal care: preparing for delivery

- In the early 3rd trimester, women are seen monthly and, at each visit, BP, urinalysis, and fundal height measurement, as well as enquiry about maternal well-being and fetal activity, are recorded.
- FBC and antibody screen is repeated at 28 and 34wks gestation, and rhesus –ve women are given anti-D prophylaxis at these times.
- From 36wks onwards, fetal presentation, as well as growth are assessed, and an ultrasound assessment performed if indicated.
- Preparation for labour and delivery should be discussed.
- The final routine visit between 40 and 41wks includes discussions on induction of labour after 41wks gestation.
- In women who wish to avoid induction, the risks of prolonging pregnancy should be discussed and a plan for increased fetal surveillance with cardiotocography (CTG) and ultrasound assessment of fetal growth and liquor volume can be made.

Pregnancy complications

Minor symptoms of pregnancy: gastrointestinal

Minor symptoms of pregnancy are mostly related to hormonal, physiological, and increased weight-bearing aspects of pregnancy. Although usually mild and self-limiting, some women may experience severe symptoms, which can affect their ability to cope with activities of daily living (see Further reading).

Nausea and vomiting (morning sickness)
- Most common complaint, especially in the 1st trimester: nausea—80–85%; vomiting—52%.
- Believed to be caused by hormones of pregnancy especially hCG.
- Increased in multiple and molar pregnancies.
- May be severe enough to warrant hospital admission—hyperemesis gravidarum (see 📖 Hyperemesis gravidarum, p. 546).
- Not usually associated with poor pregnancy outcome.
- Tends to resolve spontaneously by 16–20wks.
- *Management*:
  - lifestyle modification (e.g. eat small meals, increase fluid intake)
  - take ginger
  - acupressure (P6)
  - antiemetics (prochlorperazine, promethazine, metoclopramide).

Gastro-oesophageal reflux (heartburn)
- Very common complaint at all stages of pregnancy: 1st trimester—22%; 2nd trimester—39%; 3rd trimester—72%.
- Progesterone relaxes oesophageal sphincter allowing gastric reflux, which gradually worsens with increasing intra-abdominal pressure from the growing fetus.
- *Management*:
  - lifestyle modification (e.g. sleep propped up, avoid spicy food)
  - alginate preparations and simple antacids
  - if severe, H2 receptor antagonists (ranitidine).

Constipation
- Common complaint that appears to decrease with gestation:
  - 1st trimester 39%
  - 2nd trimester 30%
  - 3rd trimester 20%.
- Progesterone reduces smooth muscle tone, affecting bowel activity.
- Often made worse by iron supplementation.
- *Management*:
  - lifestyle modification (e.g. increasing fruit, fibre, and water intake)
  - fibre supplements
  - osmotic laxatives (lactulose).

Further reading
NICE. (2008). *Antenatal care: routine care for the healthy pregnant woman*. Antenatal care CG62. 🔊 www.nice.org.uk/CG62

Minor symptoms of pregnancy: musculoskeletal and vascular

Symphysis pubis dysfunction (SPD) or pelvic girdle pain (PGP)

- Describes a collection of signs and symptoms producing pelvic pain.
- Usually mild, but can present with severe and debilitating pain.
- Incidence up to 10%.
- *Management:*
  - physiotherapy advice and support
  - simple analgesia
  - limit abduction of legs at delivery
  - CS not indicated.

See ᗡ www.pelvicpartnership.org.uk

Backache and sciatica

- Common complaint, attributed to hormonal softening of ligaments exacerbated by altered posture due to the weight of the uterus.
- Prevalence estimated between 35% and 61%.
- Pressure on the sciatic nerves may also produce neurological symptoms (sciatica).
- *Management:*
  - lifestyle modification (e.g. sleeping positions)
  - alternative therapies including relaxation and massage
  - physiotherapy input (e.g. back care classes)
  - simple analgesia.

Carpal tunnel syndrome

- Occurs due to oedema compressing the median nerve in the wrist.
- Usually resolves spontaneously after delivery.
- *Management:*
  - sleeping with hands over the side of the bed may help
  - wrist splints may be of benefit
  - if evidence of neurological deficit, surgical referral may be indicated.

Haemorrhoids

- Tend to occur in the 3rd trimester.
- Incidence 8–30% of pregnant women.
- *Management:*
  - avoid constipation from early pregnancy
  - ice packs and digital reduction of prolapsed haemorrhoids
  - suppositories and topical agents for symptomatic relief
  - if thrombosed, may require surgical referral.

Varicose veins
- Common complaint, which increases with gestation.
- Thought to be due to progesterone relaxing the vasculature and the fetal mass effect decreasing pelvic venous return.
- *Management:*
  - regular exercise
  - compression hosiery
  - consider thromboprophylaxis if other risk factors are present.

Minor symptoms of pregnancy: genitourinary and others

Urinary symptoms

- Frequency in the 1st trimester results from increased glomerular filtration rate and the uterus pressing against the bladder.
- Stress incontinence may occur in the 3rd trimester as a result of pressure on the pelvic floor.

⚠ Urinary tract infections (UTI) are common in pregnancy.
- *Management:*
  - screen for UTI (urine dipstick testing: nitrite analysis is best)
  - avoid caffeine and fluid late at night.

Vaginal discharge

- Increases due to increased blood flow to the vagina and cervix.
- Should be white/clear and mucoid;
  - offensive, coloured, or itchy may indicate an infection
  - profuse and watery may indicate ruptured membranes.
- *Management:*
  - exclude ruptured membranes
  - exclude sexually transmitted infection (STI) and candidiasis (common in pregnancy)
  - reassurance.

Itching and rashes

- Skin changes and itching are common in pregnancy.
- Rashes are usually self-limiting and not serious.
- *Management:*
  - full history and examination to exclude infectious causes (e.g. varicella (📖 Varicella (chickenpox), p. 164) and obstetric cholestasis (see 📖 Obstetric cholestasis, p. 216)
  - emollients and simple over-the-counter 'anti-itch creams'
  - reassurance—most will resolve after delivery
  - referral to dermatologist if severe.

Other common minor symptoms of pregnancy

- *Breast enlargement and pain:* may be helped with supportive underwear.
- *Mild breathlessness on exertion:* important to exclude pulmonary embolus and anaemia.
- *Headaches:* important to exclude pre-eclampsia or (rare) neurological cause.
- Tiredness.
- Insomnia.
- Stretch marks.
- Labile mood.
- Calf cramps.
- Braxton Hicks contractions.

Antepartum haemorrhage: overview

Women with placenta praevia or placental abruption may present with typical symptoms and signs and with recognized risk factors. However, there may be minimal or no per vaginum (PV) loss in a large abruption and an abruption is usually, but not always, painful.

Antepartum haemorrhage (APH) is bleeding from the genital tract in pregnancy at ≥24wks gestation before onset of labour.

Causes of antepartum haemorrhage
- Based on available literature the incidence of APH is 3 to 5% of which 53% has been due to placenta praevia and abruption and about 47% due to unexplained and other causes (e.g. local lesions).
- Placenta praevia (~1%).
- Placental abruption (~1%).
- Others (~1%), including:
- Maternal:
  - incidental (cervical erosion/ectropion)
  - local infection of cervix/vagina
  - a 'show'
  - genital tract tumours
  - varicosities
  - trauma.
- Fetal: vasa praevia.

⚠ There may be rapid and severe haemorrhage from a placenta praevia.

⚠ Most bleeding from an abruption is concealed.

Vasa praevia
- This occurs when the fetal vessels run in membranes below the presenting fetal part, unsupported by placental tissue or umbilical cord.
- Incidence is 1:2500 to 1:2700.
- May present with PV bleeding after rupture of fetal membranes followed by rapid fetal distress (from exsanguination).
- Reported fetal mortality ranges between 33% and 100%.
- Risk factors include:
  - low-lying placenta
  - multiple pregnancy
  - IVF pregnancy
  - bilobed and especially succenturiate lobed placentas.

Antepartum haemorrhage: assessment

Initial assessment

Rapid assessment of maternal and fetal condition is a vital first step as it may prove to be an obstetric emergency.

> **History**
>
> A basic clinical history should establish:
> - Gestational age.
> - Amount of bleeding (but don't forget concealed abruption).
> - Associated or initiating factors (coitus/trauma).
> - Abdominal pain.
> - Fetal movements.
> - Date of last smear.
> - Previous episodes of PV bleeding in this pregnancy.
> - Leakage of fluid PV.
> - Previous uterine surgery (including CS).
> - Smoking and use of illegal drugs (especially cocaine).
> - Blood group and rhesus status (will she need anti-D?).
> - Previous obstetric history (placental abruption/intrauterine growth restriction (IUGR), placenta praevia).
> - Position of placenta, if known from previous scan.

Maternal assessment

This should include:
- BP.
- Pulse.
- Other signs of haemodynamic compromise (e.g. peripheral vasoconstriction or central cyanosis).
- Uterine palpation for size, tenderness, fetal lie, presenting part (if it is engaged, it is not a placenta praevia).

⚠ Remember, never perform a vaginal examination (VE) in presence of PV bleeding without first excluding a placenta praevia ('No PV until no PP').

Once a placenta praevia is excluded, a speculum examination should be undertaken to assess degree of bleeding and possible local causes of bleeding (trauma, polyps, ectropion), and to determine if membranes are ruptured. A digital examination ascertains cervical changes indicative of labour.

Fetal assessment

- Establish whether a fetal heart can be heard.
- Ensure that it is fetal and not maternal (remember, the mother may be very tachycardic).
- If fetal heart is heard and gestation is estimated to be 26wks or more, FHR monitoring should be commenced.

Placenta praevia (PP) (see Fig. 2.1)

Definition
When the placenta is inserted, wholly or in part, into the lower segment of the uterus.

Major (grade III or IV)
The placenta lies over the cervical os.

⚠ Cervical effacement and dilatation would result in catastrophic bleeding and potential maternal and therefore fetal death.

Minor (grade I or II)
The placenta lies in the lower segment, close to or encroaching on the cervical os.

Incidence
About 0.5% of pregnancies at term.

Diagnosis
Transvaginal USS is safe and is more accurate than transabdominal USS in locating the placenta.

Management
- Women with major PP who have previously bled should be admitted from 34wks gestation.
- Women with asymptomatic major PP may remain at home if they:
  - are close to the hospital
  - are fully aware of the risks to themselves and their baby
  - have a constant companion
  - have telecommunication and transport.

Delivery is likely to be by CS if the placental edge is <2cm from the internal os, especially if it is posterior or thick.

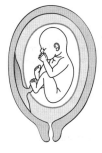
Normal placenta

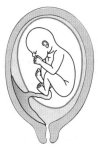
Minor placenta
praevia

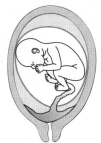
Major placenta
praevia

Fig. 2.1 Placenta praevia.

Antepartum haemorrhage: management

Limited antepartum haemorrhage (APH)
If bleeding was minor, is settling, and there are no signs of compromise, investigations in Box 2.1 should be undertaken.

Box 2.1 Assessment
Following assessment, women will fall into one of two categories:
- Bleeding heavy and continuing, mother or fetus is/soon will be compromised (see 📖 Massive obstetric haemorrhage: causes, p. 380).
- Bleeding minor, or settling, and neither mother nor fetus compromised: see section below.

Maternal management
- FBC.
- Kleihauer testing, if woman known to be RhD –ve, to determine extent of feto-maternal haemorrhage and if more anti-D is required.
- Group and save serum.
- Coagulation screen may be useful in cases of suspected abruption.

▶ In the event of APH, all RhD –ve women require 500IU of anti-D immunoglobulin, unless they are already sensitized. More anti-D may be required based on the result of the Kleihauer test.

Fetal management
- Ultrasound to establish fetal well-being (growth/volume of amniotic fluid) and to confirm placental location.
- Umbilical artery Doppler measurement (the function of the placenta may be compromised by small abruptions).

Ongoing antenatal management
- Most units admit women who have had an APH for 24h, as the risk of further bleeding is estimated to be greatest during that time.
- If the bleeding settles and mother is discharged, a clear plan for the remaining pregnancy should be made including extra fetal surveillance of growth and well-being.
- Surveillance after due date may need to be increased.

▶ Management must be individualized according to suspected cause of bleeding, gestation, fetal assessment, and continuing maternal risk factors.

✦ Management of women with a minor placenta praevia and minimal or no ongoing PV bleeding at an early gestation is controversial.

⚠ All women who have had an APH are high-risk. ↑ Surveillance of both mother and fetus.

⚠ History of APH ↑ risk of bleeding at delivery 'APH=post-partum haemorrhage (PPH)'.

Placental abruption

Definition
Placenta separates partly or completely from uterus before delivery of fetus. Blood accumulates behind placenta in uterine cavity or is lost through cervix.

Types
- *Concealed:* no external bleeding evident (<20%).
- *Revealed:* vaginal bleeding.

Presentation
- Usually present with abdominal pain.
- Typically sudden onset, constant, and severe.
- Posterior placentas may give rise to severe backache.
- The uterus is tender on palpation.
- Uterine activity is common.
- Uterus may later become hard (often described as 'woody').
- Many will be in labour (up to 50% on presentation).
- Bleeding is very variable, often dark.
- Maternal signs of shock.
- Fetal distress is common and precedes fetal death.

⚠ Remember, extent of the maternal haemorrhage may be much greater than apparent vaginal loss.

Incidence 0.5–1.0% of pregnancies.

Diagnosis Made clinically. Ultrasound is of use to confirm fetal well-being and exclude placenta praevia.

Management
- Admit all women with vaginal bleeding or unexplained abdominal pain.
- Establish immediate fetal well-being with CTG. Arrange USS as soon as possible.
- Access and bloods (see 📖 Massive obstetric haemorrhage: causes, p. 380).
- If fetal distress or maternal compromise, resuscitate and deliver.
- If no fetal distress, and bleeding and pain cease, consider delivery by term.

Further reading
RCOG. (2011). Green-top guideline 27. *Placenta praevia, placenta praevia accreta and vasa praevia: diagnosis and management.* ℘ www.rcog.org.uk

Blood pressure in pregnancy: physiology

Basic physiology

BP is directly related to systemic vascular resistance and cardiac output, and follows a distinct course during pregnancy:

- ↓ In early pregnancy until 24wks due to ↓ in vascular resistance.
- ↑ After 24wks until delivery via ↑ in stroke volume.
- ↓ After delivery, but may peak again 3–4 days post-partum.

⚠ Most women book in 1st or 2nd trimester. Be aware of the pregnant woman with a high booking BP, who may have previously undetected chronic hypertension—especially important in older pregnant women.

Blood pressure measurement

- BP must be measured correctly to avoid falsely high or low readings that may influence clinical management.
- BP should be measured sitting or in the supine position with a left sided tilt (to avoid compression of the inferior vena cava by the pregnant uterus, which reduces blood flow to the heart and consequently stroke volume and leads to falsely low BP) with the upper arm at the level of the heart.
- Use the correct cuff size (a normal adult cuff is usually for an upper arm of 34cm or less). A cuff too small may lead to a falsely high reading.
- The diastolic BP should be taken as Korotkoff V (the absence of sound), rather than Korotkoff IV (muffling of sound), which was previously used, unless the sound is heard all the way down to 0.

⚠ Be aware of automated BP monitors. They may under-record BP especially in pre-eclampsia. If unsure, check with sphygmomanometer.

Blood pressure in pregnancy: hypertension

Pre-eclampsia
See 📖 Pre-eclampsia: overview, p. 64.

Pregnancy-induced hypertension (PIH)

Defined as hypertension (>/=140/90) in the second half of pregnancy in the absence of proteinuria or other markers of pre-eclampsia.

- Affects 6–7% of pregnancies.
- At ↑ risk of going on to develop pre-eclampsia (15–26%).
- The risk ↑ with earlier onset of hypertension.
- Delivery should be aimed at the time of the EDD.
- BP usually returns to pre-pregnancy limits within 6wks of delivery.

Chronic hypertension
- It complicates 3–5% of pregnancies.
- Pregnant women who have a high booking BP (130–140/80–90 or more) are likely to have chronic hypertension.
- Increased risk of developing pre-eclampsia.
- Delivery should be planned at around the time of the EDD.

▶ Now more common because of an older pregnant population.

⚠ If BP very high, important to exclude a 2° cause, rather than attributing it to essential hypertension.

Post-partum hypertension
- New hypertension may arise in the post-partum period.
- It is important to determine whether this is physiological, pre-existing chronic hypertension, or new-onset pre-eclampsia.

▶ Remember, BP peaks on the 3rd to 5th day post-partum.

⚠ Symptoms such as epigastric pain or visual disturbance and new-onset proteinuria are suggestive of post-partum pre-eclampsia.

Postnatal management of hypertension
- Postnatally methyldopa should be changed to a β-blocker because of the risk of postnatal depression (see Table 2.1).
- Captopril can be used (up to 50mg PO tds).
- Nifedipine (10mg PO bd up to 30mg PO qds) may also be used.

▶ Women should be told that breast-feeding is safe with these drugs.
- The GP can follow up the BP in the community and titrate the medication to the BP.
- Women on medication should be offered a postnatal follow-up appointment 6wks postnatally.
- The BP usually resolves by 6wks.
- If still raised after this it is important to look for secondary causes of hypertension.

Table 2.1 Antihypertensive medications

Medication	Dose	Side effects	Breast-feeding
Labetalol	100mg bd up to 600mg qds	Avoid in asthma	Yes
	IV infusion for severe refractory hypertension		Yes
Methyldopa	250mg bd up to 1g tds	Depression change postnatally	Yes
Nifedipine	10mg bd up to 30mg tds	Tachycardia, flushing, headache	Yes
Hydralazine	25mg tds up to 75mg qds	Tachycardia, pounding heartbeat, headache, diarrhoea	Yes
Atenolol	50–100mg od	Avoid in asthma	Yes
ACE inhibitors	Postpartum only, as fetotoxic		Captopril safe

Hypertension in pregnancy treatment principles

⚠ Treatment of BP is urgently required for maternal safety at levels of ≥160/110.

• Escalation of treatment is required until levels are below this (see Table 2.1).

• Treatment should aim for BP levels not <120/80.

▶ Treatment of BP protects women from the adverse effects of ↑ BP but does not alter the course of pre-eclampsia.

Definition of pre-eclampsia

Due to its heterogeneous nature it can be difficult to define clinically.

• It is usually taken to be a BP ≥140/90 *and* ≥300mg proteinuria in a 24h collection.

• In those women who are already hypertensive, a rise in the systolic BP ≥30mmHg or diastolic BP ≥15mmHg is used.

• There may be other clues such as abnormal biochemistry or fetal growth restriction.

▶ Several individual features may indicate diagnosis of pre-eclampsia.

Pre-eclampsia: overview

Pre-eclampsia is a multisystem disorder characterized by hypertension and proteinuria and is thought to arise from the placenta. However, it can present in a wide variety of ways and not always in the classical fashion. It has a wide spectrum of severity ranging from mild to severe (eclampsia). It is a leading cause of maternal morbidity and mortality in the UK. It is a common cause of prematurity and hospital admission and has huge economic implications.

Incidence

- Pre-eclampsia affects about 5% of pregnancies (usually in mild form).
- Severe pre-eclampsia affects up to 1% of pregnancies.

Prediction of pre-eclampsia

History:

- There is an increased (x7) chance of pre-eclampsia in subsequent pregnancies in women who have had pre-eclampsia before.
- The risk increases with earlier onset (see Box 2.2), increasing severity, and after haemolysis, elevated liver enzymes, and low platelets (HELLP) syndrome (see ▣ Eclampsia and haemolysis, elevated liver enzymes, and low platelets (HELLP) syndrome, p. 70).
- Presence of other risk factors, e.g. medical disease, family history.
- *Blood tests:*
  - low pregnancy-associated plasma protein-A (PAPP-A) (▣ Common screening tests, p. 112) associated with ↑ risk.
  - raised uric acid, low platelets, and high Hb may help differentiate pre-eclampsia from PIH before proteinuria occurs.
  - interest is growing in vascular endothelial growth factor (VEGF) and placental growth factor (PlGF) (↓ before pre-eclampsia develops), and soluble FM-like tyrosine kinase 1 (sFlt-1) (↑ before pre-eclampsia is manifest).
- *Ultrasound:* uterine artery Dopplers at 11–13 or 22–24wks are predictive of early-onset or severe pre-eclampsia.

Integrated testing: the combination of independent risk factors such as history, PAPP-A, and uterine arteries at 12wks is the most effective early predictive test.

Prevention of pre-eclampsia

Women who have had severe early-onset pre-eclampsia should be offered low-dose aspirin (75mg PO od) before 16wks in the next pregnancy as it may reduce (by ~20%) the incidence of repeat severe pre-eclampsia.

Secondary causes of hypertension

- Renal disease.
- Cardiac disease, e.g. coarctation of the aorta.
- Endocrine causes, e.g. Cushing's syndrome, Conn's syndrome, or rarely a phaeochromocytoma.

Women with chronic hypertension are at risk of:

- Superimposed pre-eclampsia.
- Fetal growth restriction.
- Placental abruption.

Box 2.2 Risk factors for pre-eclampsia

- Previous severe/early-onset pre-eclampsia x7.
- Age >40 or teenager.
- Family history (mother or sister) x4.
- Obesity (BMI >30) x2.
- Primiparity x2–3.
- Multiple pregnancy x5.
- Long birth interval (>10yrs) x2–3.
- Fetal hydrops.
- Hydatidiform mole.
- Pre-existing medical conditions:
  - hypertension
  - renal disease
  - diabetes
  - antiphospholipid antibodies
  - thrombophilias
  - connective tissue disease.

Further reading

Action on Pre-Eclampsia (APEC). ♒ www.apec.org.uk

Pre-eclampsia: clinical features and investigations

Pre-eclampsia can present with a wide variety of signs and symptoms. It presents to the clinician a diagnostic dilemma and never ceases to surprise. However, most women with pre-eclampsia are asymptomatic.

Symptoms

- Headache (esp. frontal) (but very common without pre-eclampsia toxaemia (PET)).
- Visual disturbance (esp. flashing lights) (but very common without PET).
- Epigastric or right upper quadrant (of abdomen) (RUQ) pain.
- Nausea and vomiting.
- Rapid oedema (esp. face).

⚠ Symptoms usually occur only with severe disease.

Signs

- Hypertension (>140/90; severe if >/=160/110).
- Proteinuria (>300mg in 24h).
- Facial oedema.
- Epigastric/RUQ tenderness is a sign of liver involvement and capsule distension.
- Confusion.
- Hyperreflexia and/or clonus (>3 beats) is a sign of cerebral irritability.
- Uterine tenderness or vaginal bleeding from a placental abruption.
- Fetal growth restriction on ultrasound, particularly if <36wks.

Laboratory investigations

FBC

- Relative high Hb due to haemoconcentration.
- Thrombocytopaenia.
- Anaemia if haemolysis (📖 Eclampsia and haemolysis, elevated liver enzymes, and low platelets (HELLP) syndrome, p. 70).

Coagulation profile

Mildly prolonged prothrombin time (PT) and activated partial thromboplastin time (APTT).

Biochemistry

- ↑ Urate.
- ↑ Urea and creatinine.
- Abnormal LFTs (↑ transaminases).
- ↑ Lactate dehydrogenase (LDH; a marker for haemolysis).
- ↑ Proteinuria (>300mg protein/24h).

Pre-eclampsia: management

Pre-eclampsia has a number of severe complications (see Box 2.3). Cure is delivery of placenta. Management depends on several issues, including maternal and fetal well-being and gestational age.

Box 2.3 Severe complications of pre-eclampsia

- Eclampsia.
- HELLP.
- Cerebral haemorrhage.
- IUGR and fetal compromise.
- Renal failure.
- Placental abruption.

Outpatient management of pre-eclampsia

- Appropriate if:
  - BP <160 systolic and <110 diastolic and can be controlled
  - no or low (≤1+/<300mg/24h) proteinuria
  - asymptomatic.
- Difficult to distinguish from gestational hypertension.
- Warn about development of symptoms.
- 1–2/wk review of BP and urine.
- Weekly review of blood biochemistry.

Mild–moderate pre-eclampsia:

- BP <160 systolic and <110 diastolic with significant proteinuria and no maternal complications.
- Once significant proteinuria occurs, admission is advised:
  - ≥2+ protein
  - >300mg proteinuria/24h
  - a split protein:creatinine ratio can be a useful screening test for proteinuria—check with your lab for their normal values, but in general >30 equates to >300mg proteinuria/24h.
- 4-hourly BP.
- 24h urine collection for protein.
- Daily urinalysis.
- Daily fetal assessment with CTG.
- Regular blood tests (every 2–3 days unless symptoms or signs worsen).
- Regular ultrasound assessment (fortnightly growth and twice weekly Doppler/liquor volume depending on severity of pre-eclampsia).

▶ If BP increases (>160 systolic *or* >110 diastolic) antihypertensive therapy should be started (see Table 2.1). Medication does not cure the condition, but aims to prevent hypertensive complications of pre-eclampsia.

Severe pre-eclampsia: management

⚠ Defined as the occurrence of BP ≥160 systolic or ≥110 diastolic in the presence of significant proteinuria (≥1g/24h *or* ≥2+ on dipstick), *or* if maternal complications occur.

▶ Senior obstetric, anaesthetic, and midwifery staff should be informed and involved in the management of a woman with severe pre-eclampsia.

Treatment
- The only treatment is delivery, but this can sometimes be delayed with intensive monitoring if <34wks.
- Pre-eclampsia often worsens for 24h after delivery.

Indications for immediate delivery
- Worsening thrombocytopaenia or coagulopathy.
- Worsening liver or renal function.
- Severe maternal symptoms, especially epigastric pain with abnormal LFTs.
- HELLP syndrome or eclampsia.
- Fetal reasons such as abnormal CTG or reversed umbilical artery end diastolic flow.

Management
Blood pressure
- ⚠ BP needs to be stabilized with antihypertensive medication (must aim for <160 systolic *and* <110 diastolic).
- Initially use PO nifedipine 10mg: can be given twice 30min apart.
- If BP remains high after 2–3 nifedipine doses:
  - start IV labetalol infusion
  - ↑ infusion rate until BP is adequately controlled.
- Start maintenance therapy, usually labetalol; methyldopa if asthmatic.

Other management
- Take bloods for FBC, urea and electrolytes (U&E), LFTs, and clotting profile.
- Strict fluid balance chart: consider a catheter.
- CTG monitoring of fetus until condition stable.
- Ultrasound of fetus:
  - evidence of IUGR, estimate weight if severely preterm
  - assess condition using fetal and umbilical artery Doppler.

⚠ If <34wks, steroids should be given and the pregnancy may be managed expectantly unless the maternal or fetal condition worsens.

Eclampsia and haemolysis, elevated liver enzymes, and low platelets (HELLP) syndrome

Eclampsia

Eclampsia is defined as the occurrence of a tonic-clonic seizure in association with a diagnosis of pre-eclampsia.

- Complicates approximately 1–2% of pre-eclamptic pregnancies.
- May be the initial presentation of pre-eclampsia, and may occur before hypertension or proteinuria.
- Fits may occur antenatally (38%), intrapartum (18%), or postnatally usually within the first 48h (44%).

⚠ Eclampsia is an obstetric emergency. Every hospital in the UK should have an eclampsia protocol and eclampsia box with all the drugs for treatment.

⚠ When new to a hospital, familiarize yourself with protocol and whereabouts of the drug box.

⚠ Eclampsia is a sign of severe disease: most women who die with pre-eclampsia or eclampsia do so from other complications, such as blood loss, intracranial haemorrhage, or HELLP.

HELLP syndrome

This is a serious complication regarded by most as a variant of severe pre-eclampsia which manifests with haemolysis (H), elevated liver enzymes (EL), and low platelets (LP).

- Incidence is estimated at 5–20% of pre-eclamptic pregnancies.
- Maternal mortality is estimated at 1%, with perinatal mortality estimates of 10–60%.
- Liver enzymes ↑ and platelets ↓ before haemolysis occurs.
- Syndrome usually self-limiting, but permanent liver or renal damage may occur.
- Symptoms include:
  - epigastric or RUQ pain (65%)
  - nausea and vomiting (35%)
  - urine is 'tea-coloured' due to haemolysis.
- Signs include:
  - tenderness in RUQ
  - ↑ BP and other features of pre-eclampsia.
- Eclampsia may co-exist.
- Delivery is indicated.
- Treatment is supportive and as for eclampsia (magnesium sulfate ($MgSO_4$) is indicated).
- Although platelet levels may be very low, platelet infusions are only required if bleeding, or for surgery and <40.

⚠ Beware of epigastric pain in any pregnant and immediately postnatal women: always check the BP, urine, and liver enzymes.

Management of eclampsia

▶▶ Call for help—obstetric specialist registrar (SpR), senior house officer (SHO), and consultant, anaesthetic SpR and consultant, delivery suite coordinator.

- Basic principles of airway, breathing, and circulation plus IV access.
- Most eclamptic fits are short-lasting and terminate spontaneously.
- $MgSO_4$ is the drug of choice for both control of fits and preventing (further) seizures.
- A loading dose of 4g should be given over 5–10min followed by an infusion of 1g/h for 24h.
- If further fits occur a further 2g can be given as a bolus (the therapeutic range for Mg is 2–4mmol/L).
- In repeated seizures use diazepam (if still fitting the patient may need intubation and ventilation and imaging of the head to rule out a cerebral haemorrhage).
- Strict monitoring of the patient is mandatory.
- Pulse, BP, respiration rate, and oxygen saturations every 15min.
- A urometer and hourly urine.
- Assessment of reflexes every hour for Mg toxicity (usually knee reflexes, but use biceps if epidural in situ).
- Mg toxicity is characterized by confusion, loss of reflexes, respiratory depression, and hypotension.
- Half/stop infusion if oliguric (<20mL/h) or raised creatinine and seek senior/renal advice.
- If toxic give 1g calcium gluconate over 10min.
- If hypertensive (BP >160/110) give BP-lowering drugs:
  - oral nifedipine
  - IV labetalol (avoid in asthmatics).
- Fluid restrict the patient to 80mL/h or 1mL/kg/h due to the risk of pulmonary oedema (even if oliguric the risk of renal failure is small); monitor the renal function with the creatinine.
- A CVP line may be needed if there has been associated maternal haemorrhage and fluid balance is difficult or if the creatinine rises.
- The fetus should be continuously monitored with CTG.
- Deliver fetus once the mother is stable.
- Vaginal delivery is not contraindicated if cervix is favourable.
- If HELLP syndrome coexists, consider high-dose steroids and involvement of renal and liver physicians.

Third stage should be managed with 5–10U oxytocin, rather than syntometrine® or ergometrine because of increase in BP.

Further reading

NICE. (2010). *The management of hypertensive disorders during pregnancy*. Hypertension in pregnancy, CG107. ℘ www.nice.org.uk/cg107

Multiple pregnancy: overview

Incidence

- About 1 in 34 babies born in the UK is a twin or triplet. Incidence of multiple pregnancy was rising, but now appears to be stable at:
  - twins—15:1000
  - triplets—1:5000
  - quadruplets—1:360 000.
- Higher multiples than this are extremely rare, but do occur: a surviving set of quintuplets was born in the UK in 2007.

Aetiology

Multiple predisposing factors including:
- Previous multiple pregnancy.
- Family history.
- Increasing parity.
- *Increasing maternal age:*
  - <20yrs: 6:1000
  - >35yrs: 22:1000
  - >45yrs: 57:1000.
- *Ethnicity:*
  - Nigeria: 40:1000
  - Japan: 7:1000.
- Assisted reproduction—incidence of multiple pregnancy:
  - clomiphene—10%
  - intrauterine insemination (IUI)—10–20%
  - IVF with 2-embryo transfer—20–30%.

▶ In an attempt to decrease this complication, the Human Fertilization and Embryology Authority (HFEA) recommend that no more than two embryos should be transferred per IVF cycle.

Further reading

℘ www.hfea.gov.uk
℘ www.multiplebirths.org.uk

Multiple pregnancy: types

Dizygotic twins

Dizygotic twins result from two separate ova being fertilized by different sperm, simultaneously implanting and developing. Consequently, these fetuses will have separate amniotic membranes and placentas (dichorionic and diamniotic—DCDA). Twins may be different sexes. This mechanism of twinning accounts for two-thirds of multiple pregnancies; this type is most affected by predisposing factors, such as age and ethnicity.

Monozygotic twins

Monozygotic twins result from division into two of a single, already developing, embryo and will be genetically identical and, therefore, always the same sex. Whether they share the same amniotic membrane and/or chorion depends on the stage of development when the embryo divides. About two-thirds are monochorionic diamniotic.

See Fig. 2.2 for an explanation of the mechanism of twinning.

Timing of division in monozygotic twins
- <3 days → DCDA 30%.
- 4–7 days → monochorionic, diamniotic (MCDA) 70%.
- 8–12 days → monochorionic, monoamniotic (MCMA) <1%.
- >12 days → conjoined twins (very rare).

The worldwide monozygotic twining rate appears to be constant at about 3.5 per 1000. However, the rate is slightly greater than expected with IVF treatment.

Diagnosis

There are several signs and symptoms associated with multiple pregnancy including:
- Hyperemesis gravidarum.
- Uterus is larger than expected for dates.
- Three or more fetal poles may be palpable at >24wks.
- Two fetal hearts may be heard on auscultation.

However, the vast majority are diagnosed on ultrasound in the 1st trimester (at a dating or nuchal translucency scan). As most women in the UK now have USS at some stage in their pregnancy, diagnosis is rarely missed.

Chorionicity

Determining chorionicity allows risk stratification for multiple pregnancy and is best done by ultrasound in the 1st trimester or early in the 2nd. The key indicators are:
- Obviously widely separated sacs or placentae—DC.
- Membrane insertion showing the lambda (λ) sign—DC.
- Absence of λ sign <14wks diagnostic of MC.
- Fetuses of different sex—DC (dizygotic).

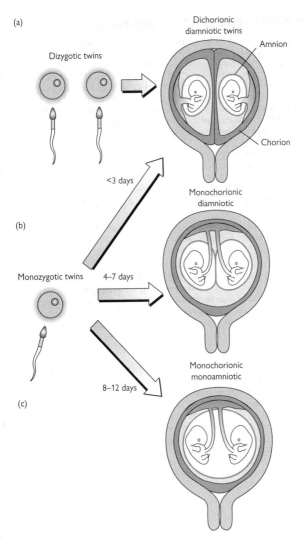

Fig. 2.2 Mechanism of twinning. Dizygotic twins (a) are always DCDA, but with monozygotic twins (a, b, and c), the type will depend on the time of the division of the conceptus.

Multiple pregnancy: antenatal care

- All multiple pregnancies are by definition 'high risk' and the care should be consultant led.
- Establish chorionicity—most accurately diagnosed in 1st trimester (absence of λ sign diagnostic), so an early USS should be considered with any indications of multiple pregnancy (e.g. fundus palpable before 12wks or exaggerated symptoms of early pregnancy).
- Routine use of iron and folate supplements should be considered.
- A detailed anomaly scan should be undertaken.
- Advise aspirin 75 milligrams (mg) od if additional risk factors for pre eclampsia.
- Serial growth scans at 28, 32, and 36wks for DC twins.
- More frequent antenatal checks because of ↑ risk of pre-eclampsia.
- Discuss mode, timing and place of delivery.
- Establish presentation of leading twin by 34wks.
- Offer delivery at 37–38wks: induction or lower segment Caesarean section (LSCS).

⚠ Surveillance needs to be more intensive for MC twins particularly <24wks, or higher multiples, so referral to a specialist fetal medicine team is advisable.

Preterm delivery and multiple pregnancy

See 📖 Preterm labour: prevention and prediction, p. 100).
- Incidence increased: principal cause of morbidity and mortality.
- Predictable with transvaginal cervical scanning.
- Not thought to be preventable by cervical cerclage.
- Beneficial effect of progesterone limited at best.

Maternal risks associated with multiple pregnancy

The risks of pregnancy appear to be heightened with twins compared with singletons, leaving mothers at increased risk of:
- Hyperemesis gravidarum.
- Anaemia.
- Pre-eclampsia (5× greater risk with twins than singletons).
- Gestational diabetes.
- Polyhydramnios.
- Placenta praevia.
- Antepartum and post-partum haemorrhage.
- Operative delivery.

Fetal risks associated with multiple pregnancy

- All fetal risks increased with MC twins.
- ↑ *Risk of miscarriage:* especially with MC twins.
- Congenital abnormalities more common only in MC twins including:
  - neural tube defects
  - cardiac abnormalities
  - gastrointestinal atresia.
- IUGR: up to 25% of twins.
- *Preterm labour:* main cause of perinatal morbidity and mortality:
  - 40% twins deliver before 37wks
  - 10% twins deliver before 32wks.
- ↑ *Perinatal mortality:*
  - singletons 5:1000
  - twins 18:1000
  - triplets 53:1000.
- ↑ Risk of intrauterine death (stillbirth):
  - singletons 8:1000
  - twins 31:1000
  - triplets 84:1000.
- ↑ Risk of disability (mainly, but not entirely, due to prematurity and low birth weight).
- ↑ *Incidence of cerebral palsy (CP):*
  - singletons 2:1000
  - twins 7:1000
  - triplets 27:1000.
- *Vanishing twin syndrome:* one twin apparently being reabsorbed at an early gestation (1st trimester).

Monochorionic, diamniotic twins

The shared circulation of MC twins can lead to several problems.

Twin-to-twin transfusion syndrome (TTTS)

This affects about 5–25% of MC twin pregnancies and left untreated has an 80% mortality rate. It may occur acutely at any stage or more commonly take a chronic course, which, at its worst, leads to severe fetal compromise at a gestation too early to consider delivery. It is caused by aberrant vascular anastamoses within the placenta, which redistribute the fetal blood. Effectively, blood from the 'donor' twin is transfused to the 'recipient' twin.

▶ MC twins require intensive monitoring, usually in the form of serial USS every 2wks from 16–24wks and every 3wks until delivery. This is best performed in a specialist fetal medicine unit. The treatment options potentially available include:

- Laser ablation of the placental anastamoses. This method is associated with lowest risk of neonatal handicap.
- Selective feticide by cord occlusion is reserved for refractory disease.

TTTS managed by laser treatment leads to survival of at least one in 80% and both in 50%.

Selective intrauterine growth restriction

- Growth discordance, even without TTTS, is more common.
- A very variable pattern of umbilical artery Doppler signals (intermittent absent/reversed end diastolic flow: ↑ AREDF) indicates a high risk of sudden demise.
- Treatment: if >28wks—delivery is safest; if <28wks, selective termination or laser ablation should be considered.

Termination of pregnancy issues

- Although MC twins may be discordant for structural abnormalities, genetically they are identical.
- Selective termination of pregnancy requires closure of the shared circulation so is normally performed using diathermy cord occlusion.

Twin reversed arterial perfusion (TRAP)

In this rare condition, one of an MC twin pair is structurally very abnormal with no or a rudimentary heart, and receives blood from the other (umbilical artery flow direction is reversed), which is called the 'pump twin'.

This normal twin may die of cardiac failure, and unless the abnormal twin is very small or flow to it ceases, selective termination using radiofrequency ablation or cord occlusion is indicated.

Effects of twin-to-twin transfusion on the fetus

Donor twin
- Hypovolaemic and anaemic.
- Oligohydramnios: appear 'stuck' to the placenta or uterine wall.
- Growth restriction.

Recipient twin
- Hypervolaemic and polycythaemic.
- Large bladder and polyhydramnios.
- Cardiac overload and failure.
- Evidence of fetal hydrops (ascites, pleural, and pericardial effusions).
- This twin is often more at risk than the donor.

Intrauterine death of a twin

- Dichorionic: the death of one twin in the 1st trimester or early part of the 2nd does not appear to adversely affect the remaining fetus. Loss in the late part of the 2nd or 3rd trimester usually precipitates labour, with 90% having delivered within 3wks.
- Monochorionic: because of the shared circulation, subsequent death or neurological damage from hypovolaemia follows in up to 25%, where one of the pair dies. Delivery does not decrease the risk of brain injury.

Further reading
🐁 www.eurofoetus.org

Multiple pregnancy: labour

- For all multiple pregnancies mode of delivery is debated.
- The second twin is at increased risk of perinatal mortality, but it is not currently the case that all twins are delivered by CS.
- For labour, the leading twin should be cephalic (~80%), and there should be no absolute contraindication (e.g. placenta praevia).
- Triplets and higher-order multiples are usually delivered by CS.
- Some authorities advise CS for MC twins.

For management of labour and delivery see Box 2.4.

Intrapartum risks associated with multiple pregnancy
- Malpresentation.
- Fetal hypoxia in second twin after delivery of the first.
- Cord prolapse.
- Operative delivery.
- Post-partum haemorrhage.
- Rare:
  - cord entanglement (MCMA twins only)
  - head entrapment with each other: 'locked twins'
  - fetal exsanguination due to vasa praevia.

Box 2.4 Management of labour and delivery for twins

- Twins are usually induced at ~38wks gestation, but many will have delivered spontaneously before then.
- The woman should have IV access and a current Group and Save.
- Fetal distress is more common in twins; continuous fetal monitoring with CTG is important throughout labour.
- This becomes imperative after the first twin has delivered to avoid hypoxia in the second.
- It may be helpful to monitor the leading twin with a fetal scalp electrode and the other abdominally.
- An epidural may be helpful, especially if there are difficulties delivering the second twin, but is not essential.
- Many units choose to deliver twins in theatre as there is more space available and it provides immediate recourse to surgical intervention if required.
- Importance of support for mother cannot be overestimated.
- Leading twin should be delivered as for a singleton, but with care to ensure adequate monitoring of the second throughout.
- After delivery of first baby, the lie of the second twin should be checked and gently 'stabilized' by abdominal palpation while a VE is performed to assess the station of the presenting part.
- It may be helpful to have an ultrasound scanner available in case of concerns about malpresentation of the second twin.
- Once the presenting part enters the pelvis the membranes can be broken and the second twin is usually delivered within 20min of the first.
- Judicious use of oxytocin may help if the contractions diminish after delivery of the first twin.
- If fetal distress occurs in the second twin, delivery may be expedited with either forceps or ventouse.
- If this is inappropriate, the choice is between CS and breech extraction (often after internal podalic version).
- Breech extraction involves gentle and continuous traction on one or both feet, and must only be performed by an experienced obstetrician.

⚠ It is never used to deliver singleton breeches.
- As there is an increased risk of uterine atony, syntometrine and prophylactic oxytocin infusion is recommended.

Breech presentation: overview

Breech presentation occurs when the baby's buttocks lie over the maternal pelvis. The lie is longitudinal, and the head is found in the fundus. This becomes decreasingly common with gestation, such that breech presentation at term occurs with only 3–4% of fetuses, but is much more common preterm.

Types of breech

- Extended breeches (70%):
  - both legs extended with feet by head; presenting part is the buttocks.
- Flexed breeches (15%):
  - legs flexed at the knees so that both buttocks and feet are presenting.
- Footling breeches (15%):
  - one leg flexed and one extended.

Causes and associations of breech presentation

- Idiopathic (most common).
- Preterm delivery.
- Previous breech presentation.
- Uterine abnormalities, e.g. fibroids and Müllerian duct abnormalities.
- Placenta praevia and obstructions to the pelvis.
- Fetal abnormalities.
- Multiple pregnancy.

Consequences of breech presentation

Fetal

- There is an increased risk of hypoxia and trauma in labour.
- Irrespective of the mode of delivery, neonatal and longer-term risks are increased. The reasons for this are incompletely understood but may be due in part to:
  - association with congenital abnormalities
  - many preterm babies are breech at the time of delivery.

Maternal

Most breeches are delivered by CS.

Diagnosis of breech presentation

- Before 36wks breech presentation is not important unless the woman is in labour.
- Breech presentation is commonly undiagnosed before labour (30%).
- On examination:
  - lie is longitudinal
  - the head can be palpated at the fundus
  - the presenting part is not hard
  - the fetal heart is best heard high up on the uterus.
- Ultrasound confirms the diagnosis and should also assess growth and anatomy because of the association with fetal abnormalities.

External cephalic version

External cephalic version (ECV) is a method for manually turning a breech or transverse presentation into a cephalic one. It is performed from 36wks in nulliparous women and 37wks in multiparous ones. The intention is to reduce the need for delivery by CS.

- *Method:* after USS, a forward roll technique is used. The breech is elevated from the pelvis, and pushed to the side where the back is; the head is then pushed forward and the roll completed. Excessive force must not be used. After the attempt, CTG is performed and anti-D given if the mother is Rh −ve. See Fig. 2.3.
- *Efficacy:* the success rate is about 50%. Spontaneous reversion to breech presentation occurs in 3%. Attempting ECV halves the chance of non-cephalic presentation at delivery and greatly reduces the risk of CS. Nulliparity, difficulty palpating the head, high uterine tone, an engaged breech, less amniotic fluid, and white ethnicity are associated with more difficulty.
- *Facilitation:* success rates are increased by the use of tocolysis, such as salbutamol, given either electively or if a first attempt fails. Epidural or spinal analgesia are not usually used.
- *Safety:* approximately 0.5% will require immediate delivery by CS due to fetal heart rate abnormalities or vaginal bleeding. Theoretical or minor risks include pain, precipitation of labour, placental abruption, fetomaternal haemorrhage, and cord accidents. The chances of CS during labour are slightly higher than with a fetus that has always been cephalic.
- *Other methods:* so-called natural methods of version (postural methods, acupuncture, moxabustion) remain unproven.

Contraindications to ECV

Absolute

- Caesarean delivery already indicated.
- Antepartum haemorrhage.
- Fetal compromise.
- Oligohydramnios.
- Rhesus isoimmunization.
- Pre-eclampsia.

Relative

- One previous CS.
- Fetal abnormality.
- Maternal hypertension.

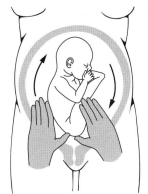

1. Gently disimpact the breech from the pelvis, guiding it towards the iliac fossa.

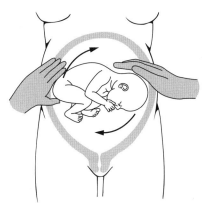

2. Continue to guide the breech upwards until the baby is transverse, then gentle pressure on the occiput helps to complete the forward roll.

Fig. 2.3 External cephalic version.

Breech presentation: delivery

Mode of delivery of breech presentation

- If ECV is declined or fails, or the breech is undiagnosed, the parents should be appraised of the evidence about breech birth.
- Most breech deliveries in the UK, USA, and Europe are by CS, because meta-analysis of RCTs has shown this to reduce neonatal mortality and short-term morbidity, although not longer-term morbidity.
- Elective CS appears protective even where the ideal conditions for vaginal delivery are present and the attendant is highly experienced.
- This policy does not increase maternal morbidity because attempting a vaginal delivery still carries a considerable risk of emergency CS, which is a more risky procedure.
- These findings have been criticized because of the trials' methodology and the way that breech labours were managed; nevertheless this is the best evidence currently available.
- The breech in advanced labour, or who is a second twin, or preterm is not necessarily best delivered by CS.

Vaginal delivery of the breech fetus

Knowledge and experience of this remains important because breech delivery requires skill and will occasionally be inevitable because of diagnosis in advanced labour or because of the mother's wishes.

Ideal selection for vaginal breech delivery
- Fetus is not compromised.
- Estimated fetal weight is <4kg.
- Spontaneous onset of labour.
- Extended breech presentation.
- Non-extended neck.

⚠ There is a risk of cord prolapse which is greatest in footling breeches (15%).

⚠ Oxytocin augmentation is not advised and failure of the buttocks to descend after full dilatation is a sign that delivery may be difficult.

Vaginal breech delivery technique

- Maternal effort should be delayed until the buttocks are visible.
- After delivery of the buttocks the baby is encouraged to remain back upwards but should not otherwise be touched until the scapula is visible.
- The arms are then hooked down by the index finger at the fetal elbow, bringing them down the baby's chest.
- The body is then allowed to hang.
- If the arms are stretched above the chest and cannot be reached, *Lovset's* manoeuvre is required.
    - This involves placing the hands around the body with the thumbs on the sacrum and rotating the baby 180° clockwise and then counterclockwise with gentle downward traction.
    - This allows the anterior shoulder and then the posterior shoulder to enter the pelvis and for the arm to be delivered from below the pubic arch.
- When the nape of the neck is visible, delivery is achieved by placing two fingers of the right hand over the maxilla and two fingers of the left at the back of the head to flex it (*Mauriceau–Smellie–Veit* manoeuvre) and maternal pushing is encouraged.
- If this fails to deliver the head, forceps should be applied before the next contraction.
- Delivery of the head should be gentle and controlled to avoid rapid decompression which could cause intracranial bleeding.
- The upright position for delivery is advocated by some experienced attendants but there is no proof that this makes delivery safer.

Further reading

Hannah ME, Hannah WJ, Hewson SA, *et al.* (2000). Planned Caesarean section versus planned vaginal birth for breech presentation at term: a randomized multi-centre trial. *Lancet* **356**: 1375–83.

Transverse, oblique, and unstable lie

Definition

- A **transverse** or **oblique** lie occurs when the axis of the fetus is across the axis of the uterus. This is common before term, but occurs in only 1% of fetuses after 37wks.
- **Unstable** lie occurs when the lie is still changing, usually several times a day, and may be transverse or longitudinal lie, and cephalic or breech presentation. See Fig. 2.4.

Assessment

- Ascertain stability from the history: has the presentation been changing?
- Ascertain fetal lie by palpation.
- Neither the head nor buttocks will be presenting.
- Also assess the laxity of the uterine wall.
- Does the presenting part move easily?
- Ultrasound should be performed to help ascertain the cause.

Management of abnormal lie

- Admission to hospital from 37wks is usually recommended with unstable lie, so that CS can be carried out if labour starts or the membranes rupture and the lie is not longitudinal.
- Whilst the lie remains unstable, the woman should remain in hospital.
- With increasing gestation the lie will usually revert to longitudinal and in these circumstances she can be discharged.
- If the lie does not stabilize, a CS is usually performed at 41wks.
- Some advocate a stabilizing induction whereby the fetus is turned to cephalic and an amniotomy immediately performed. This requires expertise.
- If the lie is stable but not longitudinal, a CS should be considered at 39wks.

Risks of abnormal lie

- Labour with a non-longitudinal lie will result in obstructed labour and potential uterine rupture.
- Membrane rupture risks cord prolapse because with longitudinal lie, the presenting part usually prevents descent of the cord through the cervix.

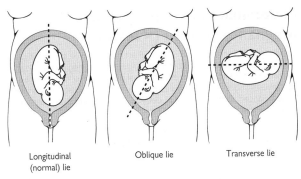

Longitudinal   Oblique lie   Transverse lie
(normal) lie

Fig. 2.4 Longitudinal, oblique, and transverse fetal lie.

Causes and associations of abnormal fetal lie

- Multiparity (particularly >para 2) with lax uterus (common).
- Polohydramnios.
- Uterine abnormalities, e.g. fibroids and Müllerian duct abnormalities.
- Placenta praevia and obstructions to the pelvis.
- Fetal abnormalities.
- Multiple pregnancy.

Abdominal pain in pregnancy: pregnancy related (<24wks)

The diagnosis of acute abdominal pain in pregnancy can be challenging. It is often difficult to differentiate between gynaecological, non-gynaecological, and pregnancy-related causes of abdominal pain. Some of the routine surgical investigations and procedures carry a risk to the fetus but this needs to be balanced against the risk of delayed diagnosis and treatment which would be harmful to both mother and child.

Miscarriage (see ☐ Chapter 15, p. 530)

- Can be associated with lower abdominal dull ache to severe continuous or colicky pain.
- Vaginal bleeding is present in most cases.
- Positive urine pregnancy test, pelvic examination, and USS are helpful in diagnosis.

Ectopic pregnancy (see ☐ Chapter 15, p. 534)

- Usually unilateral lower abdominal pain at <12wks gestation.
- Associated with brownish vaginal bleeding.
- Shoulder tip pain is suggestive of haemoperitoneum (bleeding ectopic).
- Serum hCG, USS, and laparoscopy are diagnostic.

Constipation

Physiological changes in pregnancy result in the slowing of gut peristalsis.

Signs and symptoms Varied but colicky lower abdominal pain (L>R) is the most common.

Management
- High-fibre diet.
- Osmotic laxatives.
- Glycerin suppositories.

Round ligament pain

This pain is attributed to stretching of the round ligaments.

Incidence 20–30% of pregnancies.

Signs and symptoms
- Commonly presents in 1st and 2nd trimester.
- Pain is often bilateral and located on the outer aspect of the uterus.
- Radiating to the groin.
- Aggravated by movement (especially getting up from a chair or turning over in bed).

Treatment
- Reassurance.
- Simple analgesia.
- Support belts may help.

Urinary tract infection

UTIs are more common in pregnancy and are an important association of preterm labour.

Signs and symptoms
- Suprapubic/lower abdominal pain.
- Dysuria, nocturia, and frequency.

Investigations
- Urine dipstick:
  - nitrites strongly suggest a UTI
  - blood, leucocytes, and protein raises index of suspicion.
- Midstream sample urine (MSU).

Management
- Antibiotics.
- Analgesia.
- ↑ Fluid intake.

Fibroids—red degeneration

Uterine fibroids occur in 20% of women of reproductive age. They may increase in size during pregnancy, compromising blood supply to central areas and causing pain. This is known as red degeneration.

Incidence
15% of pregnant women who have fibroids.

Signs and Symptoms
- Usually occurs between the 12th and 22nd week of pregnancy.
- Constant pain localized to one area of the uterus coinciding with the site of the fibroid (may be severe pain).
- May have a low-grade pyrexia.

Investigations
- USS (identifies fibroids but cannot confirm red degeneration).
- FBC (may show leucocytosis).

Treatment
- Analgesia (pain should resolve in 4–7 days; however, it may be severe and prolonged, so advice from pain specialists should be sought).

▶ Placental abruption differs in that the fibroid uterus is soft except at the site of the fibroid and the FH is normal.

⚠ Myomectomy must not be performed in pregnancy as it will bleed ++ (the only exception being for a torted pedunculated fibroid).

Abdominal pain in pregnancy: pregnancy related (>24wks)

Labour

Signs and symptoms
- Usually presents with regular painful contractions.
- Preterm labour may present with a history of vague abdominal pain which the woman may not associate with uterine activity.

△ Consider a VE in pregnant women with abdominal pain.

Braxton Hicks contractions

These are spontaneous benign contractions of the uterus, commonly occurring in the 3rd trimester.

Signs and symptoms
- Painless and infrequent tightenings of the uterus.
- VE reveals uneffaced and closed cervix.

Investigations
- Exclusion of precipitants of preterm labour (dipstick/MSU for UTI).
- Fibronectin assay if uncertain whether preterm labour (see 📖 Preterm labour: overview, p. 98).

Treatment
- Reassurance.

Symphysis pubis dysfunction

Signs and symptoms
Pubic pain relating to upper thighs and perineum.
- Aggravated by movement.
- Difficulty walking resulting in a waddling gait.

Treatment
- Analgesia and physiotherapy.

Reflux oesophagitis

Relaxation of the oesophageal sphincter occurs in pregnancy and the pressure of the gravid uterus on the distal end of the oesophagus results in an increased incidence of reflux oesophagitis. Gastric ulceration is less common due to decreased gastric acid secretion.

Incidence
60–70% of pregnant women.

Risk factors
- Polyhydramnios.
- Multiple pregnancy.

Signs and symptoms
- Epigastric/retrosternal burning pain exacerbated by lying flat.

Management
- Exclude pre-eclampsia.
- Antacids, H$_2$ receptor antagonists.
- Dietary and lifestyle advice (avoidance of supine position).

Uterine rupture

This usually occurs during labour but has been reported antenatally.

Risk factors
- Previous CS or other uterine surgery.
- Congenital abnormalities of the uterus.
- Induction or use of oxytocin in labour.
- Failure to recognize obstructed labour.

Signs and symptoms
- Tenderness over sites of previous uterine scars.
- Fetal parts may be easily palpable.
- Fetus not palpable on VE.
- Vaginal bleeding may be evident.
- Signs of maternal shock may be present.

⚠ CTG may show fetal distress and change in apparent uterine activity (contractions may seem to disappear on the tocograph).

Investigations
- FBC.
- Cross-match blood.

Management
- Maternal resuscitation.
- Urgent laparotomy to deliver fetus and repair uterus.

Other causes of abdominal pain in pregnancy
- Placental abruption.
- Pre-eclampsia/HELLP.

Abdominal pain in pregnancy: bowel related

Appendicitis

This is the most common surgical emergency in pregnant patients. Its incidence is 1:1500–2000 pregnancies with equal frequency in each trimester. Pregnant women have the same risk of appendicitis as non-pregnant women.

Signs and symptoms

- Classically periumbilical pain shifting to right lower quadrant.

⚠ Pain moves towards the right upper quadrant during the 2nd and 3rd trimesters due to displacement of the appendix by a gravid uterus.
- Nausea and vomiting.
- Anorexia.
- Guarding and rebound tenderness present in 70% of patients.

⚠ Rovsing's sign and fever are often absent in the pregnant patient.

Investigations

- White cell count (WCC) and C-reactive protein (CRP) are often ↑.
- USS: to exclude other causes of pain; CT/MRI may be considered.

Management

Diagnostic laparoscopy/laparotomy and appendicectomy.

⚠ Fetal loss is 3–5% with an unruptured appendix, ↑ to 20% if ruptured.

Intestinal obstruction

It is the third most common non-obstetric reason for laparotomy during pregnancy. It complicates 1:1500–3000 pregnancies. Incidence increases as the pregnancy progresses. Adhesions are the commonest cause.

Signs and symptoms

- Acute abdominal pain.
- Vomiting.
- Constipation.
- Pyrexia.

Diagnosis

- Erect abdominal X-ray (AXR) showing gas-filled bowel with little gas in large intestine.
- USS (abdominal and pelvic).

Treatment

- Conservative treatment ('drip and suck').
- Surgery for any acute obstructive cause or when not responding to conservative management.

Causes of intestinal obstruction
- Adhesions.
- Volvulus.
- Intussusception.
- Hernia.
- Neoplasm.

Abdominal pain in pregnancy: other causes

Acute cholecystitis

This is the second most common surgical condition in pregnancy (progesterone diminishes smooth muscle tone and predisposes to cholestasis leading to gallstone formation). The incidence of gallstones is 7% in nulliparous and 19% in multiparous women. The incidence of acute cholecystitis is 1–8:10 000 pregnancies.

Signs and symptoms
- Colicky epigastric/right upper quadrant pain.
- Nausea and vomiting.
- Murphy's sign may be positive in acute cholecystits.
- Jaundice (indicating obstruction of the common bile duct).
- Signs of systemic infection (fever and tachycardia).

Investigations
- FBC, LFTs, CRP (WCC and alkaline phosphatase are ↑ in pregnancy).
- ↑ Bilirubin (identify patients with concomitant biliary tree obstruction).
- USS biliary tract (may demonstate calculi or a dilated biliary tree).

Management
- Conservative approach is the most common management.
- Analgesics and antiemetics.
- Hydration.
- Antibiotics.
- Cholecystectomy preferably by laparoscopic approach may be indicated in patients with recurrent biliary colic, acute cholecystitis, and obstructive cholelithiasis (usually after delivery).

Adnexal torsion

This occurs when an enlarged ovary twists on its pedicle.

⚠ Torsion of the ovary and other adnexal structures is more common in pregnant than non-pregnant women.

Signs and symptoms
- Sudden-onset unilateral colicky lower abdominal pain.
- Nausea and vomiting.
- There may be systemic symptoms such as fever.

Investigations
- WCC and CRP: may be elevated.
- USS of pelvis may show an adnexal mass and Doppler studies may show impaired blood flow.

Management

If suspected, urgent laparotomy should be performed to either remove or untwist the adnexa. This may either preserve the ovary or present a non-viable ovary from becoming gangrenous.

Pancreatitis

This occurs more frequently in the 3rd trimester and immediate post-partum period. It can occur in early pregnancy associated with gallstones.

⚠ Although rare, it is more common in pregnancy than in non-pregnant women of a similar age.

Incidence 1:5000 pregnancies.

Risk factors
- Gallstone disease.
- High alcohol intake.
- Hyperlipidaemia.

Signs and symptoms
- Epigastric pain commonly radiating to the back.
- Pain exacerbated by lying flat and relieved by leaning forwards.
- Nausea and vomiting.

Investigations
- Serum amylase and lipase levels.
- USS to establish presence of gallstones.

Management
Conservative treatment is the mainstay:
- IV fluids.
- Electrolyte replacement.
- Parenteral analgesics, e.g. morphine (pethidine is contraindicated).
- Bowel rest with or without nasogastric suction.

⚠ Early surgical intervention is recommended for gallstone pancreatitis in all trimesters as >70% of patients will relapse before delivery.
- Laparoscopic/open cholecystectomy.
- Endoscopic reterograde cholangio-pancreatography (ERCP) has a limited role in pregnancy because of radiation exposure to the fetus.

⚠ If pancreatitis is severe, liaise with high dependancy unit/intensive care unit (HDU/ITU).

Non-abdominal causes of abdominal pain

Other conditions unrelated to abdominal structures may also present with abdominal pain:
- Lower lobe pneumonia.
- Diabetic ketoacidosis.
- Sickle cell crisis.

▶ Women with social problems and domestic abuse may repeatedly attend with undiagnosable pain and it is important to ask them about this directly but sympathetically.

Preterm labour: overview

Preterm birth is defined as delivery between 24 and 37wks.

- Delivery <34wks is more useful as adverse outcomes are rare after then.
- 1/3 is medically indicated (e.g. PET), and 2/3 spontaneous.
- Accounts for 5–10% of births but ~50% of perinatal deaths.
- It also causes long-term handicap—blindness, deafness, and cerebral palsy. The risk is higher the earlier the gestation.
- The incidence is ↑ over the years.
- >50% of women with painful preterm contractions will not deliver preterm: fetal fibronectin/transvaginal USS may help in diagnosis.

Risk factors for preterm delivery
- Previous preterm birth or late miscarriage.
- Multiple pregnancy.
- Cervical surgery.
- Uterine anomalies.
- Medical conditions, e.g. renal disease.
- Pre-eclampsia and IUGR (spontaneous and iatrogenic).

Acute preterm labour
- Preterm labour associated with cervical weakness (avoid the term 'incompetence') classically presents with increased vaginal discharge, mild lower abdominal pain, and bulging membranes on examination.
- Preterm labour associated with factors such as infection, inflammation, or abruption presents with lower abdominal pain, painful uterine contractions, and vaginal loss.
- Spontaneous rupture of membranes (SROM) is a common presentation of/antecedent for preterm labour.

▶ In practice it is often less clear-cut than this, and infection and cervical weakness are related and often coexist.

History
- Ask about pain/contractions—onset, frequency, duration, severity.
- Vaginal loss: SROM or PV bleeding.
- Obstetric history (check hand-held notes).

Examination
- Maternal pulse, temperature, respiratory rate.
- Uterine tenderness (suggests infection/abruption).
- Fetal presentation.
- Speculum: look for blood, discharge, liquor. Takes swabs.
- Gentle VE.

Investigations
- FBC, CRP (raised WCC and CRP suggest infection).
- Swabs, MSU.
- USS for fetal presentation (malpresentation common) and estimated fetal weight (EFW).
- Consider fetal fibronectin/transvaginal USS if available (see 📖 Methods for prediction of preterm labour, p. 101).

Management of preterm labour

- Establish whether threatened or 'real' preterm labour:
  - transvaginal cervical length scan (>15mm unlikely to labour)
  - fibronectin assay: if –ve, unlikely to labour.
- Admit if risk high.
- Inform neonatal unit.
- Arrange *in utero* transfer if no suitable beds available.
- Check fetal presentation with USS.
- Steroids (12mg betametasone IM—two doses 24h apart).

▶ Antenatal steroids reduce rates of respiratory distress, intraventricular haemorrhage, and neonatal death (Royal College of Obstetricians and Gynaecologists (RCOG)) grade A recommendation).

- Consider tocolysis (drug treatment to prevent labour and delivery) not >24hrs.
  - Allow time for steroid administration and/or *inutero* transfer.
  - Currently used tocolytics include nifedipine, and atosiban IV.

🖎 Aim should be not just prolongation of gestation (a surrogate measure) but improvement in perinatal morbidity and mortality. Trials of tocolysis have not shown improvement in these substantive outcome measures, so some prefer to avoid them.

- Liaison with senior obstetricians and neonatologists is essential, especially at the margins of viability (23–26wks). A clear plan needs to be made about:
  - mode of delivery
  - monitoring in labour
  - presence of pediatrician/appropriate intervention at delivery.
- Give IV antibiotics but only if labour confirmed.

Further reading

RCOG. (2004). Green-top guideline no.7. *Antenatal corticosteroids to prevent respiratory distress syndrome.* 🖜 www.rcog.org

Preterm labour: prevention and prediction

Prevention

Treatment of bacterial vaginosis (BV)

Some evidence suggests this may reduce the incidence of preterm prelabour rupture of membranes (PPROM) and low birth weight in women with previous preterm birth. Clindamycin rather than metronidazole is used.

Progesterone

- In high risk women (e.g. previous history of late miscarriage/preterm birth), reduces recurrence.
- In low risk women with a short cervix, reduces preterm birth by about 50%. As a result, screening for preterm birth with cervical scanning may become universal.
- Effect absent/very limited in twin pregnancies.
- Cream or pessaries used.

Cervical sutures (cerclage)

🖎 May be of benefit in selected cases. Can be inserted vaginally or, in extreme cases, abdominally. Not thought to be useful in multiple pregnancies.

- Elective (women with previous loss from cervical weakness).
- Ultrasound-indicated (in response to short cervix on transvaginal scan (TVS)).
- Rescue (in response to cervical dilatation).

Cervical pessary

These are used more often in Europe but evidence suggests they are effective.

Reduction of pregnancy number

Selective reduction of triplet or higher-order multiple pregnancies (to 2) reduces the risk of preterm labour while slightly increasing the risk of early miscarriage.

Methods for prediction of preterm labour

Transvaginal USS of cervix
- In asymptomatic women with a singleton pregnancy:
  - risk of delivering before 32wks is 4% if cervix is >15mm long at 23wks
  - increasing exponentially to 78% if cervix is 5mm.
- In symptomatic women with a singleton pregnancy:
  - cervix <15mm, risk of delivery within 7 days is 49%
  - cervix >15mm, risk of delivery within 7 days <1%.

Fetal fibronectin (FFN)
- FFN is a protein not usually present in cervicovaginal secretions at 22–36wks.
- Those with a +ve FFN test are more likely to deliver (test for FFN with swab and commercially available kit).
- Predicts preterm birth within 7–10 days of testing (+ve likelihood ratio (LR) of 5.42 and –ve LR of 0.25).

Preterm prelabour rupture of membranes: overview

- This complicates 1/3 of preterm deliveries.
- About 1/3 is associated with overt infection (more common at earlier gestations).

History

- Ask about vaginal loss.
  - Gush.
  - Constant trickle or dampness.

⚠ Chorioamnionitis may cause few symptoms but is associated with significant neonatal morbidity and mortality.

⚠ Chorioamnionitis is also associated with significant risks to the mother.

Features suggestive of chorioamnionitis

History:
- Fever/malaise.
- Abdominal pain, including contractions.
- Purulent/offensive vaginal discharge.

Examination:
- Maternal pyrexia and tachycardia.
- Uterine tenderness.
- Fetal tachycardia.
- Speculum: offensive vaginal discharge—yellow/brown.

▶ Avoid VE as this increases the risk of introducing infection.

Investigations

- FBC, CRP (raised WCC and CRP indicate infection).
- Swabs (high vaginal swab (HVS), low vaginal swab (LVS)).
- MSU.
- USS for fetal presentation, EFW, and liquor volume.

Preterm prelabour rupture of membranes: management

- If evidence of chorioamnionitis:
  - steroids (betametasone 12mg IM)
  - deliver whatever the gestation
  - broad spectrum antibiotic cover.
- If no evidence of chorioamnionitis, manage conservatively:
  - admit
  - inform special care baby unit (SCBU) and liaise with neonatologists
  - steroids (12mg betametasone IM—two doses 24h apart)
  - antibiotics (erythromycin).

▶ Use of antibiotics reduces major markers of neonatal morbidity but without long-term benefits. The ORACLE trial showed erythromycin to be beneficial.

⚠ Co-amoxiclav is associated with an increased risk of necrotizing enterocolitis (NEC) and should be avoided.

Prognosis

Depends on:
- Gestation at delivery.
- Gestation at PPROM:
  - PPROM at <20wks—few survivors
  - PPROM at >22wks—survival up to 50%.
- Reason for PPROM:
  - prognosis better if PPROM secondary to invasive procedure (e.g. amniocentesis), rather than spontaneous.

Risks to fetus from PPROM

- Prematurity.
- Infection.
- Pulmonary hypoplasia.
- Limb contractures.

Table 2.2 Data from EPICure study (cohort of babies born in the UK and Ireland in 1995)

Gestation (weeks)	Survival to discharge (as % of live births)	Survival (severe disability) (as % of live births)
<23	1	50
23–23+6	11	31
24–24+6	26	24
25–25+6	44	22

Further reading

Costeloe K, Hennessy E, Gibson AT, *et al.* (2000). The EPICure study: outcomes to discharge from hospital for babies born at the threshold of viability. *Pediatrics* **106(4)**: 659–71.

Kenyon SL, Taylor DJ, Tarnow-Mordi W; ORACLE Collaborative Group. (2001). Broad-spectrum antibiotics for preterm, prelabour rupture of fetal membranes: the ORACLE 1 randomised trial. *The Lancet* **357(9261)**: 979–88.

Prolonged pregnancy: overview

Prolonged pregnancy is a cause of anxiety for both women and obstetricians. It is a common occurrence and is a recognized cause of increased fetal morbidity and mortality.

> **Definition of prolonged pregnancy**
> According to the International Federation of Gynaecology and Obstetrics (FIGO), prolonged pregnancy is defined as any pregnancy that exceeds 42wks (294 days) from the first day of the LMP in a woman with regular 28-day cycles. Different terminologies are used generally in day-to-day practice, such as postdates, post-term, and postmaturity.

Incidence

The incidence of pregnancy lasting 42wks or more is 3–10%. With one previous prolonged pregnancy there is a 30% chance of another one. With a history of two this rises to 40%. Incidence also varies depending on whether EDD is based on LMP or dating USS. Women who book in the 1st trimester and have an early dating scan have an incidence of prolonged pregnancy of <5%.

Dates cannot be relied upon in the following circumstances:
- Uncertainty of LMP (10–30% of women).
- Irregular periods.
- Recent use of COCP.
- Conception during lactational amenorrhea.

Maternal risks
- Maternal anxiety and psychological morbidity.
- Increased intervention:
  - induction of labour
  - operative delivery with ↑ risk of genital tract trauma.

Fetal risks of prolonged pregnancy

Perinatal mortality ↑ after 42wks of gestation
- Intrapartum deaths are 4 times more common.
- Early neonatal deaths are 3 times more common.

Other risks
- Meconium aspiration and assisted ventilation.
- Oligohydramnios.
- Macrosomia, shoulder dystocia, and fetal injury.
- Cephalhaematoma.
- Fetal distress in labour.
- Neonatal—hypothermia, hypoglycaemia, polycythaemia, and growth restriction.

Fetal postmaturity syndrome
- This is used to describe post-term infants who show signs of intrauterine malnutrition.
- The neonate has a scaphoid abdomen, little subcutaneous fat on the body or limbs, peeling skin over the palm and feet, overgrown nails, and an anxious, alert look.
- The baby's skin is also stained with meconium.
- This condition constitutes only a small proportion of babies born after 42wks.

⚠ These features can be seen at an earlier gestation in babies with IUGR. Hence, the term prolonged pregnancy is preferred to postmaturity for pregnancy beyond 42wks.

Prolonged pregnancy: management

- Attempt to confirm the EDD as accurately as possible: EDD based on 1st trimester USS is accurate to within a week.
- Assess any other risk factors which may be an indication to induce close to the EDD:
  - pre-eclampsia
  - diabetes
  - antepartum haemorrhage
  - IUGR associated with placental insufficiency.
- Offer 'stretch and sweep' at 41wks.
- Offer induction of labour between 41 and 42wks:
  - this slightly reduces perinatal mortality
  - it also reduces the risk of CS
  - but it 'medicalizes' many labours
  - if declined, ensure adequate fetal surveillance.

Fetal monitoring

This should include an initial USS assessment of growth and amniotic fluid volume. Women should be offered daily CTGs after 42wks. They should also be advised to report any decrease in fetal movements.

(See 📖 Monitoring the high-risk fetus: cardiotocography, p. 153.)

Counselling

Most units in the UK advise induction of labour by 42wks because of the increased perinatal mortality and morbidity beyond this time. However, many women regard elective induction of labour as interference with the natural phenomenon of childbirth. It is therefore important to discuss the issue sensitively and respect the woman's decision. Written information should be provided clearly outlining the arguments for and against induction to ensure the woman is able make an informed decision. Any specific risk factors complicating her pregnancy, such as pre-eclampsia, should be clearly explained and the conversation carefully documented in the notes.

Those mothers who prefer to await spontaneous onset of labour should have appropriate counselling regarding increased fetal mortality and morbidity. They should also have adequate fetal surveillance, which should include a USS assessment of fetal growth and liquor volume.

Further reading

Department of Health (1993). *Changing childbirth, report of the Expert Maternity Group.* Cumberledge Report. HMSO, London.

Fetal medicine

Prenatal diagnosis: overview

Benefits

Congenital abnormalities affect approximately 2% of newborn babies in the UK, and account for around 21% of perinatal and infant deaths, as well as causing significant disability and morbidity later in life. Although some pregnancies are known to be at high risk, e.g. for mothers with type I diabetes or parents with a previously affected child, the vast majority of congenital defects occur unexpectedly in otherwise uncomplicated pregnancies. Prenatal identification in such situations can help in a multitude of ways:

- Enabling decision on timing, mode, and place of delivery (e.g. in a unit that provides paediatric surgery).
- Preparing parents to cope with an affected child.
- Introducing parents to specialist neonatal services.
- Ensuring fetal surveillance, such as later USSs to monitor the condition and ensure the best possible outcome.
- Potentially allowing *in utero* treatment (rarely available at present).
- Giving parents the option of terminating the pregnancy in severe cases.

Counselling

The news that there is a problem with their unborn child is often devastating for parents. How they respond to the situation will vary with such factors as age, social background, and religious belief. Not all parents will wish to terminate the pregnancy: many will choose to go on, even in the face of abnormalities incompatible with life. Some parents report that the opportunity to hold their child enabled them to grieve. Counselling must be supportive, informative, and non-directional. Care must also be taken to counsel adequately before any screening tests. If parents have no intention of having the riskier diagnostic tests performed then there is little benefit in screening and much anxiety may be generated. Detailed written information should always be provided beforehand.

Trisomy 21 (Down's syndrome)

Commonest identifiable cause of learning disability. Usually occurs as a result of non-disjunction of chromosome 21 at meiosis (95%). May also be due to balanced translocation in parents (4%). 1% estimated due to mosaicism. Variable penetrance, which explains wide range of features and characteristics seen in people with Down's syndrome. Around 50% will have one or more serious congenital abnormality. Around 10% will die before age of 5yrs, and current life expectancy is 50–55yrs.

Risk of trisomy 21 ↑ with maternal age

- *<25yrs:* 1:1500
- *30yrs:* 1:910
- *35yrs:* 1:380
- *40yrs:* 1:110
- *45yrs:* 1:30

- Natural prevalence 1:600 live births, but incidence is now 6:10 000 due to termination of pregnancy.
- *Typical appearance:*
  - flat nasal bridge
  - epicanthic folds
  - single palmar crease.
- *Intellectual impairment:*
  - 80% profound or severe
  - mean mental age at 21yrs is 5yrs
  - increased risk of early-onset dementia.
- *Congenital malformations:*
  - cardiac abnormalities (46%, e.g. VSD, atrial septal defect (ASD), and tetralogy of Fallot)
  - gastrointestinal atresias are common (e.g. duodenal atresia).
- Increased risk of other medical conditions, including:
  - leukaemia
  - thyroid disorders
  - epilepsy.

Genetic counselling after diagnosis of trisomy 21

- If the karyotype indicates straightforward trisomy 21 from non-disjunction, the risk of recurrence is ~1% above the risk from maternal age alone.
- If a chromosomal translocation is demonstrated, the recurrence risk is 1:10 if the mother, and 1:50 if the father, is carrying the abnormality.

Support groups

Down Syndrome Medical Interest Group. ✆ www.dsmig.org.uk

Other types of aneuploidy

Trisomy 18 (Edwards' syndrome)
Second-most common autosomal trisomy. Most due to non-disjunction at meiosis. Vast majority will die soon after birth; survival to 1yr is anecdotal.
- Incidence 1:6000 live births (prevalence estimated at 1:3000).
- Risk increases with increasing maternal age.
- *Features:*
  - craniofacial abnormalities including small facial features, small chin, and low-set ears
  - rocker bottom feet.
- *Congenital malformations:*
  - cardiac abnormalities in almost all fetuses (usually VSD)
  - gastrointestinal abnormalities
  - urogenital abnormalities.

Trisomy 13 (Patau's syndrome)
Least common autosomal trisomy; ~75% due to non-disjunction. Babies die soon after birth.
- Incidence 1:10 000 live births.
- Risk increases with increasing maternal age.
- *Features:* craniofacial, including cyclopia with proboscis located on forehead; microcephaly.
- *Congenital malformations (midline):*
  - holoprosencephaly (failure of cleavage of the embryonic forebrain)
  - gastrointestinal abnormalities, especially exomphalos
  - cleft lip and palate (midline).

See ℗ www.rarechromo.org

Turner's syndrome (45 XO)
This affects only females and is due to the loss of an X chromosome. It is one of the few chromosomal abnormalities that does not result in mental impairment. Almost all women with Turner's syndrome will have short stature and loss of ovarian function, but the extent of the other features varies enormously.
- Incidence 1:2500 live female births.
- *Features:*
  - short stature, webbed neck, and wide carrying angle
  - non-functioning 'streak' ovaries
  - coarctation of the aorta.

See ℗ www.tss.org.uk

Klinefelter's syndrome (47 XXY)
Affects only males and caused by non-disjunction of the X chromosomes. The individual is almost always sterile and may have hypogonadism. They are phenotypically tall with occasionally reduced IQ. Incidence 1:700 live male births.

Screening for chromosomal abnormalities

Ideally, screening should be offered to all women at the time of booking. In the UK, almost all units use the 'combined test' to screen for Down's syndrome, the most common chromosomal abnormality. This has a detection rate of 75% with a false +ve rate (FPR) of no more than 3%. This means that a risk of 1 in 150 or less is considered 'high risk'.

Counselling

Detailed, unbiased, written information should be provided about the condition itself, types of test available, and the implications of the results. It is important for a woman to understand that a negative result does not guarantee that her baby does not have an abnormality.

Screening relies on the integration of different independent risk factors, such as maternal age, blood hormone levels, and scan findings. These findings are slightly dependent on other factors including maternal weight, ethnicity, IVF pregnancies, smoking, multiple pregnancy, and diabetes, and calculations are modified according to these.

Screening versus diagnostic tests

Care must always be taken to explain the difference between the types of test available including their advantages, disadvantages, and limitations.

Screening tests

- Should be cheap and widely available.
- Non-invasive, safe, and acceptable.
- Have good sensitivity (high detection rate) and specificity (low FPR).
- Provide a measure of the risk of being affected by a certain disorder (e.g. 1 in 100 risk of Down's syndrome).
- Must have a suitable diagnostic test for those identified as 'high risk'.

Diagnostic tests

- Need to definitely confirm or reject the suspected diagnosis (e.g. the fetus does, or does not, have Down's syndrome).
- Must be as safe as possible.
- Must have high sensitivity and specificity.
- The implications of the disorder tested for must be serious enough to warrant an invasive test.

Common screening tests

Combined test

When
Scan and blood test at 11–13+6wks.

How
- Ultrasound (nuchal) scan measurement of the subcutaneous (SC) tissue between the skin and the soft tissue overlying the cervical spine with the fetus in the neutral position (see Fig. 3.1).
- A blood test measuring:
  - PAPP-A
  - β-human chorionic gonadotrophin (hCG).

Summary
- Now the recommended and most commonly used screening test.
- Performance enhanced by use of additional risk factors: nasal bone, tricuspid regurgitation.
- Careful ultrasound can identify many structural abnormalities.

Risk of trisomy 21
Calculated by multiplying the background maternal age and gestation-related risk by a likelihood ratio derived from the nuchal translucency (NT) measurement and the two blood tests.

Combined test

Advantages
- Performance ~90% detection for 5% FPR (75% for 3%).
- May detect other abnormalities such as anencephaly.
- An increased NT is also a marker for structural defects, e.g. cardiac malformations.
- Result usually available in 1st trimester, allowing surgical termination of pregnancy (TOP).
- Acceptable detection rate for all trisomies.

Disadvantages
Expensive and difficult to perform nuchal scan.

Triple and quadruple tests

When
Blood tests at 16wks.

How
- Dating scan (but not nuchal scan).
- Blood tests at 15wks measuring:
  - oestriol
  - hCG
  - alpha-fetoprotein (AFP)
  - inhibin A (not if triple).

Summary
- Recommended if NT scan not possible or gestation too advanced.
- Less operator dependent (scan) than the combined test.

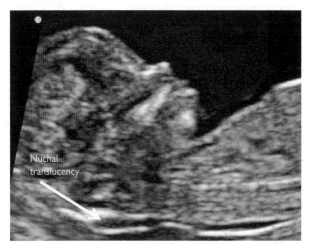

Fig. 3.1 Nuchal translucency at 11–14wks USS.

Nasal bone or tricuspid regurgitation
- Fetuses with Down's syndrome are more likely to have an absent or hypoplastic nasal bone and have significant tricuspid regurgitation at 11–13+6wks.
- Only in conjunction with a nuchal scan can the presence or absence of these be used to modify the risk of a combined test.
- They may considerably increase the accuracy of the combined test.
- These are not commonly used because they require skill and time to detect accurately.

Other screening tests

Integrated test

When
- Nuchal scan and blood tests (10–13+6wks).
- Blood tests again at 15wks.

How
- Nuchal scan.
- PAPP-A at 10wks.
- Quadruple test at 15wks measuring:
  - oestriol
  - hCG
  - AFP
  - inhibin A.

Summary
Best screening test (see Table 3.1), but expensive and seldom used.

Serum integrated test

When
Blood test at 10wks, then again at 15wks.

How
- Dating scan (but not nuchal scan).
- PAPP-A at 10wks.
- Quadruple test at 15wks measuring:
  - oestriol
  - hCG
  - AFP
  - inhibin A.

Summary
Less operator dependent (scan) than the combined test and probably as accurate; not recommended despite this (see Table 3.1).

Table 3.1 Comparison of screening tests available for Down's syndrome

	Combined	Serum integrated test	Integrated test	Triple test	Quadruple test
Trimester	1st	1st and 2nd	1st and 2nd	2nd	2nd
Type	Scan and blood test	Two blood tests	Scan and two blood tests	Blood test	Blood test
Detection rate	90%	85%	85%	71%	75%
For a given false +ve rate	5%	2.7%	1.2%	6%	5%

Significance of raised serum AFP

An elevated level of maternal serum AFP (greater than 2.2 multiples of median (MoM)) can also be used as a screening tool for open neural tube defects. It is also elevated in other conditions, including:
- Abdominal wall defects.
- Congenital nephrosis.
- Upper fetal bowel obstruction.
- Placental or umbilical cord tumours.
- Sacrococcygeal teratoma.
- Multiple pregnancy.
- After bleeding in early pregnancy.

An elevated AFP should trigger closer fetal and maternal surveillance as it is also a marker of adverse perinatal outcomes including:
- Fetal death.
- IUGR.
- Late pregnancy bleeding.
- Preterm delivery.

Diagnosis of structural abnormalities

This should be offered to all women in the UK at the time of booking and usually takes the form of the 'anomaly scan', a detailed USS undertaken at around 18–21wks gestation. The aim is to identify specific structural malformations.

The detection of malformations may vary and is dependent on:
• The anatomical system affected.
• Gestational age at the time of the scan.
• Skill of the operator.
• Quality of the equipment.
• BMI of the mother.

Percentage of abnormalities detected by routine anomaly scan (these figures are better under optimum conditions)
• Central nervous system: 76%.
• Urinary tract: 67%.
• Pulmonary: 50%.
• Gastrointestinal: 42%.
• Skeletal: 24%.
• Cardiac: 17%.

NHS Screening Programmes: fetal anomaly 2010. ℘ http://fetalanomaly.screening.nhs.uk

Minimum standards required for 18–21wk anomaly scan

Fetal normality
• Skull shape and internal structures:
  • cavum pellucidum
  • cerebellum
  • ventricular size at atrium <10mm
  • nuchal fold.
• Spine—longitudinal and transverse views.
• Abdominal shape and content at the level of:
  • stomach
  • kidneys
  • umbilicus/abdominal wall.
  • bladder.
• Arms (three bones and hand).
• Legs (three bones and foot).
• Heart:
  • four-chamber view
  • outflow tracts—pulmonary artery and aorta
  • lungs.
• Face and lips.

Neural tube defects

Craniospinal defects occur early in development when the neural tube fails to close properly. Type and severity depend on degree and site of defect. There is growing evidence that prevalence is declining, possibly due to increased use of folate supplementation.
- Spina bifida and anencephaly make up over 95% of neural tube defects (NTDs).
- Incidence 2:1000 in England (3:1000 in Scotland).

Anencephaly

Absence of skull vault and cerebral cortex. It is incompatible with life, with babies rarely living more than a few hours if they are not stillborn.

Spina bifida

Incomplete fusion of vertebrae potentially allowing herniation of all or part of spinal cord. The malformation falls into three categories:
- *Spina bifida occulta (mildest):*
  - split in vertebrae with no herniation of spinal cord
  - varies from asymptomatic to mild neurological symptoms.
- *Meningocele (least common):*
  - split in vertebrae with herniation of meninges and cerebrospinal fluid (CSF)
  - varies from normal neurological function to moderate symptoms.
- *Myelomeningocele (most severe):*
  - split in vertebrae allows herniation of spinal cord and meninges
  - invariably have abnormal neurology at and below the lesion
  - usually have an abnormal cerebellum and hydocephalus, which may result in mental impairment.

⚠ Dietary supplementation with folic acid decreases the incidence of NTDs. Recommended doses are:
- 400 micrograms/day for 3mths before conception, continued to 12wks.
- 5mg/day for women with previously affected child or those taking anticonvulsants.

Specific USS findings with some neural tube defects
- *Anencephaly:*
  - absence of cranium and bulging eyes ('frog-like' appearance)
  - 99% will be detected by 20wks (see Fig. 3.2).
- *Spina bifida:* findings vary according to the severity of the lesion:
  - defect seen in the vertebral bodies or tissue overlying the spine
  - frontal bone scalloping ('lemon sign')
  - abnormal shaped cerebellum ('banana sign')
  - up to 95% detection rate for major defects

Association for Spina Bifida and Hydrocephalus. ℘ www.asbah.org

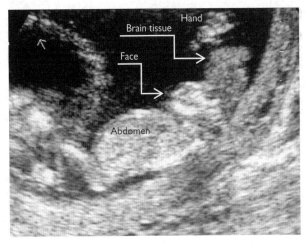

Fig. 3.2 Ultrasound of anencephaly.

Cardiac defects (congenital heart disease)

Cardiac defects are the most common major malformation in children, with an estimated incidence of 6–8:1000. They may be associated with a chromosomal abnormality, commonly trisomy 21 or 18, and with many other congenital abnormalities. Where isolated, many can be surgically corrected at birth, leading to a good quality of life. The most commonly seen abnormalities are VSDs (Fig. 3.3).

Risk factors for cardiac abnormalities
- Family history of congenital heart disease (CHD) in first-degree relative (recurrence risk 3%).
- Previous affected child (risk depends on type).
- Drug exposure, particularly anticonvulsants and lithium.
- Maternal diabetes mellitus.
- Other congenital abnormalities.
- Increased nuchal translucency (risk related to thickness).

Timing of cardiac scans
- In skilled hands many cardiac abnormalities can be seen at 12–13wks.
- Most cardiac abnormalities are missed at routine anomaly scans. The detection rate improves with training and specifically if 'three-vessel' and 'outflow tracts' views are found in addition to the four-chamber view (Fig. 3.4).
- Cardiac abnormalities may be better detected at 22wks than at 20wks. Evolution of defects change and later scanning, e.g. at 32wks, may be beneficial.

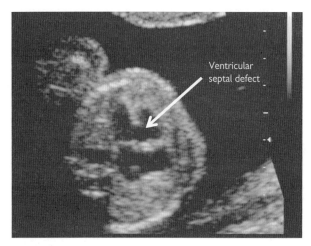

Fig. 3.3 USS of ventricular septal defect.

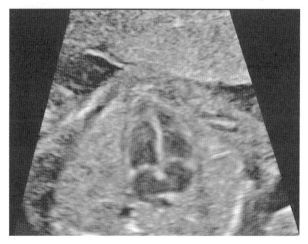

Fig. 3.4 USS of a normal cardiac four-chamber view.

Urinary tract defects

Renal agenesis
- Bilateral renal agenesis is lethal because of anhydramnios causing lung hypoplasia.
- It may not be evident until >16wks because amniotic fluid is not all urinary before this time.

Posterior urethral valve syndrome
- This occurs in male fetuses where folds of mucosa block the bladder neck causing outflow obstruction.
- The severity is variable; back pressure may cause irreversible renal damage and oligohydramnios.

Hydronephrosis
- Accounts for 75% of fetal renal abnormalities.
- At least 40% resolve spontaneously in the neonatal period.
- It is usually due to pelviueretric obstruction, vesicoureteric reflux, utereocele, or posterior urethral valves (Fig. 3.5).
- Most cases can be treated postnatally so the prognosis is excellent.

Specific USS findings with some urinary tract defects
- *Posterior urethral valves:*
  - thick walled dilated bladder with 'keyhole' sign of upper urethral dilatation
  - hydronephrosis
  - variable degrees of oligohydramnios according to severity.
- *Ureterocele:* cystic area of prolapsed ureter in bladder.

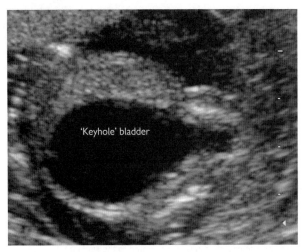

Fig. 3.5 Ultrasound of posterior urethral valve syndrome (keyhole bladder).

Lung defects

Lung hypoplasia

- Failure to develop sufficient alveoli to permit adequate gas exchange at delivery.
- Often due to mid-trimester oligohydramnios from very preterm rupture of membranes or renal anomalies.
- May be due to compression (e.g. diaphragmatic hernia).
- Severity is increased with:
  - preterm rupture of membranes at less than 25wks gestation
  - severe oligohydramnios (amniotic fluid index (AFI) <4) for more than 2wks
  - earlier delivery.

⚠ Estimated mortality rate 71–95%.

Diaphragmatic hernia

- A defect in the diaphragm results in the abdominal contents herniating into the chest.
- There is a 30% incidence of aneuploidy and a strong association with other malformations.
- The degree of compromise is correlated to the amount of compression of the original chest contents; prognosis is worse if the liver is in the chest and if little contralateral lung tissue is visible.
- Approximately 40% will die postnatally of lung hypoplasia; the others will require postnatal surgery.
- *In utero* treatment for severe cases involving tracheal obstruction (fetoscopic tracheal occlusion (FETO)) should be considered.

Congenital cystic adenomatoid malformation

- A rare form of lung disease where the normal alveolar tissue is replaced by a proliferation of cysts resembling bronchioles.
- The prognosis is good, but occasional very severe cases may cause hydrops.

💧 Postnatal surgery in asymptomatic cases is contentious.

Specific ultrasound findings with some lung defects

Diaphragmatic hernia

- Stomach or liver is seen within chest cavity.
- With a left-sided hernia, the heart may be deviated to the right.
- Abdominal circumference is often smaller than expected.
- Usually detectable at 20wks.

Congenital cystic adenomatoid malformation (CCAM)

- Cystic mass present within the lung parenchyma.
- Usually detectable at 20wks (Fig. 3.6).

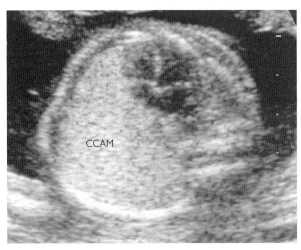

Fig. 3.6 USS of (solid) congenital cystic adenomatoid malformation (CCAM)—it appears as a bright, space occupying lesion in the chest and can be solid, cystic, or a combination of both.

Gastrointestinal defects

Exomphalos (omphalocele)

- Failure of the gut to return into the abdominal cavity after the normal embryological extrusion and rotation; the bowel, and sometimes other viscera, are contained within a sac and the umbilical cord arises from the apex of this sac (see Table 3.2).
- Approximately 1/3 occur with chromosomal abnormalities and up to 50% of the remainder have other malformations (e.g. cardiac).
- Prognosis depends on karyotype, presence of co-existing malformations, and presence of bowel ischaemia.
- Requires referral to a fetal medicine centre and postnatal surgery.
- Exomphalos alone is not an indication for delivery by CS.

Gastroschisis

- This involves protrusion of the gut through an anterior abdominal wall defect, usually to the right of the umbilical cord; the bowel is not covered by a sac and floats freely (see Table 3.2).
- Usually occurs in very young women. Rare after 25yrs.
- There is no increased risk of chromosomal abnormalities.
- The fetal gastrointestinal tract may become obstructed or atretic.
- Approximately 1 in 10–20 will die *in utero* or postnatally, but in the remainder the prognosis is good.
- Requires referral to a fetal medicine centre and postnatal surgery.
- Vaginal delivery is not necessarily contraindicated.

Gastrointestinal obstruction

- *Duodenal atresia:* 30% have trisomy 21.
- *Oesophageal atresia:* 15% have aneuploidy.
- *Other atresias:* may occur with syndromes or gastroschisis.
- *Cystic fibrosis:* common with bowel obstruction.

Table 3.2 Comparison of the features of exomphalos and gastroschisis

	Exomphalos	Gastroschisis
Viscera contained within a sac	Yes, unless ruptured	No
Insertion of umbilical cord	At apex of sac	Next to the defect
Evisceration of:	Liver ± intestinal loops, spleen	Intestinal loops only
Chromosomal abnormalities	30%	<1%
Other malformations	50%	<5%
Mortality	40%	5–10%

Specific USS findings with some gastrointestinal defects

Anterior abdominal wall defects
- Bowel is seen outside the abdominal wall.
- Detection rates >95%.

Duodenal atresia
- Distension of stomach and proximal duodenum ('double bubble') (Fig. 3.7).
- May not be apparent by 20wks, but usually seen by 25wks.
- Polyhydramnios.

Oesophageal atresia
- Absence of stomach bubble and polyhydramnios.
- Often not seen due to presence of a tracheo-oesophageal fistula.

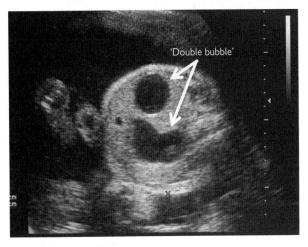

Fig. 3.7 USS of duodenal atresia ('double bubble').

Soft markers/normal variant screening

Some ultrasound features at 20wks may themselves be of little signifi-cance, but are nevertheless slightly more common in chromosomally abnormal fetuses. They have therefore been used to modify the risk of aneuploidy. However, these features may cause considerable parental anxiety as they are often, mistakenly, seen as abnormalities. Furthermore, they may increase the false +ve rate of screening.

Choroid plexus cysts
- Small benign cysts in the choroid plexus (Fig. 3.8), seen in about 1% of 20wk scans.
- Weakly associated with trisomy 18.
- NSC recommends these are not considered significant.

Echogenic intracardiac foci
- 1 or more small echogenic foci ('golf balls') in the cardiac ventricles.
- No significance for cardiac defects.
- Slight increase (~1.5-fold) in risk of chromosomal abnormalities.
- NSC recommends these are not considered significant.

Two-vessel umbilical cord
- Cord contains only one umbilical artery.
- Slight increase in chromosomal abnormalities.
- Slight increase in perinatal risk, and renal tract, and cardiac abnormalities.
- NSC recommends these are not considered significant.

Mild renal pelvic dilatation
- Dilatation of >7mm at 20wks.
- Slightly increased (~1.5-fold) risk of chromosomal abnormalities.
- Repeat scan in 3rd trimester (to ensure not enlarged) and neonatal follow-up is recommended.

Echogenic bowel
- Bowel with areas of echogenicity similar in brightness to bone.
- Moderate association (~5-fold increase) with chromosomal abnormalities.
- Although usually benign, occasionally associated with increased perinatal risk, cystic fibrosis, and bowel obstruction.
- Consider referral for expert opinion.

Increased nuchal fold
- 20wk equivalent of nuchal translucency (>6mm in transverse section).
- Increased risk of chromosomal abnormalities (~10-fold).
- Amniocentesis for chromosomal abnormalities is usually offered.
- Sign of early hydrops.

See 🔗 www.fetalanomaly.screening.nhs.uk/fetalanomalyresource/whats-in-the-hexagons1/about-the-scan/normal-variant-screening.

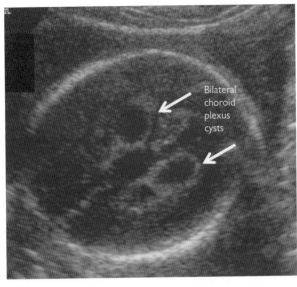

Fig. 3.8 USS of choroid plexus cysts.

Diagnostic tests

Chorionic villus sampling (CVS)

Diagnostic test usually performed between 10 and 13wks and involves aspiration of some trophoblastic cells. The amount of tissue obtained is small, but sufficient for karyotyping, and with the development of fluorescent *in situ* hybridization (FISH) and polymerase chain reaction (PCR), rapid analysis is possible (see Fig. 3.9). It requires ultrasound guidance and is usually performed transabdominally, occasionally transcervically.

Indications
- For karyotyping if 1st trimester screening test suggests high risk for aneuploidy.
- For DNA analysis if parents are carriers of an identifiable gene mutation such as cystic fibrosis or thalassaemia.

Benefits
Allows 1st trimester TOP if an abnormality is detected:
- Can be performed surgically.
- Can be done before the pregnancy has become physically apparent.

Risks
- Miscarriage as a result of CVS is estimated at 1%.
- Increases risk of vertical transmission of blood-borne viruses such as HIV and hepatitis B.
- False negative results (rare) from contamination with maternal cells—especially with DNA analysis requiring PCR.
- Placental mosaicism producing misleading results—estimated at <1%.

Amniocentesis

This is only undertaken from 15wks onwards. It involves aspiration of amniotic fluid which contains fetal cells shed from the skin and gut. It is performed transabdominally with ultrasound guidance (see Fig. 3.10).

Indications
- For karyotyping if screening tests suggest aneuploidy.
- For DNA analysis if parents are carriers of an identifiable gene mutation, such as cystic fibrosis or thalassaemia.
- For enzyme assays looking for inborn errors of metabolism.
- For diagnosis of fetal infections such as CMV and toxoplasmosis.

Benefits
- Lower procedure-attributed miscarriage rate than CVS (~1%).
- Less risk of maternal contamination or placental mosaicism.

Risks

- Miscarriage as a result of amniocentesis is estimated at 1%, although recent data suggest that the risk of miscarriage after amniocentesis is very little higher than would occur naturally.
- Failure to culture cells ~0.5%.
- Full karyotyping may take 3wks (results for certain chromosomal abnormalities may be available more rapidly using FISH or PCR).

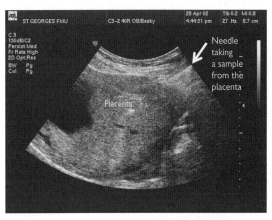

Fig. 3.9 Chorionic villus sampling.

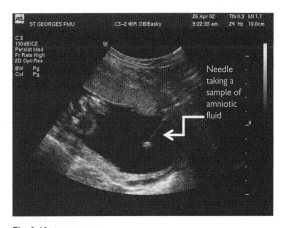

Fig. 3.10 Amniocentesis.

Fetal hydrops: overview

Definition
Fetal hydrops is the abnormal accumulation of serous fluid in two or more fetal compartments. This may be pleural or pericardial effusions, ascites, skin oedema, polyhydramnios, or placental oedema. It may be divided into non-immune and immune causes.

Pathophysiology
The mechanism for the development of hydrops appears to be due to an imbalance of interstitial fluid production and inadequate lymphatic return. This can result from congestive heart failure, obstructed lymphatic flow, or decreased plasma osmotic pressure.
- *Immune hydrops:* results from blood group incompatibility between the mother and the fetus causing fetal anaemia.
- *Non-immune hydrops:* results from other causes, including fetal anaemia that is due to other causes such as fetal infection.

Incidence
Occurs in ~1:2000 births.

Non-immune fetal hydrops: diagnosis and investigations
Ultrasound
- The diagnosis is made by USS.
- Associated structural abnormalities may be seen.
- Fetal echocardiography is required to diagnose cardiac lesions.
- Peak systolic velocity in middle cerebral artery shows fetal anaemia.

Fetal blood or amniotic fluid sampling
- Fetal blood sampling if anaemia is suspected (with blood ready for *in utero* transfusion).
- Amniotic fluid or fetal blood for chromosome analysis +/– virology.

Maternal blood testing
- Kleihauer test for feto-maternal haemorrhage.
- Antibody screen must be performed to exclude immune hydrops.
- Virology (parvovirus, CMV, toxoplasmosis).
- Consider haemoglobin electrophoresis for α-thalassaemia trait.

Non-immune fetal hydrops: principal causes

Severe anaemia
- Congenital parvovirus B19 infection.
- α-Thalassaemia major (common in areas such as South-east Asia).
- Massive feto-maternal haemorrhage.
- Glucose-6-phosphate dehydrogenase deficiency.

Cardiac abnormalities
- Structural abnormalities.
- Fetal tachyarrhythmia (supraventricular tachycardia (SVT) or atrial flutter).
- Congenital heart block.

Chromosomal abnormalities
- Trisomies 13, 18, and 21.
- Turner's syndrome (45 XO).

Other genetic syndromes
Multiple other syndromes, e.g. achondrogenesis, Noonan's syndrome, Fryn's syndrome, myotonic dystrophy.

Other infections
- Toxoplasmosis (📖 Toxoplasmosis, p. 168).
- Rubella (📖 Rubella (German measles), p. 156).
- CMV (📖 Cytomegalovirus, p. 162).
- Varicella (📖 Varicella (chickenpox), p. 164).

Other structural abnormalities
- Congenital cystic adenomatoid malformation (CCAM).
- Diaphragmatic hernia.
- Pleural effusions.

Twin-to-twin transfusion syndrome
Recipient from volume overload and donor from anaemia (see 📖 Twin-to-twin transfusion syndrome, p. 78).

Placental
Chorioangioma.

Non-immune hydrops: treatment

The prognosis depends on the underlying cause. Where treatment is not possible, the option of TOP should be discussed. In the 3rd trimester, delivery may be a better alternative than *in utero* treatment.

If severe polyhydramnios is present, removal of excess amniotic fluid (amnioreduction) may reduce the risk of preterm labour. Consider giving steroids before the procedure as it carries a small risk of triggering preterm labour.

Treatable causes of non-immune fetal hydrops

Fetal anaemia

In utero blood transfusion may be performed.

Pleural effusions or large cystic CCAM

In utero percutaneous drainage and subsequent insertion of shunt into amniotic fluid may be possible.

Twin-to-twin transfusion syndrome

Laser photocoagulation of placental anastomoses.

Cardiac

- Tachyarrhythmias may be treated with maternal digoxin and flecainide.
- Valvotomy of stenotic cardiac valves is technically possible, but is usually too late if hydrops has already developed.

Rhesus isoimmunization (immune hydrops)

Definition Occurs when a maternal antibody response is mounted against fetal red cells. These immunoglobulin (IgG) antibodies cross the placenta and cause fetal red blood cell destruction. The ensuing anaemia, if severe, precipitates fetal hydrops, which is often referred to as immune hydrops.

Rhesus blood groups Consists of three linked gene pairs; one allele of each pair is dominant—C/c, D/d, and E/e. There are only five antigens (d is not an antigen; it merely implies absence of D). Inheritance is Mendelian. D gene is the most significant cause of isoimmunization, because ~16% of white mothers are rhesus D −ve (d/d). Incidence lower in Afro-Caribbean and Asian populations. Other significant antigens include c, E, and atypical Kell antibody. Because of success of anti-D prophylaxis, these account for up to 1/2 of cases.

Pathophysiology of rhesus disease

- Fetal cells cross into the maternal circulation in normal pregnancy; the amount is increased during particular 'sensitizing events'.
- The fetus may carry the gene for an antigen which the mother does not have—with rhesus D, the fetus may be D/d (rhesus D +ve), but the mother d/d (rhesus D −ve).
- Individuals exposed to a 'foreign' antigen mount an immune response (sensitization); initially, this is immunoglobulin (IgM), which cannot cross the placenta so this pregnancy is not at risk.
- Re-exposure in a subsequent pregnancy causes the primed memory B cells to produce IgG, which actively crosses into fetal circulation.
- IgG binds to fetal red cells, which are destroyed in the reticulo-endothelial system.
- Causes a haemolytic anaemia (if erythropoesis is inadequate to compensate, severe anaemia causes high output cardiac failure, 'fetal hydrops,' and, ultimately, death).
- In milder cases, haemolysis leads to neonatal anaemia or jaundice from increased bilirubin levels.

Potential sensitizing events for rhesus disease

- TOP or evacuation of retained products of conception (ERPC) after miscarriage.
- Ectopic pregnancy.
- Vaginal bleeding >12wks, or earlier if heavy.
- ECV.
- Blunt abdominal trauma.
- Invasive uterine procedure, e.g. amniocentesis or CVS.
- Intrauterine death.
- Delivery.

Rhesus disease: management

- All women should be checked for antibodies (rhesus and atypical) at booking, 28, and 34wks.
- If antibodies are detected, identifying the partner's status will help determine the potential fetal blood group and risk to the fetus.
- PCR of fetal cells in maternal blood may also determine the fetus's blood group, if the father is heterozygous or paternity is uncertain.
- Positive, but low levels of antibodies (<10IU/mL) should prompt repeat testing every 4wks.
- If levels are >10IU/mL, assessment for fetal anaemia is required.

▶ Amniocentesis or fetal blood sampling based on antibody levels or history alone is now obsolete.

- The peak systolic velocity (PSV) of the fetal middle cerebral artery (MCA) should be measured, about once a week. The MCA PSV will become abnormal before the baby is so anaemic as to be hydropic.
- If it is increased (>1.5 MoM), normograms for gestation are available) fetal blood sampling is indicated, with blood available for transfusion.

Treatment

- If the fetal haematocrit is <30, irradiated, Rh −ve, CMV −ve packed red cells are transfused into the umbilical vein at the cord insertion, or into the hepatic vein.
- This can be performed from 18wks onwards (beyond 35wks, delivery is preferable).
- Haemolysis will continue and the transfusion is repeated either every 2wks or when the MCA becomes abnormal again.

⚠ The risk of fetal loss, or need for urgent delivery if >26wks, is 1–3% per transfusion in skilled hands.

Postnatal management

- Anaemia can be corrected by blood transfusion.
- Severe anaemia may be accompanied by a coagulopathy from decreased platelets and clotting factors.
- Hyperbilirubinaemia and jaundice occur because *in utero* the mother cleared this red blood cell breakdown product, but the immature neonatal liver is unable to cope (this usually needs phototherapy, but may require exchange transfusion).

⚠ Antibodies may persist for weeks, causing continued haemolysis in the neonate; this requires careful monitoring with haematocrit measurements.

Prevention of rhesus (D) disease

If sufficient anti-D immunoglobulin is given to the mother it will bind to any fetal red cells in her circulation carrying the D antigen. This prevents her own immune system from recognizing them and therefore becoming sensitized.

- Anti-D (1500IU) is given to all women who are rhesus −ve (d/d):
  - routinely at 28wks
  - within 72h of any potentially sensitizing event
  - after delivery if the neonate is found to be rhesus +ve (D/d).
- Occasionally, large feto-maternal haemorrhages occur during sensitizing events. If this is suspected a Kleihauer test should be performed as the standard dose of anti-D may not be sufficient. This should be routinely undertaken at delivery if the neonate is RhD +ve.
- Other antibodies, particularly anti-Kell and anti-c, now account for about half of all cases of fetal haemolysis.
- The use of anti-D, together with smaller family sizes, mean that rhesus disease is now rare. Only about 2% of RhD −ve women in the UK have been sensitized.

Oligohydramnios

Amniotic fluid after 20wks largely consists of fetal urine. The volume depends on urine production, fetal swallowing, and absorption. Normal volume varies with gestation, and is highest between 24 and 36wks. The volume is measured by ultrasound, either by measuring the deepest vertical pool, or by adding up the deepest pools in the four quadrants of the uterus (AFI).

In oligohydramnios, the amniotic fluid volume is reduced. Normograms of both measures are available, but, as a general rule, a deepest pool of <2cm or an AFI of <8cm is considered low.

Complications
- Related to cause:
  - preterm rupture of the membranes is commonly followed by delivery and/or intrauterine infection
  - IUGR is an important cause of fetal and neonatal mortality and long-term morbidity.
- Related to reduced volume:
  - lung hypoplasia if occurs <22wks
  - limb abnormalities, e.g. talipes, if prolonged
  - oligohydramnios before 22wks has a very poor prognosis.

Investigations
- USS of fetus, including Doppler.
- Speculum examination to look for ruptured membranes.
- If suspected spontaneous rupture of membranes (SROM): CRP, FBC, and vaginal swabs should be taken.

Management of oligohydramnios

If SROM at 34–36 or more weeks
Induce labour unless CS is indicated for another reason.

If SROM before 34–36wks
- Give prophylactic oral erythromycin.
- Monitor for signs of infection (4-hourly temperature and pulse).
- Daily CTG.
- Consider induction by 34–36wks.

If IUGR
Manage according to umbilical artery Doppler and CTG.

If apparently isolated oligohydramnios
- Reconsider cause.
- Intervention is not usual if umbilical artery Dopplers are normal.

If fetal renal tract abnormality
Refer to fetal medicine centre.

Causes of oligohydramnios
- Leakage of amniotic fluid: SROM.
- Reduced fetal urine production:
  - IUGR
  - fetal renal failure or abnormalities
  - post-dates pregnancy.
- Obstruction to fetal urine output: fetal abnormalities such as posterior urethral valves.

Polyhydramnios

The amniotic fluid is increased. In general a deepest pool of >8cm or an AFI >22 is abnormal.

Causes of polyhydramnios

Increased fetal urine production
- Maternal diabetes.
- Twin–twin transfusion syndrome (recipient twin).
- Fetal hydrops.

Fetal inability to swallow or absorb amniotic fluid
- Fetal gastrointestinal (GI) tract obstruction (e.g. duodenal atresia, tracheo-oesophageal fistula).
- Fetal neurological or muscular abnormalities (e.g. myotonic dystrophy, anencephaly).
- Other rare abnormalities or syndromes (e.g. facial obstruction).
- Idiopathic (usually mild).

Complications
- Preterm delivery, probably because of uterine stretch.
- Of the cause, e.g. duodenal atresia is associated with trisomy 21.
- Malpresentation at delivery because of increased room for fetus.
- Maternal discomfort because of abdominal distension.

Investigations
- Exclude maternal diabetes with a glucose tolerance test (GTT).
- Ultrasound examination of fetus.

Polyhydramnios: management
- Severe polyhydramnios is usually associated with fetal abnormality, if massive (e.g. AFI >40), amnioreduction (drainage of excess fluid with a needle), or non-steroidal anti-inflammatory drugs (NSAIDs).
- If fetal abnormality, refer to fetal medicine centre.
- Twin–twin transfusion syndrome is best managed in a fetal medicine centre, usually with laser ablation of placental anastomoses.
- If preterm, assess risk of delivery with cervical scan and/ or fibronectin assay, and consider steroids.
- If unstable or transverse lie at term, admit to hospital: CS if labour ensues with an abnormal lie.

⚠ NSAIDs cause fetal oliguria and can constrict the ductus arteriosus: close supervision is therefore indicated.

Intrauterine growth restriction: overview

The fetus is believed to have an inherent growth potential which under ideal conditions should produce a healthy baby of the appropriate size. Attaining this potential relies on such factors as a healthy mother, well-functioning placenta, and the absence of pathology. If the *in utero* circumstances are less than ideal, the fetus will fail to achieve its full potential growth and fetal well-being may be compromised. This problem is analogous to 'failure to thrive' in children and is termed intrauterine growth restriction (IUGR).

Definition
▶ The term IUGR implies a fetus that is pathologically small.

Most epidemiological studies use *small for gestational age* (SGA) as a surrogate marker. The most commonly used method of identification of SGA is where the estimated weight of the fetus is below the 10th percentile for its gestational age.

This method is not perfect as it includes small, but healthy babies, and average-sized unhealthy babies that should have been born big.

Identifying inherent growth potential
To identify actual pathology and to improve detection of IUGR it is important to try to define the inherent growth potential of each individual fetus. Physiological factors known to affect growth and birth weight include:
• Maternal height and, to a lesser extent, paternal height.
• Maternal weight in early pregnancy.
• Parity.
• Ethnic origin.
• Gender of the fetus.

Some of these factors have been used to generate customized growth charts which aim to identify the optimal growth curve for an individual fetus. These are freely available at ℘ www.gestation.net. They appear to reduce the rate of constitutionally small babies being classed as IUGR (false +ve rate) while helping to increase detection of pathologically small babies.

Defining expected growth also requires accurate dating of pregnancy, ideally by USS in the 1st trimester between 8 and 13wks gestation.

Further reading
℘ www.gestation.net
Perinatal Institute. (2011). *Fetal growth assessment & implementation of customised charts.* ℘ www.pi.nhs.uk/growth/index_growth.htm

Importance of IUGR

For IUGR fetuses compared with normally grown population:

- Perinatal mortality is 6–10 times greater.
- Incidence of cerebral palsy is 4 times greater.
- 30% of all stillborn infants are growth restricted.

IUGR fetuses are also more likely to have:

- Intrapartum fetal distress and asphyxia.
- Meconium aspiration.
- Emergency CS.
- Necrotizing enterocolitis.
- Hypoglycaemia and hypocalcaemia.

Intrauterine growth restriction: causes

Causes of growth restriction may be grouped into maternal, utero-placental, and fetal.

⚠ By far the most common cause is utero-placental insufficiency.

Causes of IUGR

Maternal
- Chronic maternal disease:
  - hypertension
  - cardiac disease
  - chronic renal failure.
- Substance abuse:
  - alcohol
  - recreational drug use.
- Smoking.
- Autoimmune diseases, including: antiphospholipid antibody syndrome.
- Genetic disorders, including: phenylketonuria.
- Poor nutrition.
- Low socio-economic status.

Placental (placental insufficiency)
- Abnormal trophoblast invasion:
  - pre-eclampsia
  - placenta accreta.
- Infarction.
- Abruption.
- Placental location: placenta praevia.
- Tumours: chorioangiomas (placental haemangiomas).
- Abnormal umbilical cord or cord insertion: two-vessel cord.

Fetal
- Genetic abnormalities, including:
  - trisomy 13, 18, or 21
  - Turner's syndrome
  - triploidy.
- Congenital abnormalities, including:
  - cardiac, e.g. tetralogy of Fallot, transposition of the great vessels
  - gastroschisis.
- Congenital infection, including:
  - CMV
  - rubella
  - toxoplasmosis.
- Multiple pregnancy.

Intrauterine growth restriction: management and outcome

Symmetric and asymmetric IUGR

IUGR is often classified into symmetric and asymmetric, although the two groups overlap substantially

- *Symmetric growth restriction:* describes a fetus whose entire body is proportionally small and tends to be seen with very early onset IUGR and also with chromosomal abnormalities.
- *Asymmetric growth restriction:* is seen with an undernourished fetus who is compensating by directing most of its energy to maintaining the growth of vital organs such as the brain and heart at the expense of the liver, fat, and muscle. This 'head-sparing effect' results in a normal head size with small abdominal circumference and thin limbs. It is most often seen with IUGR secondary to placental insufficiency.

Management

Early identification and intensive fetal monitoring are the key to managing IUGR. The aim is to continue the pregnancy safely for as long as possible, thereby decreasing the problems associated with prematurity, but deliver before the fetus becomes excessively compromised. This is covered in depth in 🕮 Antenatal fetal surveillance, p. 146.

Long-term outcome

Most congenitally normal IUGR babies will go on to grow normally in infancy and childhood, but there may be more subtle long-term consequences, including up to 1/3 of children not reaching their predicted adult height, and having childhood attention and performance deficits.

The effects appear to last into adulthood, with a stimulus or insult at a critical, sensitive period of early life having permanent effects on structure, physiology, and metabolism. People who were small or disproportionate (thin or short) at birth have been found to have higher rates of coronary heart disease, high blood pressure, high cholesterol concentrations, and abnormal glucose-insulin metabolism (Barker hypothesis).

Further reading

Godfrey KM, Barker DJ. (2000). Fetal nutrition and adult disease. *Am J Clin Nutr* **71**(5 Suppl.): 1344–52S.

Antenatal fetal surveillance: overview

Facts

The fetus is vulnerable to any strain in the uteroplacental unit—its supply line for nutrition and gas exchange. Nearly 1/100 babies in developed countries are stillborn and 1/3 of all stillbirths occur in babies that are small for dates.

Any uteroplacental shortfall becomes more critical as the fetus gets bigger, and there is an extraordinary rate of growth during the last weeks of pregnancy. The stillbirth risk rises at the same stage.

▶ There are no treatments to reverse uteroplacental insufficiency but, potentially, delivering the baby at the right time can prevent death and disability.

⚠ The only intervention is delivery so monitoring is not useful if the fetus could not survive if it were delivered, i.e. if it is <24wks or <500g.

Stages in fetal surveillance

Antepartum fetal monitoring is done in two stages.

- *Stage 1—assigning risk:* finding normal babies developing in an abnormal situation.
- *Stage 2—timing delivery:*
  - preterm babies should be delivered only if they show signs of distress, ensuring maximum maturity while avoiding any harm.
  - after 36wks babies at high risk should be delivered.

Assigning risk

- No method of antenatal monitoring is perfect—all 'miss' affected fetuses (false negatives) and 'pick up' normal fetuses (false positives).
- Potential problems with such screening include increasing the rate of major interventions (such as CS) without benefit (see Fig. 3.11).
- Given the low prevalence of fetal compromise, the +ve predictive value of all tests when applied to low-risk populations is poor, but they perform better when applied to high-risk populations and therefore an estimation of the background risk must be made.
- Risk is assigned considering the mother's health (e.g. pre-eclampsia) and the outcome of any previous pregnancy.

✒ In the future, screening for placental function using serum markers, history, and ultrasound could establish itself as a routine test, in the same way as screening for Down's syndrome.

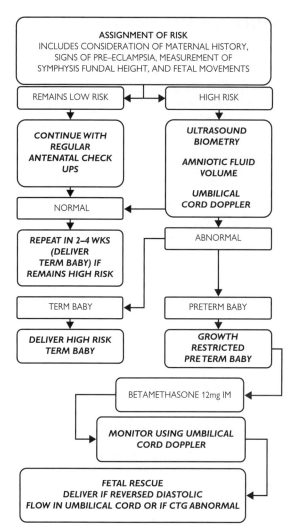

Fig. 3.11 Assigning risk in antenatal monitoring.

Identifying the high-risk fetus

Symphysis fundal height
- Measurement of the symphysis fundal height (centimetres).
- Sequential measurements can reveal changes in fetal growth.
- The detection rate of small for gestational age babies is improved by using 'customized' fundal height charts displaying curves that are specific to the mother's height, weight, parity, and ethnic group (see 📖 Intrauterine growth restriction: overview, p. 142).
- If growth is suspected to be abnormal, a USS should be organized.

Ultrasound assessment of fetal growth
Accurate knowledge of the age of the fetus is required. The fetal head circumference (HC) and abdominal circumference (AC) are measured together with the deepest pool of amniotic fluid using ultrasound and the results are charted against gestational age. Serial measurements are useful to assess the pattern of the fetal growth.

Late ultrasound aims to detect:
- Growth problems in the baby.
- Abnormalities in the amount of fluid around the baby.
- Problems with the placenta.
- Problems with the baby's position.

It should be used only where growth abnormality is suspected (SFH outside the normal range) or the patient is at high risk of uteroplacental insufficiency, because its usage has not been proven to improve outcome in unselected patients.

Uterine artery Doppler
- Resistance within the placenta can be measured from the maternal side, usually as a screening test at 23wks.
- High resistance/pulsatility in the uterine artery indicates that the mother is at increased risk of developing early onset pre-eclampsia or having a baby with IUGR; therefore she should be offered extra monitoring in pregnancy.

Routine monitoring of fetal movement
- The +ve predictive value of maternal perception of reduced fetal movements is extremely low.
- Mothers should be advised to contact their midwife or the hospital for further assessment if there is a reduction in fetal movement.

Auscultation of the fetal heart
Auscultation of the fetal heart merely confirms the fetus is alive. It provides no predictive information done (with hand-held Doppler or a Pinard stethoscope) as part of a standard antenatal examination.

Monitoring the high-risk fetus: Doppler ultrasound

Doppler ultrasound uses sound waves to study blood circulation in the baby, uterus, and placenta.

Umbilical artery Doppler

- Increasing resistance/pulsatility in the umbilical artery is an indicator of placental failure. Using this in high-risk pregnancies reduces risk of fetal death and the need for interventions around birth, such as CS.
- *Diagnostic:*
  - a high resistance/pulsatility can help to differentiate a normal, but small baby from one that is not reaching its full growth potential
  - abnormal waveforms in the umbilical artery are an early sign of fetal impairment and tend to precede changes in CTG.
- *Monitoring:*
  - in very preterm babies Doppler can be used to time fetal rescue
  - decision to deliver will depend on gestation as well as degree of abnormality.

Middle cerebral artery Doppler

- In addition to screening for anaemia, this vessel will demonstrate a reduced resistance/pulsatility in the compromised baby as a result of head sparing.
- It may be more useful than umbilical artery Doppler at term.
- It is not usually used alone in deciding timing of delivery.

Ductus venosus Doppler

- Waveform in this vein is a surrogate for cardiac function and used in monitoring for twin–twin transfusion syndrome.
- It can also be used to time delivery in severely compromised babies as an adjunct to CTGs and umbilical artery.

Understanding umbilical artery Dopplers

- When the placenta is functioning normally, flow through the umbilical artery is not impeded by end organ resistance; therefore blood continues to flow forwards (away from the heart) during cardiac diastole, seen on Doppler waveform as 'end diastolic flow' (Fig. 3.12).
- As the uteroplacental unit begins to fail, the vascular resistance rises and the forward flow in diastole begins to be reduced (this can be numerically quantified and used for monitoring).
- When the resistance is very high, blood no longer flows forwards in diastole: this is called 'absent end diastolic flow' (AEDF) (Fig. 3.13).
- When the situation is critical, the resistance is so great that blood may flow back towards the heart during diastole: this is called 'reversed end diastolic flow' (REDF) (Fig. 3.14).

⚠ These signs are used to differentiate those fetuses that are coping in an adverse situation from those that need immediate delivery.

Uterine artery Doppler

This is most used for identification of risk pregnancy.

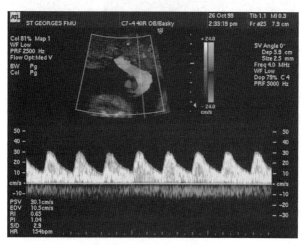

Fig. 3.12 Example of normal umbilical artery Doppler waveform.

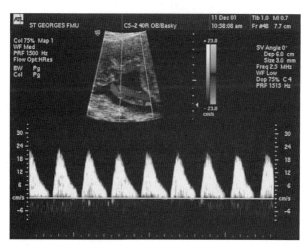

Fig. 3.13 Example of umbilical artery Doppler waveform with absent end diastloic flow (AEDF).

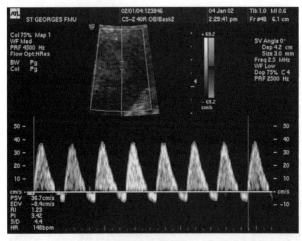

Fig. 3.14 Example of umbilical artery Doppler waveform with reversed end diastolic flow (REDF).

Monitoring the high-risk fetus: cardiotocography

- CTG is the output of electronic monitoring of the fetal heart rate, correlated with any uterine contractions.
- Analysis by inspecting the CTG is difficult, but it is more reproducible when done by computer systems, e.g. Oxford Sonicaid.

Normal cardiotocography

- The baseline fetal heart rate is between 110 and 160 beats/min and varies from that baseline by 5–25beats/min.
- The heart rate should speed up by at least 15 beats/min for at least 15s (accelerations). Two accelerations should be seen in 20min (reactive).
- There should be no slowing of the fetal heart rate from the baseline (decelerations).

▶ The most useful features in assessing the fetus's health are the variability and presence or absence of accelerations.

Abnormal cardiotocography

Caused by a failure of autonomic regulation of the heart rate, this is an end-stage event, so the lead-time between uteroplacental insufficiency causing an abnormal CTG and fetal death or long-term damage is short, and this limits its usefulness in antenatal screening.

☞ Routine antenatal CTG has not been found to be useful in low-risk populations.

CTG is used to exclude current compromise:

- In acute conditions known to cause fetal compromise, e.g. abruption and in women reporting reduced fetal movements.
- Daily in the surveillance of chronic conditions that are associated with uteroplacental insufficiency such as pre-eclampsia, and in IUGR when there is AEDF.

⚠ Because the CTG only becomes abnormal at a very late stage in IUGR, less frequent than daily CTGs should not be relied upon as a method of monitoring.

Further reading

NICE. (2008). Antenatal care: routine care for the healthy pregnant woman. In: *Fetal growth and wellbeing*. London: NICE. ♫ www.nice.org.uk/guidance/CG62

Infectious diseases in pregnancy

Rubella (German measles)

Epidemiology
- RNA togavirus.
- Spread by respiratory droplets—person to person (highly infectious).
- Incubation 14–21 days.
- Infectious for 7 days before and after appearance of rash.
- Re-infection can occur mostly with vaccine-induced immunity.

Symptoms
- Mild, febrile illness.
- Maculopapular rash.
- Arthralgia.
- Lymphadenopathy.
- Symptoms only present in 50–75% of cases.

Diagnosis
Requires serological confirmation with paired samples; acute and convalescent phase (10–14 days later). Diagnosis is based on:
- Appearance of IgM antibodies.
- ≥4-fold ↑ in IgG antibody titres or increasing IgG avidity.

Rubella-associated congenital defects
The virus disrupts mitosis, retarding cellular division and causing vascular damage. Major malformations are most likely during organogenesis with severity decreasing with advancing gestation (Table 4.1). Defects include:
- Sensorineural deafness.
- Cardiac abnormalities including VSD and patent ductus arteriosus (PDA).
- Eye lesions (congenital cataracts, microphthalmia, and glaucoma).
- Microcephaly and mental retardation.

Late-developing sequelae include:
- Diabetes.
- Thyroid disorders.
- Progressive panencephalitis.

Prevention
'Herd immunity' is maintained by widespread childhood vaccination, although the recent concern over the safety of the mumps, measles, and rubella (MMR) vaccine has decreased the uptake in the UK. Ideally, women should be tested before pregnancy to ensure immunity, but routine screening at booking identifies those at risk and in need of postnatal vaccination.

⚠ The vaccine is a live attenuated virus and therefore contraindicated in pregnancy. Women are counselled to avoid pregnancy for 10–12wks after vaccination although there is little evidence of association with congenital infection.

Table 4.1 Risk of congenital defects by gestation in primary rubella infection

Gestation	Risk of transmission	Risk of congenital abnormality	Treatment
<13wks	80%	Almost all infected fetuses	TOP may be offered without invasive prenatal diagnosis
13–16wks	50%	About 35% of those infected (mainly deafness)	Fetal blood sampling may be later offered to confirm infection
>16wks	25%	Rarely causes defects	Reassurance

Pregnant women in contact with rubella

▶ Rapidly confirm rubella in the contact. (This can be readily achieved through notification to the local Health Protection Unit (HPU)).

Reassure if the woman has had:
• 2 documented doses of rubella vaccine.
• 1 documented dose of vaccine followed by at least 1 test that has detected rubella antibody ≥10IU/mL.
• At least 2 previous rubella screening tests that have detected antibody, in at least one of which rubella antibody is ≥10IU/mL.

⚠ However, she must be advised to return if she develops a rash.

If these criteria are not met, test for IgM and IgG.

▶ Rubella IgG is detected and IgM is NOT detected:
• Reassure.
• Advise to return if she develops a rash.

▶ Rubella IgM is detected (irrespective of IgG result):
• Obtain further serum for IgG and IgM plus avidity.
• Reference testing is recommended.
• Diagnose and advise on results.

▶ Neither Rubella IgG nor IgM is detected.
• Send further sample 1mth after contact or if illness develops.
• Diagnose and advise on the results of the second sample.
• Immunize with the MMR vaccine after delivery.

Further reading

Health Protection Agency. (2011). *Guidance on viral rash in pregnancy.* ⌕ http://www.hpa.org.uk/webc/HPAwebFile/HPAweb_C/1294740918985

Measles

Indigenous measles was rare in the UK after the introduction of the MMR vaccine in 1988. Unfortunately, measles has seen an increase recently due to decreased uptake of routine vaccination. 2007 saw 971 cases in England and Wales, the biggest rise in reported measles cases since records began in 1995.

Epidemiology
- RNA paramyxovirus.
- Spread by respiratory droplets—person to person (highly infectious).
- Incubation 9–12 days.
- Infectious for 2–5 days before and after appearance of rash.

Symptoms
- Significant fever.
- Generalized maculopapular erythematous rash (appears 2–4 days after onset of symptoms).
- Koplik's spots seen inside the mouth (pathognomonic).
- The four C's: cough, coryza, conjunctivitis and ('C') Koplik's spots.

Maternal complications
- Pneumonia.
- Acute encephalitis (rarely subacute sclerosing panencephalitis).
- Corneal ulceration leading to corneal scarring.

⚠ Measles in pregnancy can be associated with maternal mortality, as well as severe morbidity.

Diagnosis
Requires serological confirmation with paired samples; acute and convalescent phase (10–14 days later). Diagnosis is based on:
- IgM in serum taken >4 days but <1mth after the onset of rash.
- Viral RNA detected in the saliva.

The effect of maternal measles on the fetus
Although associated with fetal loss and preterm delivery, no congenital infection or damage would be anticipated in a surviving fetus.

Neonatal measles has been associated with subacute sclerosing panencephalitis. Therefore, administration of human normal immunoglobulin (HNIG) immediately after birth or exposure is recommended for neonates born to mothers in whom the rash appears 6 days before to 6 days after birth.

Pregnant women in contact with measles

▶ Try to rapidly confirm measles in the contact. (This can be readily achieved through notification to the local HPV.)

Factors ↑ likelihood of the contact having measles include:
- The contact took place when the woman was abroad.
- The contact with suspected measles had travelled abroad.
- The contact had not been vaccinated against measles.
- The contact has recently been hospitalized.

Reassure measles risk is remote if the woman has had:
- 2 documented doses of measles vaccine or
- A previous test demonstrating immunity.

⚠ However, she must be advised to return if she develops a rash.

If these criteria are not met then send serum for IgG.
- Measles IgG detected—reassure.
- Measles IgG not detected—arrange HNIG through the local HPU.

▶▶ Women found to be IgG –ve should be immunized with 2 doses of the MMR vaccine after delivery.

Further reading

Health Protection Agency. (2011). *Guidance on viral rash in pregnancy.* ℜ http://www.hpa.org.uk/webc/HPAwebFile/HPAweb_C/1294740918985

Parvovirus B19

Epidemiology
- DNA virus.
- Spread by respiratory droplets—person to person.
- Incubation 4–20 days.
- Seroprevalence: ~50% of UK women immune.
- Incidence of primary infection in pregnancy <1:100.

Symptoms
- Often asymptomatic.
- Typical 'slapped cheek' rash (erythema infectiosum).
- Maculopapular rash.
- Fever.
- Arthralgia.

Diagnosis
Requires serological confirmation with paired samples; acute and convalescent phase (>10 days later). Recent infection is confirmed by:
- Appearance of IgM antibodies.
- ↑ IgG antibodies.

Maternal risks
Minimal in fit and healthy women. However, immunocompromised individuals are at risk of sudden haemolysis potentially severe enough to require blood transfusion.

Fetal risks
- Fetal infection rate is thought to be ~30%.
- The virus causes suppression of erythropoiesis sometimes with thrombocytopenia and direct cardiac toxicity, eventually resulting in cardiac failure and hydrops fetalis.
- There are no congenital defects associated with parvovirus infection.

⚠ About 10% of fetuses infected at <20wks gestation will die.

Management
Serial USS, measuring the peak systolic velocity of the fetal middle cerebral artery, are required to monitor for anaemia as this may develop many weeks after the initial infection. *In utero* red blood cell transfusion should be considered to prevent fetal demise in severely anaemic, hydropic fetuses. These patients should be cared for in a specialist fetal medicine unit.

▶ Many of these fetuses will also be significantly thrombocytopenic and, therefore, a platelet transfusion must be considered to reduce the risk of fetal bleeding at the time of the *in utero* transfusion.

Pregnant women in contact with parvovirus B19

Send serum for parvovirus B19 IgM and IgG.

▶ Parvovirus B19 IgG is detected and IgM is not detected:
- Reassure.
- Advise to return if mother develops a rash.

▶ Parvovirus B19 IgM is detected (irrespective of IgG result):
- Send the sample for confirmatory testing.
- Obtain further serum (reference testing is recommended).
- Refer for specialist advice.

▶ Neither parvovirus B19 IgG nor IgM is detected:
- Send further sample 1mth after contact or if illness develops.
- Diagnose and advise on the results of the second sample.
- Refer for specialist advice.

Further reading

Health Protection Agency. (2011). *Guidance on viral rash in pregnancy.* ℜ http://www.hpa.org.uk/webc/HPAwebFile/HPAweb_C/1294740918985

Cytomegalovirus

Epidemiology
- Herpes virus.
- Transmitted in bodily fluids—low infectivity.
- Can remain dormant within host for life; reactivation common.
- Seroprevalence: ~50% of UK women.
- Incidence of 1° infection in pregnancy ~1:100.

Symptoms
Asymptomatic in 95% of cases. May present with:
- Fever.
- Malaise.
- Lymphadenopathy, atypical lymphocytosis, and mononucleosis.

Diagnosis
Maternal infection
Usually requires serological confirmation with paired samples; acute and convalescent phase (14 days later). Recent infection confirmed by:
- Significant ↑ in IgM antibodies (may persist for up to 8mths).
- ↑ IgG antibody titres.
- Culture/PCR of maternal urine (not widely available).

Fetal infection
Culture/PCR of amniotic fluid (after 20wks).

CMV-associated congenital defects
- IUGR.
- Microcephaly.
- Hepatosplenamegaly and thrombocytopenia.
- Jaundice.
- Chorioretinitis.
- Later-developing sequelae include:
  - psychomotor retardation—reported to account for as much as 10% of mental retardation in children <6yrs old
  - sensorineural hearing loss.

Outcome
- With a primary maternal infection 40% of fetuses will be infected, irrespective of gestation. Of these: 90% are normal at birth, of which 20% will develop late, usually minor sequelae.
- 10% are symptomatic, of which:
  - 33% will die
  - 67% will have long-term problems.

Management
As most fetuses will be unaffected, counselling about management (including TOP) is very difficult, even in the face of confirmed fetal infection. However, close monitoring of fetal growth and well-being is clearly indicated, with appropriate paediatric follow-up.

Non-vesicular rashes in pregnancy

Investigation will be directed by clinical features and epidemiological information. Causes may include:
- Streptococcal infection.
- Meningococcal infection.
- Enteroviruses.
- CMV.
- Epstein–Barr virus (EBV).
- Syphilis.

△ Special consideration must be given to the possibility of:
- Rubella.
- Measles.
- Parvovirus B19.

▶ If features are compatible with rubella, measles, or parvovirus B19 appropriate laboratory investigation must be initiated irrespective of past testing or immunization.

▶ Rubella and measles diagnosed on the basis of clinical suspicion are notifiable diseases and should be reported to the local HPU.

Further reading

Health Protection Agency. (2011). *Guidance on viral rash in pregnancy*. ℘ http://www.hpa.org.uk/webc/HPAwebFile/HPAweb_C/1294740918985

Varicella (chickenpox)

Epidemiology
- Varicella zoster virus (VZV)—DNA virus.
- Spread by respiratory droplets and contact with vesicle fluid.
- Incubation 10–21 days.
- Infectious from 2 days before rash until all vesicles are crusted.
- Seroprevalence: ~90% of UK women immune.
- Incidence of 1° infection in pregnancy ~3:1000.

Symptoms
- Fever.
- Malaise.
- Maculopapular rash which becomes vesicular then crusts over.

Diagnosis
If there has been exposure without a good history of previous infection, serum should be tested for VZV IgG antibodies. If antibodies are detected within 10 days of contact, immunity can be assumed and reassurance given. If not, varicella-zoster immunoglobulin (VZIG) should be given as soon as possible. Diagnosis of varicella itself is usually made on the history of contact and appearance of the typical rash.

> **Maternal risks**
> ⚠ Varicella in pregnancy is often more severe and may be life-threatening as a consequence of:
> - Varicella pneumonia.
> - Hepatitis.
> - Encephalitis.

Fetal risks
Fetal infection rate is thought to be ~25% in all trimesters: if <20wks there is a 2% risk of fetal varicella syndrome with congenital defects (Table 4.2) including:
- Skin scarring.
- Limb hypoplasia.
- Eye lesions (congenital cataracts, microphthalmia, chorioretinitis).
- Neurological abnormalities (mental retardation, microcephaly, cortical atrophy, and dysfunction of bladder and bowel sphincters).

Neonatal risks
▶ Neonatal varicella is seen in babies whose mothers contracted it in the last 4wks of pregnancy. Severe infection, which may be fatal, is most likely to occur if the rash appears 5 days before delivery or 2 days after. These babies should all receive VZIG as soon as possible.

Treatment
Oral aciclovir reduces the duration of symptoms if given within 24h of the rash appearing. Its effect on the incidence of serious sequelae is unknown.

Table 4.2 Risk to fetus from primary maternal varicella infection by gestation

Gestation	Risk to fetus	Management
<20wks	2% will develop fetal varicella syndrome (FVS)	Detailed ultrasound examination at 16–20wks, may consider TOP if evidence of FVS seen. Neonatal ophthalmic examination
>20wks	Not associated with congenital abnormality	Fetal and neonatal surveillance
Within 4wks of delivery	About 20% will develop neonatal varicella infection	VZIG as soon as possible, 14 days monitoring for signs of infection, and aciclovir if varicella develops

RCOG. *Green-top guidelines.* www.rcog.org.uk

Herpes simplex

Epidemiology

- Herpes simplex virus (HSV)—type 2 causes >70% genital infections.
- Spread by sexual contact.
- Incubation ~2–7 days.
- Individual may be infectious even when apparently asymptomatic.
- Seroprevalence of HSV 2: ~20% of UK women.

Symptoms

Primary HSV infection is the most severe and usually results in:
- Mild flu-like illness.
- Inguinal lymphadenopathy.
- Vulvitis; pain sometimes severe enough to cause urinary retention.
- Small, characteristic vesicles on the vulva.

Diagnosis Usually made on the history appearance of the typical rash, but viral culture of vesicle fluid is the gold standard. Acute and convalescent antibody levels may sometimes be helpful.

Maternal risks

In pregnancy a primary attack may be severe. Complications include:
- Meningitis.
- Sacral radiculopathy—causing urinary retention and constipation.
- Transverse myelitis.
- Disseminated infection.

Fetal risks Primary infection may lead to miscarriage or preterm labour, but no related congenital defects have been identified.

Neonatal risks

Transmission rate from vaginal delivery during 1° maternal infection may be as high as 50%, but is relatively uncommon during a recurrent attack (<5%). Neonatal herpes appears during the first 2wks of life.
- 25% limited to eyes and mouth only.
- 75% widely disseminated, of which:
  - ~70% will die
  - many of the survivors will have long-term problems including mental retardation.

Management

Aciclovir may decrease severity and duration of the primary attack if given within 5 days of onset of symptoms. If labour is within 6wks of primary infection then delivery by CS is recommended provided the membranes have not been ruptured for >4h. With active vesicles from a recurrent attack, the risk of surgery must be carefully weighed against the very small risk of neonatal infection.

Malaria

Epidemiology
- Protozoan infection (75% *Plasmodium falciparum*).
- Not endemic in the UK, but commonly imported (~1500 cases in 2008).
- Spread by the bite of a sporozite-bearing female mosquito.

Symptoms
There are often no specific symptoms or signs, with the infection presenting with a 'flu-like' illness, but may include:
- Fever (cyclical 'spiking').
- Rigors/chills/sweats.
- Muscle pain and general malaise.

Diagnosis
- Diagnosis is made from blood films.
- Rapid detection tests may miss low parasitaemia.
- 3 −ve malaria smears 12–24h apart rules out malaria.

Maternal risks
Pregnancy increases the risk of developing severe disease.

Fetal risks
Effects on pregnancy
- Miscarriage or preterm delivery.
- Stillbirth.
- Congenital malaria.
- Low birth weight (2° to prematurity or IUGR).

Management
⚠ Malaria in pregnancy should be treated as an emergency.
- Women should be admitted to hospital.
- Quinine and clindamycin is the treatment of choice for falciparum malaria (IV artesunate should be used for severe cases).
- Treat the fever with antipyretics.
- Screen for anaemia and treat appropriately.
- Uncomplicated malaria is not a reason for induction of labour.

▶ Proguanil and chloroquine are probably the safest drugs for malarial prophylaxis in pregnancy.

▶ In the UK, malaria in pregnancy must be reported to the public health authorities and the Health Protection Agency (www.hpa.org.uk) and slides, plus a blood aliquot, should be sent to the Malaria Reference Laboratory for confirmation, which is performed free of charge.

Further reading
RCOG. *Green-top guidelines.* ⌕ www.rcog.org.uk

Toxoplasmosis

Epidemiology
- Protozoan parasite *Toxoplasma gondii*.
- Spread by contact with cat faeces and eating undercooked meat.
- Incubation <2 days.
- Seroprevalence: ~20% of UK women immune.
- Incidence of 1° infection in pregnancy ~1:500. Rare in UK.

Symptoms
Asymptomatic in about 80% of cases. May present with:
- Fever.
- Lymphadenopathy.

Diagnosis
Maternal infection
Requires serological confirmation with paired samples; acute and convalescent phase (>28 days later). Recent infection is confirmed by:
- Isolated very high titres of IgM antibodies (may persist up to 1yr).
- Concurrent high IgM and IgG antibodies.
- 4-fold ↑ in IgG antibodies.

Fetal infection
May be diagnosed by the presence of IgM antibodies in amniotic fluid or fetal blood. Amniocentesis is accurate only after 20wks. Although ultrasound signs, such as cerebral ventriculomegaly, can occur, most affected fetuses have a normal scan.

Maternal risks
Minimal in fit and healthy women. However, immunocompromised individuals are at risk of severe disseminated illness with chorioretinitis and encephalitis.

Management
Starting spiramycin on diagnosis of maternal infection may decrease the risk of fetal infection. If vertical transmission occurs combination anti-toxoplasmosis therapy is used. Neonatal follow-up should include an ophthalmic review and cranial radiological studies. It is usually recommended that future pregnancies are delayed until maternal IgM antibodies have been cleared.

Fetal risks

Spontaneous miscarriage is common with infection in the first trimester (Table 4.3). Defects associated with primary infection include:
- Chorioretinitis.
- Microcephaly and hydrocephalus.
- Intracranial calcification.
- Mental retardation.

Table 4.3 Risk of congenital defects by gestation in toxoplasmosis infection

Gestation	Risk of transmission	Risk of congenital abnormality in infected fetuses
<12wks	~17%	75%
12–28wks	~25%	25%
>28wks	65%	<10%

Hepatitis B

Epidemiology
- Hepatitis B virus (HBV)—DNA virus.
- Spread by infected blood, blood products, or sexual contact.
- Incubation 2–6mths.
- Incidence of carrier status in UK women is ~1:100.

Symptoms
Prodrome of non-specific systemic and gastrointestinal symptoms followed by an episode of jaundice.

Diagnosis
Based on clinical picture and serological detection of:
- HB surface antigen (HBsAg) → current infection.
- HB E antigen (HBeAg) → active viral replication.
- Anti-HBsAg antibodies → indicates immunity from either infection or vaccination.

Maternal risks
In the developed world, hepatitis B infection in pregnancy has a similar course to that seen in the non-pregnant individual:
- 65% subclinical disease with full recovery.
- 25% develop acute hepatitis.
- 10% become chronic carriers.
- <0.5% develop fulminant hepatitis, which has a significant mortality rate.

Fetal risks
Severe acute infection may lead to miscarriage or preterm labour, but no related congenital defects have been identified.

Management
▶ In the UK all women should be routinely screened for HBV at booking.

▶ High-risk women (e.g. commercial sex workers and IV drug users) should be counselled and vaccinated before pregnancy.

⚠ Babies whose mothers have acute or chronic HBV should receive HBV IgG and HBV vaccination within 24h of delivery. This is thought to be up to 95% effective at preventing neonatal HBV infection.

Neonatal risks

Transmission usually occurs at delivery, but <5% may be due to transplacental bleeding *in utero*. Neonatal infection may be fatal, and usually results in chronic carrier status with significant lifelong risks of cirrhosis and hepatocellular carcinoma. The carrier status of the mother at delivery determines the risk of vertical transmission:

- HBsAg and HBeAg +ve: ~95% risk.
- HbsAg +ve and HBeAg −ve: <15% risk.

Group B streptococcus

Epidemiology
- *Streptococcus agalactiae.*
- Common bowel commensal.
- Up to 20% women carry it vaginally.

Symptoms
None.

Diagnosis
Culture from a lower vaginal swab (LVS) and perianal swab.

Fetal risks
Associated with preterm prelabour rupture of membranes and preterm delivery.

Management
The RCOG does not recommend routine antenatal screening for GBS. However, intrapartum antibiotic prophylaxis should be offered to women with a history of previous neonatal GBS infection. Prophylaxis should also be considered if GBS is discovered incidentally in either the vagina or urine, but there is no benefit to be gained from attempting to eradicate it antenatally. Intrapartum prophylaxis should be considered with the following risk factors:
- Prematurity (<37wks).
- Prolonged rupture of membranes (>18h).
- Pyrexia in labour.

Antibiotics
The recommended prophylaxis in labour is IV benzylpenicillin started as soon as possible after onset of labour and at least 2h before delivery (3g initially then 1.5g every 4h throughout labour). In case of penicillin allergy, IV clindamycin should be used (900mg every 8h).

Further reading
RCOG. *Green top guidelines.* ॐ www.rcog.org.uk

Neonatal risks

Most frequent cause of early-onset, severe neonatal infection (incidence 1:2000 live births). Up to 70% of babies whose mothers carry group B streptococcus (GBS) will themselves be colonized at delivery, but only 1% of these will develop symptoms of sepsis. Early-onset GBS infection (<4 days from delivery) has about a 20% mortality rate and may present with:

- Pneumonia.
- Septicaemia.
- Meningitis.

Late-onset infection (>7 days) is not associated with maternal GBS carriage.

⚠ This carries a mortality rate of about 20%. Of those surviving, 50% will have serious neurological sequelae, such as cortical blindness and deafness.

Group A streptococcus

The Centre for Maternal and Child Enquiries (CMACE) 2006–2008 identified infection as a leading direct cause of maternal death. Many deaths were from group A streptococcal (GAS) disease caught in the community, mirroring the rise in general population.

Epidemiology

- *Streptococcus pyogenes*.
- Most common bacterial cause of acute pharyngitis ('strep throat').
- Up to 30% of population are asymptomatic carriers (skin or throat).
- Easily spread—person to person or droplet.

Diseases caused by GAS

- Pharyngitis.
- Impetigo.
- Cellulitis.
- Scarlet fever.
- Rheumatic fever.
- Toxic shock syndrome.

CMACE GAS findings and recommendations

- Strep throat is one of the most common bacterial infections of childhood.
- All of the mothers who died from GAS either worked with or had young children.
- Several mothers had a history of a recent sore throat or had a family member with a sore throat or respiratory infection.
- Organism may be transferred from the throat or nose to the perineum via the hands when using the toilet or changing sanitary towels.
- Antenatal education should raise awareness of this and the importance of good personal hygiene including washing hands before, as well as after, using the toilet or changing sanitary towels.

⚠ GAS sepsis should never be underestimated; onset may be insidious with women appearing deceptively well before suddenly collapsing with little or no warning. Once established there may be rapid deterioration into septic shock, disseminated intravascular coagulation (DIC) and multi-organ failure.

Fetal risks

No congenital infection or damage would be anticipated in a fetus following maternal GAS infection.

Further reading

Cantwell R, Clutton-Brock T, Cooper G. (2011). Saving mothers' lives: reviewing maternal deaths to make motherhood safer: 2006–2008. The Eighth Report of the Confidential Enquiries into Maternal Deaths in the United Kingdom. *British Journal of Obstetrics and Gynaecology*, **118**(Suppl 1):1–203.

Other infections

Syphilis (see Chapter 17, p. 556)

- Currently relatively rare in the UK, but reported to be increasing.
- Routinely screened for at booking, but care must be taken when interpreting the results as biological false +ves are common.
- The spirochaete can cross the placenta and is associated with preterm delivery, stillbirth, and congenital syphilis defects, including:
  - 8th nerve deafness
  - Hutchinson's teeth
  - saddle nose
  - sabre shins.
- Treatment with penicillin:
  - <16wks—prevents virtually all congenital infection
  - >16wks—still effective in most cases.

Listeria monocytogenes

- Rare, affecting about 1:10 000 pregnancies in the UK.
- Found in soft cheese, pate, undercooked meat, and shellfish.
- Produces gastroenteritis often accompanied by flu-like symptoms.
- Crosses the placenta causing amnionitis, and miscarriage or preterm labour.
- Neonatal infection may be:
  - generalized septicaemia
  - pneumonia
  - meningitis.
- Treatment is with high dose amoxicillin or erythromycin.

Epstein–Barr virus

- Infectious mononucleosis is a common presentation of primary EBV.
- A generalized maculopapular rash may occur (particularly if ampicillin or a similar antibiotic has been taken).
- Primary infection in pregnancy carries no specific risk to the fetus.

Enteroviruses

- Includes Coxsackie virus groups A and B, echovirus, and enterovirus 68–71.
- Wide range of manifestations, including meningitis, rash, febrile illness, and myocarditis.
- No clear causal relationship evident for adverse fetal or neonatal outcome.

▶ Hand, foot, and mouth is caused by an enteroviral infection. Primary infection or contact with it in pregnancy is not known to have any adverse consequences for the fetus.

HIV and pregnancy

Facts
- In 2010 in the UK:
  - an estimated 91 500 people were living with HIV
  - of those about 22 000 are unaware of their infection
  - 2.1 million HIV tests were performed
  - half of newly diagnosed adults were late stage at diagnosis
  - less than 1% of people with HIV died.
- Over 1/2 have acquired their infection via heterosexual contact.
- Around 35% are of black African ethnicity.
- Highly active antiretroviral therapy (HAART) (Table 4.4) has ↑ life expectancy.
- By 2010 >98% of all diagnosed women received assisted reproductive technologies (ART) before delivery.
- Pregnancy does not alter the course of the infection.
- High viral loads (VL) and low CD4 counts indicate the likelihood of mother to child transmission (MTCT) and the need for the mother to receive therapy for her own health.
- Among women on combination antiretroviral therapy (cART) with an undectable viral load at delivery, MTCT rate is estimated at 0.1%.
- Aggregated data on antiretroviral exposure and congenital malformations are collected in the UK by the Antiretroviral Pregnancy Registry (APR).

Prepregnancy counselling
⚠ Counselling of couples already known to be discordant with regard to HIV infection is important, as the risk of HIV transmission is estimated to be 0.03–1% for each act of unprotected intercourse.
- Where the mother is +ve and the partner –ve, self-insemination with the partner's sperm is recommended.
- Sperm washing is recommended if male is +ve and female –ve.
- An alternative is donor insemination if the male partner is +ve.
- IVF should take account of the parents' viral load, CD4 counts, and any AIDS defining illness.
- Women conceiving on an effective HAART regimen should continue even if it contains efavirenz or does not contain zidovudine. Exceptions are:
  - protease inhibitor (PI) monotherapy should be intensified to include one or more agents that cross the placenta
  - the combination of stavudine and didanosine should not be prescribed in pregnancy.

Antenatal screening
Routine antenatal screening was introduced in 1999 as part of the antenatal booking investigations. This is an opt-out policy and has increased the rate of HIV diagnosis significantly. This has proved to be one of the major successes in the management of HIV-infected patients as MTCT is now a rare occurrence in the UK.

Confidentiality

⚠ It is estimated that 30–75% of the partners of HIV +ve mothers are unaware of the diagnosis.

▶ It is important to establish the need for healthcare workers and partners to be aware of the diagnosis early so that an effective care plan can be put in place. This may require establishing a local mechanism to flag notes to indicate that additional information is available on a need-to-know basis should the mother be admitted as an emergency.

▶ Women should be encouraged to have all relevant information recorded in their hand-held notes.

Table 4.4 Classes of antiretroviral drugs

Class of drug	Examples	Potential problems
Nucleoside analogue reverse transcriptase inhibitors (NRTI)	Zidovudine (ZDV, previously AZT) Lamivudine (3TC) Didanosine (ddl) Stavudine (d4T) Abacavir (ABC) Tenofovir Emtricitabine	All generally well tolerated, but reported case of: anaemia, nausea, and vomiting; elevated transaminases and hyperglycaemia. Lactic acidosis is a possibility when d4T and ddl are combined
Non-nucleoside analogue reverse transcriptase (NNRTI)	Nevirapine (NVP) Delavirdine Efavirenz inhibitors	Greatest experience is with NVP, but although well tolerated there is an association with deranged liver function in women with good CD4 counts. Rash is also reported
Protease inhibitors (PIs)	Ritinovir Indinavir Nelfinavir Saquinavir	Hyperglycaemia is a risk with new-onset diabetes or exacerbation of existing diabetes Diarrhoea, with nausea, vomiting, and altered taste Altered liver function reported
HIV-1 Integrase strand transfer inhibitor	Raltegravir	Depression Hyperglycaemia Changes in body fat distribution

Further reading

APR. (2012). ℘ www.apregistry.com

HIV: antenatal care

Social and ethical issues

- Antenatal care should be delivered by a multidisciplinary team, the precise composition of which will vary.
- As there may be social, housing, or immigration issues, the involvement of social services should be considered.
- Other support groups may be required if there are issues with regard to drug addiction.
- Testing of other children is recommended.

⚠ Failure to engage with the antenatal care plan may require the involvement of legal services to address child protection issues.

▶ Local guidelines may exist for the eligibility for free NHS care; however, it is considered unethical to deny treatment to an HIV +ve mother as this treatment would protect her unborn child and potentially her own health.

Highly active antiretroviral therapy in pregnancy

- Women requiring HAART for their own health should commence treatment as soon as possible.
- By 2011, there were over 11 000 HIV-exposed uninfected children in the UK, whose mothers took some form of ART in pregnancy.
- There is most evidence and experience with zidovudine plus lamivudine, but tenofovir plus emtricitabine or abacavir plus lamivudine are acceptable alternatives.
- The 3rd agent in HAART should be nevirapine if the CD4 count is less than 250, or efavirenz, or a boosted PI.
- No routine dose alterations are recommended for ART during pregnancy.
- Women who do not require treatment for themselves should commence temporary HAART at 14/40 if the baseline VL is >30K (consider starting earlier if VL >100 000).
- All women should have commenced HAART by 24wks.
- Zidovudine monotherapy can be used in women planning a Caesarean section who have a baseline VL of <10 000 and a CD4 of >350.

Special considerations

- Integrated screening for trisomy 21 is recommended to reduce the number of women requiring invasive testing.

⚠ If not on treatment and an invasive procedure cannot be delayed until viral suppression is achieved, it is recommended that women should commence HAART to include raltegravir and be given a single dose of nevirapine 2–4h prior to the procedure.

- Fetal USS should be performed as per national guidelines.
- If admitted 'unwell', consider complications of ART.
- ECV can be performed in women with HIV.

Monitoring of HIV +ve pregnant women

- Sexual health screening is recommended at presentation and in the 3rd trimester.
- Newly diagnosed HIV +ve pregnant women do not require any additional baseline investigations compared with non-pregnant HIV +ve women, other than those routinely performed in the general antenatal clinic.
- HIV sequence analysis should be performed prior to initiation of treatment, except for late-presenting women. Post-short-course treatment sequence is recommended to ensure that mutations are not missed with reversion during the off-treatment period.
- Women who either conceive on HAART or do not require HAART for their own health should have a minimum of one CD4 count at baseline and one at delivery.
- In women who commence HAART in pregnancy a VL should be performed 2–4wks after commencing HAART, at least once every trimester, at 36wks, and at delivery.
- In women commencing HAART in pregnancy LFTs should be performed at initiation of HAART and at each antenatal visit.
- In the event that a woman who has either conceived on or initiated HAART has not achieved a plasma VL of <50c/mL at 36wks the following interventions are recommended:
  - review adherence and concomitant medication
  - perform genotype if appropriate
  - consider therapeutic drug monitoring
  - optimize to best regimen
  - consider intensification.

British HIV Association. (2012). *Guidelines for the management of HIV infection in pregnant women.* ℰ www.bhiva.org

HIV: perinatal concerns

Delivery

Vaginal delivery

- Untreated women with a CD4 count ≥350 and a viral load of <50 can be treated with zidovudine monotherapy or HAART (including Trizivir®) and can aim for a vaginal delivery.
- Vaginal delivery is recommended for women on HAART with an HIV viral load <50 at 36wks.
- In women in whom a vaginal delivery has been recommended and labour has commenced, obstetric management should follow the same guidelines as for the uninfected population.
- Vaginal birth after Caesarean (VBAC) should be offered to women with a viral load <50.

Caesarean delivery

- Delivery by CS is recommended for women taking zidovudine monotherapy, irrespective of plasma viral load at the time of delivery and for women with viral load >400 regardless of ART.
- Where the indication for CS is the prevention of MTCT, CS should be undertaken at between 38 and 39wks gestation.

Rupture of membranes (ROM)

- In the presence of ROM ≥34wks delivery should take place immediately, by either CS or induction of labour (IOL) according to viral load.
- When PPROM occurs at <34wks:
  - steroids should be administered
  - virological control should be optimized
  - there should be multidisciplinary discussion about the timing and mode of delivery.

Intrapartum zidovudine

Intrapartum IV zidovudine (ZDV) infusion is recommended in the following circumstances:
- women with a viral load of >10 000 who present in labour, or with ruptured membranes, or who are admitted for planned CS
- untreated women presenting in labour or with ruptured membranes in whom the current viral load is not known.

Late presentation

- Women presenting in labour/with ROM/requiring delivery without a documented HIV result must be recommended to have an HIV diagnostic point of care test (POCT).
- A reactive POCT result must be acted upon immediately with initiation of the interventions to prevent MTCT without waiting for formal serological confirmation.
- A woman who presents after 28wks should commence HAART without delay.
- If the viral load is unknown or >100K, a 3 or 4 drug regimen that includes raltegravir is suggested.
- An untreated woman presenting in labour at term should be given a stat dose of nevirapine and commence fixed-dose zidovudine with lamivudine and raltegravir.
- It is suggested that intravenous zidovudine be infused for the duration of labour and delivery.

British HIV Association. (2012). *Guidelines for the management of HIV infection in pregnant women. (2012).* ℘ www.bhiva.org

HIV: postnatal concerns

Postnatal management and follow-up

- Women requiring therapy for their own health (with a history of an AIDS-defining illness or with a CD4 count <350) should continue HAART after delivery.
- ART should be continued in all women who commenced cART for MTCT with a CD4 count of between 350 and 500 during pregnancy who are co-infected with hepatitis B virus (HBV) or hepatitis C virus (HCV).
- When stopping NNRTI-based HAART post-partum the NNRTI washout period should be covered by 2wks PI-based therapy.
- All mothers and children require long-term follow-up.

Neonatal management

- Neonatal post-exposure prophylaxis (PEP) should be commenced within 4h of birth and should continue for at least 4wks.
- Zidovudine monotherapy is recommended if:
  - maternal viral load is <50 HIV RNA copies/mL at 36wks gestation/ delivery
  - mother delivered by CS whilst on zidovudine.
- Neonates <72h old should initiate 3-drug therapy immediately if:
  - their mothers are HIV +ve and untreated
  - maternal viral load at 36wks gestation/delivery is not <50 HIV RNA copies/mL.
- Primary pneumocystis pneumonia (PCP) prophylaxis, with co-trimoxazole, should be initiated from age 4wks in:
  - all HIV infected infants
  - infants with an initial +ve molecular diagnostic test result
  - infants whose mother's viral load at 36wks was >1000 or unknown (and continued until HIV infection has been excluded).

▶ All cases of HIV in pregnancy (whether diagnosed before or during pregnancy) should be reported to the National Study of HIV in Pregnancy and Childhood at the RCOG even if the pregnancy is not continued to term. Email: nshpc@ich.uci.ac.uk

Further reading

British HIV Association. (2012). *Guidelines for the management of HIV infection in pregnant women.* ℘ www.bhiva.org

Vaccination and travel

Vaccination

- Live attenuated vaccines such as rubella, polio, and MMR are contraindicated in pregnancy.
- Passive immunization with specific human immunoglobulin is safe and may provide important protection (e.g. VZIG).
- Women who are HbsAg −ve but considered at high risk should be offered HBV vaccination in pregnancy.
- Vaccinations for travel should be considered on an individual basis, and the small risk from the vaccine compared with the risk from contracting the disease:
  - cholera—limited efficacy therefore not recommended
  - hepatitis A—low risk, but consider HNIG for short periods
  - meningococcus—safety unknown, consider if high risk
  - rabies—consider immunoglobulin for post-exposure prophylaxis
  - tetanus—safe in pregnancy
  - yellow fever—safety unknown, consider if high risk.

Travel—general advice

Food

Avoid foodstuffs that may pose a potential risk of infection:
- Unwashed fruit and vegetables.
- Raw eggs.
- Undercooked meat.
- Tap water in countries with poor sanitation (beware of ice cubes).
- Shellfish in hepatitis A endemic areas.

Malaria

Appropriate antimalarials should be taken, accompanied by avoidance of exposure to mosquito bites:
- Mosquito nets.
- Long sleeves and trousers (tucked into socks).
- Insect repellents.

⚠ Recommend that the woman checks that her travel insurance will cover any health or pregnancy-related problems abroad. They may class pregnancy as a 'pre-existing condition' and therefore not cover it.

Flying in pregnancy

- Most airlines will allow pregnant women to fly up to 36wks gestation:
  - ~32wks with multiple pregnancy
  - at >28wks many will request medical certification of fitness to fly.
- The risk of venous thromboembolism (VTE) significantly ↑ with flights of >8h.
- Simple measures should be recommended to ↓ the risk of VTE:
  - avoid dehydration (and alcohol!)
  - take regular short walks around the plane
  - use graduated compression hosiery.

● Consider low dose aspirin.

⚠ Women with other risk factors for deep vein thrombosis (DVT) (such as factor V Leiden carriers) may require low molecular weight heparin for flights of 5h or more.

Medical disorders in pregnancy

Epilepsy: overview

- 0.6% of pregnancies occur in women with epilepsy.
- Most women have been diagnosed before conception.
- If the first seizure occurs in pregnancy there is a wide differential diagnosis (see Box 5.1).
- Seizure frequency can ↑ (37%), ↓ (13%), or remain unchanged (50%).
- Poorly controlled epileptics and those who stop medication are at the highest risk of ↑ seizure frequency.

⚠ The fetus usually tolerates seizures without long-term sequelae, but there is ↑ risk of fetal demise with status epilepticus.

Fetal risks

There is an increased risk of major congenital anomalies (2–5%) in women with epilepsy. Most of this risk is due to anticonvulsant medication; however, women not on antiepileptic drugs still have a higher risk than the general population. The use of multiple drugs carries a higher risk to the fetus than monotherapy. Higher doses lead to increased risk. Dividing doses and reducing peak blood levels may be beneficial. Any change in anticonvulsant therapy should be undertaken before pregnancy. Once pregnancy is diagnosed the woman should continue on her anticonvulsant drugs, and not change, as teratogenic risk exposure has already occurred. Folic acid (5mg) reduces the risk of some anomalies.

Fetal risks of anticonvulsant therapy

- Teratogenicity: congenital anomalies or fetal anticonvulsant syndrome.
- Neonatal withdrawal.
- Vitamin K deficiency (enzyme inducers) → haemorrhagic disease of newborn.
- Developmental delay and behavioural problems.

Drugs used in treatment of epilepsy

These have varying risks of congenital anomalies and can be divided according to their ability to induce liver enzymes.

Enzyme-inducing anticonvulsants

- Carbamazepine.
- Phenobarbital.
- Phenytoin.
- Primidone.

Non-enzyme-inducing anticonvulsants

- Valproate.
- Lamotrigine.
- Gabapentin.
- Ethosuximide.

Box 5.1 Differential diagnosis of first seizure in pregnancy

- Eclampsia.
- Epilepsy.
- Infection:
  - meningitis
  - encephalitis
  - abscess.
- Metabolic:
  - drug or alcohol withdrawal
  - drug toxicity
  - hypoglycaemia
  - electrolyte imbalance (↑ Na, ↓ Na, ↑ Ca).
- Severe hypoxia.
- Space-occupying lesion.
- Vascular:
  - cerebral vein thrombosis
  - thrombotic thrombocytopaenic purpura (TTP)
  - cerebral infarction or haemorrhage.

✿ All patients who present with their first seizure in pregnancy should have imaging of the brain with CT or, preferably, MRI and be reviewed by a neurologist.

Main teratogenic risks of commonly used anticonvulsants

Valproate
- Neural tube defects: ↑ 10-fold (1–2%).
- Genitourinary anomalies (hypospadias).
- Cardiac anomalies.
- Facial clefts.
- Neurodevelopmental delay: ↑ 3.5-fold.

Carbamazepine
- Neural tube defects (0.5–1%).
- Cardiac anomalies.
- Facial clefts.

Phenytoin
- Facial clefts: ↑ 5-fold.
- Cardiac anomalies.

Epilepsy: management

Prepregnancy counselling
- Involve a neurologist to confirm diagnosis is epilepsy.
- Optimize treatment, achieve seizure control, and educate patient.
- Use the least number of drugs at the lowest dose to control seizures to minimize risk of congenital anomalies.
- Consider stopping drugs if seizure free for >2yrs (warn of risk of seizures and implications for driving).
- All women should take folic acid 5mg for at least 12wks before conception and continue until delivery (↓ risk of neural tube defects).
- Risk of epilepsy in the child (4% if one parent affected, 15% if both parents affected).

Antenatal care
- Do not change medication in pregnancy if well controlled, and stress the importance of compliance with medication.
- Prenatal screening:
  - α-fetoprotein (neural tube defects)
  - detailed anomaly scan (facial clefts and cardiac abnormalities).
- Consider fetal echocardiography at 22–24wks.
- Consider vitamin K 10mg/day for the last 4wks of pregnancy (hepatic enzyme-inducing drugs may lead to neonatal coagulopathy).
- General advice (showers rather than baths, avoid sleep deprivation).
- The levels of newer antiepileptics, particularly lamotrigine, may fall precipitously and usually require a 30–50% rise in dose by 30wks.

✏ There is no role for routine monitoring of drug levels (it may be useful in women with increased seizure frequency, suspected non-compliance, concern over toxic side effects, or polypharmacy).

Intrapartum care
- Aim for vaginal delivery (CS should be for obstetric indications; seizures are not an indication unless in status epilepticus).
- Labour is associated with increased risk of seizures due to sleep deprivation, reduced absorption of drugs, and hyperventilation.
- Control seizures with benzodiazepines.
- Ensure usual anticonvulsants are taken at the correct time.

Postnatal care
- Neonatal vitamin K to ↓ risk of haemorrhagic disease of the newborn.
- Breast-feeding is not contraindicated (anticonvulsants reach breast milk and thus slow withdrawal occurs, although phenobarbital and benzodiazepines may cause sedation in the baby).
- If the anticonvulsant dose was increased in pregnancy it should be reduced back to prepregnancy levels slowly post-partum.
- Contraception with enzyme-inducing drugs:
  - COCP containing 50 micrograms oestrogen with a shorter pill-free interval
  - progestogen-only pill (POP) is less effective
  - intrauterine contraceptive device (IUCD) is ideal.
- General advice (bathing and feeding) to minimize risk of harm to baby from seizures.

Cerebrovascular accident

Cerebrovascular accidents (CVAs) are rare in women of reproductive age, but there is an ↑ risk in the post-partum period. There is a 9-fold ↑ risk for infarcts and 28-fold ↑ for haemorrhagic stroke in the first 6wks post-partum compared with non-pregnant women. Symptoms include:
- Abrupt onset of weakness.
- Sensory loss.
- Dysphasia.

Common risk factors for strokes at all ages include:
- Smoking.
- Diabetes.
- Hypertension.
- Hypercholesterolaemia.

Cryptogenic stoke is more common in young people often from emboli phenomenon, the origin of which is never found. Patients who have previously had a stroke are unlikely to have a further event in pregnancy, unless stoke was caused by dissection (usually vertebral artery).

Management
- Treatment depends on the cause (see Box 5.2).
- Anticoagulation may be appropriate.

Subarachnoid haemorrhage

Outside pregnancy the commonest cause is a ruptured berry aneurysm, but arteriovenous malformations (AVMs) may dilate in pregnancy due to the effect of oestrogen, resulting in a similar incidence.

Presentation
- Headache.
- Vomiting.
- Loss of or impaired consciousness.
- Neck stiffness.
- Focal neurological signs.

Management
- Early treatment is recommended to reduce the chance of subsequent bleeding (the risk is high for AVM).
- Surgery is usually recommended, excision of the AVM, coiling, or clipping.
- Interventional radiology is associated with exposure of the fetus to large doses of radiation.
- Nimodipine is used to decrease vasospasm.
- *Delivery:*
  - labour is a high-risk time for bleeding, so elective CS should be recommended if the lesion is inoperable
  - epidural anaesthesia is contraindicated with a recent subarachnoid haemorrhage (SAH) due to raised intracranial pressure
  - if the lesion has been successfully treated, vaginal delivery is recommended (a longer passive 2nd stage with early use of assisted delivery may reduce the risk of rebleeding).

Box 5.2 Causes of CVAs in pregnancy

Infarcts
- Pre-eclampsia/eclampsia.
- Central nervous system (CNS) vasculitis.
- Carotid artery dissection.
- Emboli:
  - mitral stenosis
  - peripartum cardiomyopathy
  - endocarditis
  - paradoxical emboli.
- Coagulopathies:
  - thrombophilia
  - antiphospholipid syndrome.
- Thrombotic thrombocytopaenic purpura.
- Cerebral vein thrombosis.

Haemorrhagic
- Pre-eclampsia/eclampsia.
- DIC.
- AVM.
- Ruptured berry aneurysm.
- CNS vasculitis.

Investigations

A neurologist should be involved in the investigation and management.
- MRI or CT scan of head.
- Cerebral angiography +/− venography.
- Echocardiogram.
- Carotid Dopplers.
- Thrombophilia screen and antiphospholipid antibodies.
- Homocystine level/methylenetetrahydrofolate reductase (MTHFR) screen.

Cardiac disease: management

The pattern of heart disease in pregnancy has changed over the past few decades. CHD is now more common than rheumatic heart disease and ischaemic heart disease has become a common cardiac cause of death in pregnancy.

⚠ Normal pregnancy is associated with significant haemodynamic changes. These may not be tolerated in women with heart disease.

Antenatal management

- Multidisciplinary management with an obstetrician, cardiologist, anaesthetist, and, occasionally, cardiothoracic surgeon.
- Preconception counselling should be offered to:
  - optimize maternal cardiovascular status (may involve surgery)
  - modify medication
  - discuss maternal and fetal risks of pregnancy.
- The ability of a woman to tolerate pregnancy depends on:
  - exercise tolerance (New York Heart Association (NYHA) class)
  - presence of pulmonary hypertension or left heart obstruction
  - presence of cyanosis.
- Decide if termination recommended (e.g. pulmonary hypertension).
- Correct factors that may lead to decompensation (anaemia, infection, hypertension, and arrhythmias).
- Monitor for signs of heart failure and consider serial maternal echos.
- Monitor fetal growth by serial ultrasound as risk of IUGR and death *in utero*, especially with maternal cyanosis.

⚠ Risk of CHD in fetus is 3–5% if either parent is affected. Some conditions carry higher risk. It is higher if mother rather than father is affected. Arrange for fetal echocardiography at 22wks.

Intrapartum and post-partum management

- A clear intrapartum care plan should be agreed before labour.
- Aim for a vaginal delivery usually with a short active 2nd stage (CS is indicated if aortic root >4.5cm, left ventricular ejection fraction (LVEF) <30%, aortic dissection or aneurysm).
- In labour, maternal cardiac ± invasive monitoring may be required (the fetus should be continuously monitored).
- Avoid aortocaval compression.
- Decide on need for endocarditis prophylaxis.
- Blood loss should be minimized by active management of 3rd stage followed by an infusion of oxytocin, but ergometrine and prostaglandin F2α (PGF2α, dinoprost) should be avoided.
- Epidural analgesia may reduce changes in heart rate and BP associated with pain (low-dose epidural is usually well tolerated, but may cause serious complications with restricted cardiac output).
- Strict fluid balance is mandatory as there is a much higher risk of pulmonary oedema the first few days post-partum.
- Discuss contraception before discharge.

Haemodynamic changes in normal pregnancy

- Peripheral vasodilatation leads to a fall in systemic vascular resistance.
- Cardiac output increases by:
  - 40% during pregnancy (↑ heart rate and ↑ stroke volume)
  - 15% in the 1st stage of labour
  - 50% in the 2nd stage of labour.
- Following delivery there is further increased cardiac output due to increased venous return from:
  - relief of vena caval obstruction
  - tonic uterine contraction (expels blood into systemic circulation).
- Blood pressure falls in pregnancy and reaches a nadir around 24wks.
- Colloid osmotic pressure falls leading to increased susceptibility to pulmonary oedema.
- Hypercoagulability.

▶ These changes start in early pregnancy.

---

❶ Level of risk of maternal mortality (absolute risk level depends on the degree of the condition in the individual)

High risk (red alert—mortality could be as high as 50%)
- Pulmonary hypertension.
- Aortic dissection.
- Complicated aortic coarctation.
- Marfan's syndrome with significant aortic root involvement.
- Myocardial infarction.

Moderate risk (amber alert)
- Mitral stenosis NYHA class 3 or 4.
- Severe aortic stenosis.
- Mechanical heart valves.

Minimal risk
- ASD.
- VSD.
- PDA.
- Corrected tetralogy of Fallot.
- Tissue valve prosthesis.
- Pulmonary and tricuspid valve disease.
- Mild mitral stenosis.
- Arrhythmias.

Artificial heart valves

Women with artificial heart valves often have near-normal cardiac function and therefore tolerate pregnancy well. The main maternal and fetal risk is from anticoagulation, which must be continued throughout pregnancy as without it there is a high morbidity (stroke) and mortality (valve thrombosis). The choice of anticoagulant should be made after discussion with the patient. Warfarin better protects against valve thrombosis, therefore is better for the mother, but heparin is better for the fetus.

Anticoagulant drugs and risks

Low molecular weight heparin
- Less maternal bleeding.
- No risk to fetus (does not cross the placenta).
- Increased risk of embolic events.
- Increased risk of valve thrombosis—may require emergency valve replacement and has a high mortality.
- Osteoporosis and heparin-induced thrombocytopenia.

Warfarin
- Increased risk of miscarriage.
- Risk of warfarin embryopathy (risk dose dependent: ↑ if >5mg/day).
- Maternal and neonatal bleeding.
- Long half-life.

⚠ There is a 4–12% risk of an embolic event per pregnancy.

Management
- Antenatally there are two options:
  - continue warfarin throughout pregnancy—aim for an international normalized ratio (INR) of 3.0
  - conceive on warfarin, change to LMWH from 6–12wks to minimize risk of warfarin embryopathy, then use warfarin from 12 to 37wks.
- Risk of bleeding in labour with warfarin (mother and baby) is high:
  - all patients should be changed to LMWH at 37wks
  - LMWH should be stopped in labour and restarted after delivery
  - warfarin should be restarted 7–10 days post-partum.
- Reversal in the event of life-threatening bleeding:
  - warfarin—fresh frozen plasma, vitamin K, and prothrombin complex concentrates (PCCs)
  - LMWH—protamine sulphate.
- Heparin and warfarin can safely be given to breast-feeding mothers.
- Low-dose aspirin should be given with LMWH because of its anti-thrombotic effects and relative safety.

Tissue valves
- Bio-prosthetic or homograft valves do not require anticoagulation.
- They have a shorter life expectancy than mechanical valves, so structural deterioration may occur in pregnancy (especially the mitral valve).
- Anticoagulation would still be required with arrhythmias, e.g. atrial fibrillation.

Endocarditis prophylaxis

Endocarditis prophylaxis should be given to the following two groups:

High risk
- Prosthetic heart valves (mechanical or tissue).
- Previous bacterial endocarditis.
- Complex cyanotic heart disease (Fallot's tetralogy, transposition).
- Surgically constructed systemic/pulmonary shunts.

Moderate risk
- Hypertrophic cardiomyopathy.
- Acquired valvular lesions.
- Mitral valve prolapse with severe regurgitation.
- Other congenital cardiac malformations.

Prophylaxis is not recommended for:
- Isolated secundum ASD.
- Surgically repaired ASD or VSD.
- Cardiac pacemakers.
- Mitral valve prolapse without regurgitation.

▶ Recommended antibiotics:
- Amoxicillin 1g IV plus gentamicin 120mg IV at onset of labour or rupture of membranes, then amoxicillin 500mg orally 6h later.
- Vancomycin 1g IV or teicoplanin 400mg IV if penicillin allergy with gentamicin 120mg IV.

Acquired heart disease

Mitral stenosis
- This is the most common lesion of rheumatic heart disease (90%).
- ↑ Risk of pulmonary oedema in pregnancy, greatest in labour:
  - ↑ in heart rate in pregnancy, ↓ ventricular filling time, and ↑ pulmonary blood volume leading to pulmonary oedema
  - first line treatment for pulmonary oedema in pregnancy should be diuretics. β-blockers also used to slow heart rate and improve left atrial emptying (add digoxin if in atrial fibrillation (AF)).
- Mitral stenosis is the most likely lesion to require treatment for pulmonary oedema, heart failure or surgery in pregnancy.
- With severe mitral stenosis, consider surgery before pregnancy.
- The risk of thromboembolism is ~1.5% in pregnancy, higher with left atrial enlargement and AF (treat with LMWH).

Mitral regurgitation is well tolerated in pregnancy; heart failure and endo-carditis are rare.

Aortic stenosis
- Aortic valve disease is less common than mitral valve disease (it is less likely to be 2° to rheumatic disease, more likely to be due to a congenital bicuspid valve).
- The severity and risk of complications is dependent on the gradient across the valve: >100mmHg in the non-pregnant state is severe.

⚠ Associated symptoms are chest pain, syncope, and sudden death.

Pulmonary hypertension and Eisenmenger's syndrome
1° pulmonary hypertension is an idiopathic abnormality of the pulmonary vasculature. In Eisenmenger's syndrome there is pulmonary hypertension with reversal of the initial left-to-right shunt and consequent cyanosis. There is a fixed high pulmonary vascular resistance and inability to increase pulmonary blood flow. This leads to slowly worsening hypoxaemia.

⚠ Maternal mortality is high (25%) but has improved. Death classically occurs in the first few days post-partum.
- Women should be advised to avoid getting pregnant and termination offered if pregnancy occurs.
- Pregnancy should be managed in a pulmonary hypertension centre with multidisciplinary care from cardiologists, obstetricians, and anaesthetists.
- Antenatal care includes anticoagulation, oxygen, bed rest, and serial assessment of fetal growth.
- Avoid manoevures that suddenly increase vagal tone (with resultant bradycardia) and venous return, e.g. ergometrine.
- Avoid PGF2α which is associated with pulmonary vasoconstriction and pulmonary hypertensive crisis.
- Delivery should be in a high dependency unit with tight control of blood pressure, fluid balance, and oxygen saturations.

🖝 Mode of delivery and epidural use are controversial.

Myocardial infarction and cardiomyopathy

Myocardial infarction

Remains rare in pregnancy, but incidence has been increasing due to increased age at pregnancy and lifestyle factors.

⚠ Mortality high (20% immediate, 32% overall); highest in puerperium.

- Risk factors include smoking, hypertension, diabetes, hypercholesterolaemia, family history, and obesity.
- There may be atypical symptoms, such as abdominal or epigastric pain, and vomiting or dizziness.
- Diagnosis is based on history, electrocardiograph (ECG) changes, and elevated troponin.

⚠ Single normal ECG especially in a pain-free patient does not rule out ischaemia. Serial ECGs should be considered.

- Patient should be managed on a coronary care unit by cardiologists.
- 1° percutaneous coronary intervention (PCI) is the treatment of choice in the pregnant patient.
- Thrombolysis is associated with high fetal loss rates, but should be considered if primary PCI is not available.
- *Delivery:* aim for a vaginal delivery with a short 2nd stage (avoid ergometrine as it can cause coronary artery spasm).
- Women with a past history of myocardial infarction (MI) should have a prepregnancy assessment of cardiac function (echo and exercise test) with counselling on the basis of the results, and aspirin should be continued in pregnancy.

Peripartum cardiomyopathy

- This is a rare condition—incidence <1:2000.
- It occurs between 32wks and 6mths after delivery.
- *Risk factors:*
  - increasing maternal age
  - multiparity
  - multiple pregnancy
  - Afro-Caribbean ethnicity
  - poor socio-economic class
  - hypertension in pregnancy.
- *Presentation:* breathlessness, palpitations, oedema, poor exercise tolerance, and embolic phenomena.
- *Diagnosis:* global dilatation of all four chambers of the heart (seen on echo) with exclusion of other causes of cardiomyopathy.
- *Management:* supportive; should include angiotensin-converting enzyme inhibitors (ACEIs) and anticoagulation (☞ immunosuppression has been tried).
- If the diagnosis is made antenatally, delivery is indicated.
- Consider heart transplantation if there is heart failure despite optimal medical therapy.

⚠ Mortality 25–50% (long-term survival likely if patient survives initial episode).

⚠ Recurrence risk high (up to 50%). Avoid further pregnancies if cardiac function does not return to normal.

Congenital heart disease

The most common CHDs in pregnancy are PDA, ASD, and VSD. They are generally well tolerated in pregnancy.

Marfan's syndrome

This is an autosomal dominant condition (chromosome 15) caused by a defect in fibrillin synthesis (genetic testing is available). The main risk is of aortic dissection and rupture. This risk increases if there is a family history of rupture and/or there is evidence of aortic root dilatation.

Management

- Monthly maternal echo for aortic dimensions until 8wks post-partum.
- β-Blockers should be given for hypertension or aortic dilatation as they are shown to reduce rate of dilatation and risk of dissection.
- Aim for vaginal delivery with a short 2nd stage (if aortic root dilatation is present, deliver by CS).

⚠ Mortality

- <1% if aortic root <4cm.
- >25% if aortic root >4cm.
- Pregnancy is contraindicated with an aortic root >4.5cm until aortic root replacement.

Coarctation of aorta

- This has usually been corrected before pregnancy. The main risk is of aortic dissection; this risk is highest if there is hypertension present (usually treated with β-blockers). Condition is also associated with berry aneurysms, which can bleed in pregnancy causing cerebral haemorrhage.
- If uncorrected or recurrent, coarctation risks include:
  - hypertension
  - heart failure
  - angina.
- Avoid balloon angioplasty in pregnancy (↑ risk of dissection).
- Deliver by CS if there is associated aortic dilatation.

Fallot's tetralogy

- The majority of women with Fallot's will have had surgery and the risk to their pregnancy will depend on not only the type of surgery but also its level of success.
- There are two main risks in pregnancy:
  - paradoxical emboli can pass from right-to-left through the shunt causing strokes
  - cyanosis affects the fetus leading to increased risk of miscarriage, IUGR, prematurity, and death *in utero*.
- Risks are minimized by anticoagulation (prophylactic dose LMWH), bed rest, and oxygen.

Anaemia

Physiological adaptation in pregnancy
- Plasma volume expansion (50%) greater than red cell mass ↑ (25%).
- This leads to physiological dilution with ↓ Hb and haematocrit.
- Anaemia is diagnosed if Hb <10.5 g/dL in pregnancy.
- There should be no change in mean corpuscular volume (MCV) or mean corpuscular haemoglobin concentration (MCHC) in normal pregnancies.
- Normally pregnancy has:
  - 2–3-fold increase in iron requirements
  - 10–20-fold increase in folate requirements in pregnancy.

Iron-deficiency anaemia
- The most common cause of anaemia in pregnancy (90% of cases).
- *Diagnosis:* ↓ MCV, ↓ MCHC, and ↓ ferritin.
- Often asymptomatic and detected on screening.
- Treat by oral iron supplementation: vitamin C (orange juice) ↑ absorption, tea ↓ absorption.
- Parenteral iron should be considered in those who do not tolerate the oral preparations (corrects the anaemia more rapidly).
- The expected improvement in haemoglobin is ~1g/dL/wk.
- In situations such as multiple pregnancy or known depletion of iron stores, consider prophylactic supplementation even if no anaemia.
- If severe iron-deficiency anaemia (Hb <7g/dL) is diagnosed near term, blood transfusion may be considered.

Folate deficiency
- Also common in pregnancy (5% of cases of anaemia).
- *Risk factors:*
  - poor nutritional status
  - haematological problems with a rapid turnover of blood cells, e.g. haemolytic anaemia and haemoglobinopathies
  - drug interaction with folate metabolism, e.g. antiepileptics.
- *Diagnosis:* ↑ MCV, ↓ serum, and ↓ red cell folate.
- Folic acid given preconception and in early pregnancy to reduce risk of neural tube defects (400 micrograms/day for general population).
- Women with high risk of neural tube defects should take 5mg folic acid daily. The high-risk group includes those women:
  - on anticonvulsants
  - with a previous child affected with a neural tube defect
  - with demonstrated deficiency
  - with diabetes
  - with a BMI >35
  - with sickle cell disease.

Vitamin B12 deficiency
- Occurs in pernicious anaemia, terminal ileum disease, and strict vegans.
- It is uncommon to make a new diagnosis in pregnancy.
- Women with a previous diagnosis should continue treatment throughout pregnancy.

Sickle cell disease

Inheritance is autosomal recessive. Most commonly seen in people of Afro-Caribbean origin, but also occurs in those from the Middle East, Mediterranean, and Indian subcontinent. As diagnosis has usually been made in childhood, it is rare to make a new diagnosis in pregnancy.

Pathophysiology

Results in distortion of the shape of red cells into a rigid sickle shape. This leads to microvascular blockage, stasis, and infarction in any organ in the body. Crises can be precipitated by infection, dehydration, hypoxia, and cold.

Risks in pregnancy

- Crises are more common during pregnancy.
- ↑ Risk of pre-eclampsia.
- ↑ Risk of delivery by CS 2° to fetal distress.

Clinical features of sickle cell disease

- Haemolytic anaemia.
- Painful crises.
- Hyposplenism (chronic damage to the spleen results in atrophy).
- Increased risk of infection (UTI, pyelonephritis, pneumonia, puerperal sepsis).
- Avascular necrosis of bone.
- Increased risk of thromboembolic disease (pulmonary embolism (PE), stroke).
- Acute chest syndrome (fever, chest pain, tachypnoea, ↑ WCC, pulmonary infiltrates).
- *Iron overload:* leads to cardiomyopathy.
- Maternal mortality 2%.

Management

- Multidisciplinary care with an obstetrician and haematologist.
- Prepregnancy counselling should involve screening of the partner (if the partner is a carrier, consider prenatal diagnosis).
- Stop iron-chelating agents before pregnancy.
- If there is a history of iron overload, arrange a maternal echo.
- Give folic acid 5mg/day and penicillin prophylaxis for hyposplenism.
- Monitor Hb and HbS percentage and arrange transfusion if necessary (may have red cell antibodies from multiple transfusions).
- Screen for urine infection each visit.
- Treatment of a crisis involves adequate analgesia, oxygen, rehydration, and antibiotics if infection suspected (exchange transfusion may be required in severe crises).
- Regular assessment of fetal growth with ultrasound, including Doppler.
- Aim for vaginal delivery ensuring adequate hydration and avoiding hypoxia (continuous fetal monitoring as increased risk of fetal distress).
- Consider antenatal and postnatal thromboprophylaxis.

- ✎ The use of prophylactic antibiotics is controversial.

Fetal risks in sickle cell disease
- Miscarriage.
- IUGR.
- Prematurity.
- Stillbirth.

⚠ Perinatal mortality is increased 4–6-fold compared to the general population.

Thalassaemia

Adult haemoglobin is made up from two α- and two β-globin chains associated with a haem complex. There are four genes for α-globin and two for β-globin chain production. An adult's blood is normally made up of HbA ($\alpha_2\beta_2$, 97%), HbA$_2$ ($\alpha_2\delta_2$, 1.5–3.5%), and HbF ($\alpha_2\gamma_2$, <1%). Thalassaemia is a group of genetic conditions leading to impaired production of the globin chains and resulting in red cells with inadequate haemoglobin content. Fetal haemoglobin consists of 2α and 2γ chains, so a fetus cannot be affected by β-thalassaemia.

α-Thalassaemia

- Caused by defects in 1–4 of the α-globin genes.
- Most common in individuals from South-east Asia.
- α-Thalassaemia trait has two (α0) or three (α+) normal genes: women are usually asymptomatic, but may become anaemic in pregnancy.
- In HbH there are three defective genes:
  - unstable haemoglobin is formed by tetramers of the β chain
  - chronic haemolysis results and iron overload is common
  - offspring will have either α0 or α+ thalassaemia.
- α-Thalassaemia major (Hb Barts) has no functional α genes and is incompatible with life:
  - fetuses are often hydropic and born prematurely
  - severe early-onset pre-eclampsia often complicates the pregnancy.

β-Thalassaemia

- β-Thalassaemia trait has one defective gene and women are asymptomatic but may become anaemic in pregnancy.
- It is most common in individuals from Cyprus and Asia.
- Incidence of β-thalassaemia minor is 1:10 000 in the UK compared with 1:7 in Cyprus: offspring have a 1:4 chance of β-thalassaemia major.
- β-Thalassaemia major has two defective genes and women are often transfusion dependent:
  - iron overload can occur
  - puberty is often delayed
  - there is subfertility and only very few pregnancies have been reported.
- Repeated transfusions cause iron overload, leading to endocrine, hepatic, and cardiac dysfunction:
  - heart failure is the most common cause of death
  - iron-chelating therapy can reduce the incidence of iron overload
  - the condition can be cured by bone marrow transplant.

THALASSAEMIA **203**

Management of pregnancy with thalassaemia

- Check ferritin in early pregnancy: give iron supplements only if iron deficient.
- Women need folic acid 5mg daily:
  - if failure to respond to folate PO, then IM (and oral iron if needed); a blood transfusion may be required
  - parenteral iron should be avoided.
- If the woman has thalassaemia, the partner needs screening:
  - if positive, the couple need counselling on the risk of pregnancy with thalassaemia major
  - prenatal diagnosis should be offered.

Screening for thalassaemia in pregnancy

- Screen all women of Mediterranean, Middle Eastern, Indian, Asian, African, or West Indian ethnic origin by haemoglobin electrophoresis at booking.
- In $\alpha0$ and $\alpha+$ thalassaemia no abnormal haemoglobin is made and there is no excess in HbA_2 or HbF:
  - Hb electrophoresis is normal
  - the diagnosis can be confirmed by globin chain synthesis studies or DNA analysis of nucleated cells.
- In α-thalassaemia there is a raised concentration of HbA_2 and/or HbF.
- Suspect the diagnosis of thalassaemia in the presence of:
  - low MCV
  - low MCHC
  - microcytic anaemia with normal MCHC (which differs from iron deficiency where the MCHC is also low).

Haemophilia

X-linked inherited deficiency of clotting factor VIII and IX that causes problems with bleeding. Haemophilia A (factor VIII deficiency) is 4 times more common than haemophilia B (factor IX deficiency). Can vary in severity depending on the clotting factor levels: mild (>5% to <40%), moderate (1–5%), or severe (<1%). Severity tends to be similar within members of one family. The use of prophylactic recombinant factor replacement from childhood has now drastically changed the outlook and life expectancy for affected children.

Incidence
- 15:100 000 males.
- Female carriers have one abnormal gene and do not usually have significant bleeding problems, but the clotting factor level is around 1/2 normal (occasionally clotting factors may be much lower because of lyonization).
- Female carriers have a 50% chance of having an affected son and a 50% chance of having carrier daughters.
- An affected male will produce carrier daughters and unaffected sons.
- 1/3 of newly diagnosed infants has no family history and are the result of a new mutation.

Prenatal diagnosis and antenatal care
- Manage jointly with haematologist.
- Genetic counselling and prenatal diagnosis (if the mutation is known by DNA-based family studies) should be offered to affected families.
- Fetal sexing can be done if the mutation is not known, with fetal cell free DNA testing from a maternal blood sample.
- Check hepatitis serology as previous exposure to blood products.
- Maternal coagulation factor activity should be checked at booking, 28, and 34wks, and when clinically indicated (e.g. bleeding, before surgery).
- There is increased risk of post-partum haemorrhage (factor VIII, but not factor IX, increases in pregnancy in normal women and haemophilia carriers. Therefore, women with factor IX deficiency are most at risk while pregnant. There is a rapid ↓ to prepregnancy levels after delivery).

Intrapartum and post-partum care
- Aim for vaginal delivery.
- Check maternal coagulation factor activity (factor VIII or factor IX), aiming for levels >50IU/L (give appropriate clotting factors if lower than this).
- Also send FBC, clotting screen, and group and save when in labour.
- Avoid fetal scalp electrodes, fetal blood sampling, ventouse, and rotational forceps deliveries in affected or male fetuses with unknown status.
- Epidural anaesthesia can be used if normal coagulation screen, platelet count >100 × 10^9/L, normal bleeding time, and clotting factor >50IU/L.
- Maintain clotting factors >50IU/l and give tranexamic acid for 5 days post-partum to reduce risk of post-partum haemorrhage.
- Avoid IM injections in neonate with possible clotting disorder.
- Send cord blood of males for clotting factor VIII or IX levels (refer to haemophilia centre if diagnosis is confirmed).

Von Willebrand's disease

- Autosomal dominant (types 1 and 2).
- Autosomal recessive (type 3)—more uncommon and severe.
- Stabilizes factor VIII and helps adherence of platelets to vessel wall.
- Diagnosis by measuring:
  - von Willebrand's factor (vWF) antigen
  - factor VIII
  - ristocetin cofactor activity.
- Levels of vWF and factor VIII increase in pregnancy and fall rapidly post-partum.
- Main risk is post-partum haemorrhage.
- Desmopressin can be used in some type 1 cases (it stimulates the release of vWF from endothelial cells).

Autoimmune idiopathic thrombocytopaenic purpura

- Caused by antibodies to surface antigens on platelets, leading to platelet destruction.
- Incidence 1–3:1000 pregnancies.
- Diagnosis is by exclusion of other causes of thrombocytopenia.
- Pregnancy does not affect the disease, but due to a lower median platelet count in pregnancy, the platelet count of women with idiopathic thrombocytopaenic purpura (ITP) usually falls further in pregnancy.

Fetal risks

- IgG antiplatelet antibodies can cross the placenta and cause fetal thrombocytopaenia.
- Difficult to predict which fetus will be affected (it has no relation to maternal platelet count).
- Can lead to antenatal and intrapartum intracranial haemorrhage:
  - <2% with a history of ITP before pregnancy
  - risk is highest if there has been a previously affected child.

Management

- FBC every 2–4wks.
- Bleeding is unlikely if platelet count is >50 x 10^9/L (treatment is not required at this level).
- Patients with bleeding or platelet count <50 x 10^9/L should be started on oral steroids, >75% respond within 3wks.
- Patients who fail to respond to steroids can be treated with IV immunoglobulin.
- Splenectomy is rarely performed in pregnancy.
- Platelet transfusions may be required if rapid response is needed.
- In labour, avoid:
  - fetal scalp electrodes
  - fetal blood sampling
  - ventouse delivery
  - rotational forceps delivery.
- No fetal benefit from delivery by CS, but ↑ maternal risks.
- Cord platelet count should be taken at birth:
  - the count reaches a nadir at around day 4
  - the neonate may require IV immunoglobulin.

Causes of thrombocytopaenia in pregnancy

- Spurious.
- Gestational thrombocytopaenia.
- Pre-eclampsia.
- Idiopathic thrombocytopaenic purpura.
- Thrombotic thrombocytopaenic purpura.
- Disseminated intravascular coagulopathy.
- Systemic lupus erythematosus.
- Bone marrow suppression.

Asthma

This is the most common respiratory disease encountered in pregnancy and affects 1–4% of women of childbearing age. It is caused by reversible bronchoconstriction of smooth muscle in the airways, with inflammation and excess mucus production. Diagnosis is based on recurrent episodes of wheeze, shortness of breath, chest tightness, or cough, and variation in peak expiratory flow rate (PEFR) of >15% after treatment with bronchodilators. Pregnancy outcomes in women with asthma are usually good.

Effect of pregnancy on asthma

1/3 of patients show no change in their asthma, 1/3 show improvement, and 1/3 deteriorate, usually in those with more poorly controlled asthma at conception. Deterioration occurs most often between 24 and 36wks. There may be a different effect in different pregnancies. Deterioration may be caused by cessation of maintenance therapy.

Effect of asthma on pregnancy

Usually there is no effect on the fetus or course of the pregnancy, but poorly controlled asthma may be associated with low birth weight and preterm labour.

Management

- Current therapy should continue in pregnancy, and women educated and reassured of the safety of the medication and warned not to stop their treatment.
- Women should continue to monitor their PEFR (↑ diurnal variation with ↓ PEFR in the night or early morning may be an early sign of worsening of asthma).
- Chronic and acute severe asthma should be treated as in the non-pregnant state (aim for O_2 sats >95% and administer O_2 if required).
- Magnesium sulfate is readily available in maternity services and may be used for acute severe asthma when there has not been a good initial response to inhaled bronchodilator therapy.
- Advise cessation of smoking.
- Chest radiograph (CXR) should be considered to exclude pneumothorax.
- ↑ Risk of gestational diabetes in women on long-term oral steroids.
- Asthma attacks are rare during labour; inhaled β-agonists can be used (there is no evidence that they interfere with uterine activity).
- Women on long-term oral steroids (prednisolone >7.5mg/day for >2wks) are at risk of Addisonian collapse during labour—give hydrocortisone 100mg every 8h.
- PGF2α should only be used in cases of life-threatening post-partum haemorrhage because of its bronchoconstriction action.
- Breast-feeding should be encouraged as it may give the child some protection against developing allergies in later life.

⚠ The fetus is at greater risk from undertreated asthma than from the drugs used in its treatment.

Asthma care: British Thoracic Society recommendations
- Step 1: inhaled short-acting β-agonists: salbutamol or terbutaline.
- Step 2: inhaled steroids (up to 800 micrograms/day): beclometasone, budesonide.
- Step 3: long acting beta-agonist: salmeterol or formoterol.
- Step 4: high-dose inhaled steroid (up to 2000 micrograms/day): oral slow-release theophylline, leukotriene antagonists.
- Step 5: oral steroids: review by respiratory physician if oral steroids commenced.

⚠ Leukotriene receptor antagonists should not be commenced in pregnancy but can be continued in women who have demonstrated significant improvement in asthma control that was not achievable by other medication.

Acute severe asthma: management
- *Medication:*
  - nebulized bronchodilators
  - IV steroids
  - nebulized ipratropium
  - IV aminophylline or IV salbutamol
  - +/– antibiotics if evidence of infection.
- *Clinical findings:*
  - heart rate >110 beats/min
  - respiratory rate >25/min
  - pulsus paradoxus >20mmHg
  - PEFR <50% predicted
  - accessory muscle use
  - unable to complete sentences.

⚠ Silent chest with very little wheeze may be a sign of life-threatening asthma.

Further reading
Scottish Intercollegiate Guidelines Network. (2008). *British guideline on the management of asthma.*
   ⌕ http://www.sign.ac.uk/pdf/sign101.pdf

Cystic fibrosis

This is one of the commonest genetic conditions, affecting 1:2000 people of European origin with a gene frequency of around 1:25. Transmission is autosomal recessive and disease is caused by defective function of the cystic fibrosis (CF) transmembrane conductance regulation (CFTR) chloride channel. The condition affects the lungs, gastrointestinal tract, pancreas, hepatobiliary system, and reproductive organs. Recurrent chest infections lead to bronchial damage and respiratory failure.

Life expectancy is improving (currently 41yrs) and women with CF are now having families. However, most men are infertile owing to congenital absence of the vas deferens and women are subfertile because of unfavourable mucus, reduced BMI, and anovulation.

Prenatal counselling

Offspring will definitely receive one affected gene from the mother, so paternal status should be ascertained. There are many different gene mutations, but screening will detect ~90% of mutations. Risk of an affected child is 2–2.5% for unknown paternal carrier status. If the father's screen is negative the risk of an affected child falls to 1:500. If the father is a carrier the chance of an affected child is 1:2. Chorionic villus sampling can then be performed to check the fetus for affected genes.

Management of pregnancy with CF

- Care involves a multidisciplinary team with chest physician (CF unit), obstetrician, dietitian, and physiotherapist.
- Principles of care involve control of respiratory infections, avoidance of hypoxia, maintaining nutrition, and fetal surveillance.
- Chest physiotherapy should continue as in the non-pregnant state.
- Watch for signs of chest infection; treat aggressively with antibiotics, tailored according to sputum culture results.

⚠ Avoid tetracyclines and parenteral aminoglycosides, which may cause ototoxicity in high doses.

- Cardiac status should be checked by echocardiography.
- In the later stages of pregnancy patients can become breathless even without infections (if oxygen saturations are ≤90% at rest, hospital admission for oxygen therapy is indicated).
- High calorie intake with pancreatic enzyme supplementation is required.
- 8% of pregnant women with CF have pre-existing diabetes and 20% have diabetes by term.
- Fetal monitoring with regular growth scans (fetal risks are IUGR due to maternal hypoxaemia and preterm labour).
- Aim for a vaginal delivery (limit the 2nd stage, as pneumothoraces can occur with prolonged or repeated Valsalva manoevures).
- Avoid general anaesthesia and inhalational analgesia if possible.
- Same thing applies with PGF2α as many CFs have an element of obstructive airways disease.
- Breast-feeding is recommended (ensure continued nutritional supplementation).

Predictors of poor maternal or fetal outcomes in CF
- Hypoxaemia: PaO_2 <60mmHg free from infection.
- Cyanosis.
- Pulmonary hypertension.
- Poor prepregnancy lung function: forced expiratory volume in 1s (FEV_1) <60% predicted.
- Pancreatic insufficiency (especially diabetes) and malnutrition.
- Lung colonization with *Burkholderia cepacia*.

Respiratory infections

Pneumonia

This has the same incidence as in the non-pregnant population: 1–2:1000 pregnancies.
- Risk factors include smoking, chronic lung disease, and immunosuppression.
- *Clinical features*: fever, cough, purulent sputum, chest pain, and breathlessness.
- *Investigations*: FBC, CRP, CXR, sputum culture, serology (mycoplasma, *Legionella*, and viral titres), and arterial blood gases.
- Fetal risks are preterm labour and possibly IUGR.
- Treatment involves physiotherapy, adequate oxygenation, hydration, and appropriate antibiotics.

⚠ Varicella infection (chickenpox) causes pneumonia in 10% of cases in pregnancy. Mortality is ~10% and is highest in the latter stages of pregnancy. Women who develop varicella in pregnancy should be treated with aciclovir; they should be hospitalized if respiratory signs develop (on a non-obstetric ward with barrier nursing).

Tuberculosis

- The incidence of tuberculosis (TB) is increasing in the UK, especially in the immunosuppressed (HIV) and immigrant population. It is uncommon in pregnancy, but does not adversely affect the outcome if it is diagnosed and treated appropriately in the first 20wks or so.
- *Clinical features*: cough, haemoptysis, fever, weight loss, chest pain, and night sweats.

⚠ Diagnosis may be delayed by an unnecessary reluctance to perform investigations such as CXR in pregnancy.

- *Investigations*: CXR (classically calcification and upper lobe abnormalities), sputum microscopy with a Ziehl–Nielsen stain, sputum culture (can take 6wks), bronchoscopy if no sputum, and tissue biopsies for extrapulmonary TB. A Mantoux test cannot distinguish active disease from previous disease or vaccination.
- There is increased risk of prematurity and IUGR if treatment is inadequate or delayed (transplacental spread of infection is rare).

Neonatal considerations

Transmission from mother to baby after delivery (or to other caregivers) can occur if the mother remains infective (smear +ve). Women usually become non-infectious (smear –ve) within 2wks of starting treatment. The baby should be given Bacillus Calmette–Guerin (BCG) vaccination and, if smear +ve, prophylaxis with isoniazid for 3mths.

Antibiotic recommendations for pneumonia
- Amoxicillin for community-acquired pneumonia. Use higher dose in pregnancy because of increased renal clearance (500mg tds).
- Erythromycin if penicillin allergy.
- Add erythromycin or clarithromycin if atypical organisms suspected.
Cephalosporin for hospital-acquired pneumonia.

Aetiological agents in pneumonia
- No cause found in substantial proportion of patients.
- *Streptococcus pneumoniae* (>50% of cases).
- *Haemophilus influenzae.*
- *Staphylococcus aureus* (often after a viral infection).
- *Klebsiella* (more common with chronic lung disease).
- *Pseudomonas aeruginosa* (more common with chronic lung disease).
- *Mycoplasma pneumoniae* (atypical organism).
- *Legionella pneumoniae* (atypical organism).
- *Chlamydia psittaci* (atypical organism).
- Gram −ve organisms (secondary to aspiration).
- *Pneumocystis carinii* (immunosuppressed).
- Fungal.
- *Viral:* influenza, varicella-zoster.

Management of TB in pregnancy
- Respiratory physician and microbiologist involvement is essential.
- Treatment should be supervised to encourage and confirm compliance.
- A minimum of 6mth course of treatment is required.
- A typical treatment regime for pulmonary TB would involve an initial phase of therapy with isoniazid, rifampicin, ethambutol, +/– pyrazinamide for 2mths, followed by a continuation phase of 4mths of isoniazid and rifampicin (and based on drug sensitivities):
  - *isoniazid*—can cause demyelination and peripheral neuropathy. If given with pyridoxine considered safe in pregnancy; risk of hepatitis is increased in pregnancy so monitor liver function monthly
  - *rifampicin*—can be safely used in pregnancy. It is a liver enzyme inducer; therefore, give vitamin K to the mother in the last 4wks of pregnancy to prevent haemorrhagic disease of the newborn
  - *ethambutol*—is safe in pregnancy
  - *streptomycin*—10% risk of deafness in fetus due to damage to the 8th cranial nerve; should not be used in pregnancy
  - *pyrazinamide*—considered safe after the 1st trimester, occasionally used before 14wks.

Inflammatory bowel disease

- Ulcerative colitis (UC) affects women more than men.
- Crohn's disease is equally distributed between the sexes.
- Clinical features are diarrhoea, abdominal pain, rectal bleeding, and weight loss.

Effect of inflammatory bowel disease on pregnancy

- Fertility, miscarriage, stillbirth, and fetal anomaly rates are not affected in women with quiescent or well-controlled disease.
- Active disease at conception, first presentation in pregnancy, colonic rather than small bowel disease alone, active disease after resection, and severe disease treated by surgery are all associated with increased risk of miscarriage, stillbirth, prematurity, and low birth weight.

Effect of pregnancy on inflammatory bowel disease

- If the condition is quiescent at conception the risk of relapse is the same as in non-pregnant women.
- Conception occurring at a time of active disease is associated with persistent activity during pregnancy.

Management of inflammatory bowel disease in pregnancy

⚠ Acute flares carry a high risk of adverse outcome, and are best treated aggressively.

▶ Most drugs used for inflammatory bowel disease (IBD) are considered low risk during pregnancy.

⚠ However, methotrexate and thalidomide are contraindicated.

- High-dose folic acid (2mg/day) should be given before conception to women on sulfasalazine, to protect against neural tube defects, as the drug impairs the metabolism of folate.
- Management is similar to the non-pregnant state. Maintenance therapy usually includes sulfasalazine, other 5-aminosalicylic acid derivatives, and/or steroids (available orally or rectally).
- Active disease should be investigated by stool culture to exclude infection (including parasites), inflammatory markers, and sigmoidoscopy to assess disease activity in colitis (manage by rehydration and drug therapy with sulfasalazine or steroids).
- If the active disease is refractory to steroids, then azathioprine, 6-mercaptopurine, or ciclosporin may be useful.
- The new biologic therapies such as infliximab are probably safe but little data are so far available.
- Surgery is occasionally required in pregnancy when complications occur such as intestinal obstruction, haemorrhage, perforation, fistula, abscess formation, or toxic megacolon.
- Caesarean section is usually reserved for obstetric reasons but may be considered with severe perianal Crohn's disease, as a scarred perineum is inelastic and tears may result in fistula formation.
- Caesarean section should also be considered in UC patients with a pouch or patients with poorly controlled UC that will probably need a pouch in the future.
- Breast-feeding is safe in women on steroids and sulfasalazine.

Drugs used to treat IBD in pregnancy (European evidence-based concensus rating)

Safe
- Oral 5-aminosalicylates
- Topical 5-aminosalicylates
- Sulfasalazine
- Corticosteroids
- Azathioprine
- 6-Mercaptopurine

Probably safe
- Infliximab
- Adalimumab
- Certolizumab
- Ciclosporin
- Tacrolimus
- Budesonide
- Metronidazole
- Ciprofloxacin

Contraindicated
- Methotrexate
- Thalidomide
- 6-Thioguanine (no data)

Further reading

Janneke van der Woude C, Kolacek S, Dotan I, et al. (2010). European evidenced-based consensus on reproduction in inflammatory bowel disease. *J Crohn's Colit* 4: 493–510. http://www.planapregnancy.co.uk/PP2010/static/ibd_Euro_guidelines.pdf

Obstetric cholestasis

Obstetric cholestasis affects 0.7% of pregnancies in the UK. It is more common in women of Asian ethnicity and there is geographical variation in prevalence. 1/3 of patients have a family history of the condition. It usually occurs in the 3rd trimester and resolves spontaneously after delivery.

Symptoms

- Pruritus of the trunk and limbs, without a skin rash (often worse at night).
- Anorexia and malaise.
- Epigastric discomfort, steatorrhoea, and dark urine (less common).

Diagnosis

Full investigation is required as it is a diagnosis of exclusion, but is usually made on the history, abnormal LFTs, and raised bile acids in the absence of any other cause for hepatic dysfunction.

Risks

Maternal risks
- Vitamin K deficiency (potentially leading to post-partum haemorrhage).

Fetal risks
- Preterm labour (including iatrogenic).
- Stillbirth (actual ↑ risk has yet to be determined but is likely to be small).
- ↑ Risk of meconium (delivery in a consultant-led unit is recommended).

Management of obstetric cholestasis

- Send LFTs and bile acids for all woman itching, without a rash.
- If normal, they should be repeated every 1–2wks if symptoms persist, as itching can predate abnormal LFTs.
- Exclude other causes of pruritus and liver dysfunction.
- Water-soluble vitamin K should be commenced from diagnosis.
- Symptoms may be alleviated by topical emollients (antihistamines cause sedation but do not improve pruritus).
- Ursodeoxycholic acid (8–12mg/kg daily in two divided doses) reduces pruritus between 1 and 7 days after starting, but there is no proven benefit for fetal adverse effects.
- Fetal surveillance with ultrasound and CTG monitoring are commonly used but of no proven benefit.
- Postnatal resolution of symptoms and LFTs should be established.
- Recurrence risk in subsequent pregnancy is 45–70% (it can also recur with the combined contraceptive pill).

⚠ Intrauterine death is usually sudden and cannot be predicted by biochemical results, CTG findings, or on USS.

☙ Timing of delivery is controversial as there is an increased risk of perinatal and maternal morbidity with early intervention; therefore this should be discussed with the woman on an individual basis.

Differential diagnosis of obstetric cholestasis
- Gallstones.
- Acute or chronic viral hepatitis.
- Primary biliary cirrhosis (antimitochondrial antibody +ve).
- Chronic active hepatitis (antismooth muscle antibody +ve).

Investigations for obstetric cholestasis
- *LFTs:*
  - 2–3-fold ↑ in ALT, AST, gamma-glutamyltransferase (γGT), or alkaline phosphatase
  - use pregnancy-specific reference ranges.
- Clotting screen.
- Bile acids.
- Ultrasound of the liver and biliary tree.
- Viral serology (hepatitis A, B, C, CMV, EBV).
- Autoimmune screen (antimitochondrial and antismooth muscle antibodies).

Further reading
RCOG. (2011). *Obstetric cholestasis*. Green-top guideline 43. ℘ http://www.rcog.org.uk/womens-health/clinical-guidance/obstetric-cholestasis-green-top-43

Acute fatty liver of pregnancy

This is a rare condition affecting 1:10 000 pregnancies. It typically presents in the third trimester and can occur at any parity. It is associated with twin pregnancy (9–25%), a male fetus (♂:♀ ratio 3:1), and mild pre-eclampsia (30–60%).

⚠ Acute fatty liver of pregnancy (AFLP) has a maternal mortality of 18%, higher if diagnosis is delayed, and fetal mortality of 23%.

Clinical features of AFLP
- Abdominal pain.
- Nausea and vomiting.
- Jaundice.
- Headache.
- Fever.
- Confusion.
- Coma.

- Diagnosis is based on the Swansea criteria (see Box 5.3).
- Can progress rapidly to fulminant liver failure, DIC, and renal failure.
- Hypoglycaemia is common.
- Some women have polyuria 2° to transient diabetes insipidus.
- *Investigations:* FBC and film, clotting, U&E, urate, LFT, blood gases.

Differentiating AFLP from HELLP syndrome

Distinctive features of AFLP
- Mild hypertension and proteinuria only.
- Early coagulopathy.
- Profound and persistent hypoglycaemia.
- Marked hyperuricaemia.
- Fatty infiltration on imaging the liver (may also be normal).

Management of AFLP
- This should be in a high dependency or intensive care setting with a multidisciplinary team.
- Management should involve:
  - treatment of hypoglycaemia
  - correction of coagulopathy with IV vitamin K and fresh frozen plasma (FFP)
  - strict control of BP and fluid balance.
- Delivery should follow stabilization (regional anaesthesia is contra-indicated in presence of thrombocytopaenia (<80) or deranged clotting).
- Bleeding complications are common.
- Fluid balance may require central line or even Swan–Ganz catheters.
- Following delivery, care is supportive, and most women improve rapidly after delivery with no long-term liver damage.
- Some patients with fulminant hepatic failure may require transfer to a specialist liver unit, who should be informed as soon as the diagnosis is suspected.
- Recurrence rate is unknown but may be greater than that of HELLP.

Box 5.3 The Swansea criteria for diagnosing AFL

Six or more are required in the absence of another cause:
- Vomiting.
- Abdominal pain.
- Polydipsia/ polyuria.
- Encephalopathy.
- Elevated bilirubin >14µmol/L.
- Hypoglycaemia <4mmol/L.
- Elevated urea >340µmol/L.
- Leucocytosis >11 × 10⁹/L.
- Ascites or bright liver on USS.
- Elevated transaminases aspartate aminotransferase (AAT) or alanine transaminase (ALT) >42IU/L.
- Elevated ammonia >47µmol/L.
- Renal impairment; creatinine >150µmol/L
- Coagulopathy; prothrombin time >14s or APPT >34s.
- Microvesicular steatosis on liver biopsy.

Causes of jaundice in pregnancy

Causes not specific to pregnancy
- Haemolysis
- Gilbert's syndrome
- Viral hepatitis (hepatitis A, B, C, E, EBV, CMV)
- Autoimmune hepatitis (primary biliary cirrhosis, chronic active hepatitis, sclerosing cholangitis)
- Gallstones
- Cirrhosis
- Drug-induced hepatotoxicity
- Malignancy.

Causes specific to pregnancy (10% of cases)
- Hyperemesis gravidarum
- Pre-eclampsia/HELLP syndrome
- AFLP
- Obstetric cholestasis.

Renal tract infections

More common in pregnancy because of dilatation of upper renal tract and urinary stasis. Asymptomatic bacteriuria affects 5–10% of pregnant women; untreated it can lead to symptomatic infection in 40% of cases.
- Cystitis complicates 1% of pregnancies.
- Pyelonephritis occurs in 1–2% of pregnant women and is associated with preterm labour.

Women should be screened for asymptomatic bacteriuria with MSU sample at booking. If this is −ve, the chance of developing a urinary infection in pregnancy is <2%.

Symptoms
- *Cystitis:* urinary frequency, urgency, dysuria, haematuria, proteinuria, and suprapubic pain.
- *Pyelonephritis:* fever, rigors, vomiting, loin and abdominal pain.

Consider the diagnosis of pyelonephritis in women presenting with hyperemesis or threatened preterm labour.

Investigations
- *Urinalysis:* the most useful markers are nitrites and leukocytes but they may be poor predictors of positive culture in asymptomatic bacteriuria.
- *MSU:* a positive result is confirmed with a culture of >100 000 organisms/mL. Mixed growth or non-significant culture—repeat MSU.
- *Bloods:* blood cultures, FBC, U&E, and CRP in a pyrexial patient.
- *Renal USS:* after a single episode of pyelonephritis or ≥2UTI, to exclude hydronephrosis, congenital abnormality, and calculi.

⚠ 20% of pregnant women with pyelonephritis have an abnormal renal tract.

Monthly MSU should be sent in women with culture-proven urinary infection to prove eradication. 15% develop recurrent bacteriuria and require further treatment.

Treatment
- Oral antibiotics are recommended in asymptomatic bacteriuria and cystitis to prevent pyelonephritis and preterm labour.
- Pyelonephritis should be treated with IV antibiotics until the pyrexia settles and vomiting stop. IV fluids and antipyretics should also be given (manage in hospital because of risk of preterm labour).

Duration of treatment
- *Asymptomatic bacteriuria:* 3 days.
- *Cystitis:* 7 days.
- *Pyelonephritis:* 10–14 days.

Prevention
- Increase fluid intake.
- Double voiding and emptying bladder after sexual intercourse.
- *Cranberry juice:* proven in non-pregnant population to ↓ bacteriuria.
- Prophylactic antibiotics: if ≥2 culture +ve urine infections + 1 risk factor.

Risk factors for urinary tract infection

Antenatal
- Previous infection (in previous pregnancy or outside pregnancy).
- Renal stones.
- Diabetes mellitus.
- Immunosuppression.
- Polycystic kidneys.
- Congenital anomalies of renal tract (e.g. Duplex system).
- Neuropathic bladder.

Post-partum (risk mainly associated with catheterization)
- Prolonged labour.
- Prolonged 2nd stage.
- CS.
- Pre-eclampsia.

Antibiotic options for renal tract infections

Drug of choice
Depends on antibiotic sensitivities. Options include:
- Penicillin amoxicillin.
- Cephalosporin.
- *Gentamicin:* monitor levels to minimize risk of ototoxicity.
- *Trimethoprim:* avoid in 1st trimester as it is a folate antagonist.
- *Nitrofurantoin:* avoid in 3rd trimester as risk of haemolytic anaemia in neonate with glucose-6-phosphate dehydrogenase deficiency.
- *Sulfonamides:* avoid in 3rd trimester as risk of kernicterus in neonate due to displacement of protein binding of bilirubin.

Contraindicated antibiotics
- *Tetracyclines:* cause permanent staining of teeth and problems with skeletal development.
- *Ciprofloxacin:* causes skeletal problems.

Chronic renal disease

There are increased maternal and fetal risks to pregnancy with renal disease. This is dependent upon:
- The underlying cause.
- The degree of renal impairment.
- The presence and control of hypertension.
- The amount of proteinuria.
- As renal function deteriorates, so does the ability to conceive and sustain a pregnancy. Successful pregnancies are rare with a serum creatinine >275µmol/L.

> **Risk factors**
>
> *Maternal risks*
> - Accelerated, and possibly permanent, deterioration in renal function; this is more likely if there is also hypertension and proteinuria and significant renal impairment at conception.
> - Hypertension.
> - Proteinuria.
> - Pre-eclampsia.
> - Venous thromboembolism (if nephrotic level of proteinuria).
> - UTI.
>
> *Fetal risks*
> - Miscarriage.
> - IUGR.
> - Spontaneous and iatrogenic preterm delivery.
> - Fetal death.

Management
- Multidisciplinary care involving a renal physician.
- Baseline investigations, ideally before conception, include FBC, U&E, urate, 24h protein, and creatinine clearance.
- Prepregnancy counselling (genetic counselling if a familial disorder).
- Early and regular antenatal care is advised with the following aims;
  - *control BP*—tight control lessens chance of renal function declining
  - monitor renal function and proteinuria
  - assess fetal size and well-being with serial growth scans + Doppler
  - *early detection of complication*—anaemia, UTI, pre-eclampsia, IUGR.
- Medication should be reviewed and may need altering. ACEIs should be stopped as soon as pregnancy is confirmed.
- Prophylactic low-dose aspirin may reduce the risk of pre-eclampsia.
- Erythropoetin may be required with significant renal impairment.
- Hospital admission should be considered with ↑ proteinuria or hypertension, deteriorating renal function, or symptoms of pre-eclampsia.

⚠ Look for an underlying cause of deterioration in renal function: UTI, obstruction, dehydration, pre-eclampsia, renal vein thrombosis.

⚠ It can be difficult to differentiate between pre-eclampsia and deterioration of renal impairment. Thrombocytopaenia, IUGR, and abnormal LFTs suggest the former diagnosis. Aim for vaginal delivery, but rates of CS are increased.

Commonest causes of chronic renal impairment in pregnancy

- Reflux nephropathy.[1]
- Diabetes.
- Lupus nephritis.
- Chronic glomerulonephritides.
- Polycystic kidneys.[2]

[1] Condition may be familial.
[2] Adult polycystic kidney disease is inherited in an autosomal dominant manner.

Outcomes in pregnancy dependent on renal function

Mild renal impairment (creatinine <125µmol/L)
- A successful outcome is achieved in 90% of cases.
- Increasing proteinuria is common (>50% of pregnancies) and can be in nephrotic range.

Moderate renal impairment (creatinine 125–250µmol/L)
- 25% of women experience an accelerated decline in renal function.
- Preterm delivery rate is up to 50%, and 1/3 have IUGR.
- A successful outcome is achieved in 60–90% of cases.

Severe renal impairment (creatinine >250µmol/L)
- The risk of maternal complications is significantly higher than the chance of successful pregnancy; advise against pregnancy.
- There is reduced fertility due to amenorrhoea.
- Permanent deterioration in renal function can occur in up to 25%.
- Preterm delivery rate is >70%, and the rate of IUGR is 30%.

Creatinine level is dependent on muscle mass as well as renal function so patients may have significantly different creatinine clearance on 24h urine collection, despite similar blood results. The latter is a more accurate reflection of renal function.

◆ Hypertension is an important predictor of outcome regardless of renal function.

Pregnancy after renal transplantation

Menstruation, ovulation, and fertility return after transplantation. Women should be informed of this and contraception discussed. Those who wish to conceive should be advised to wait at least 1yr after transplantation, until stabilization of renal function has been achieved and immunosuppression is at maintenance levels. The best outcomes are seen with:

• Well-controlled BP.
• No proteinuria.
• No evidence of graft rejection.
• Plasma creatinine <180, preferably <125µmol/L.

Management of pregnancy in a transplant recipient

• Multidisciplinary management with a renal physician.
• Antenatal care should be at fortnightly intervals. The aim is:
  • serial assessment of renal function: deterioration may be caused by infection, dehydration, pre-eclampsia, drug toxicity, or rejection
  • diagnosis and treatment of graft rejection
  • BP control (avoid ACEIs and β-blockers)
  • prevention, early diagnosis, and treatment of anaemia
  • detection and treatment of any infection
  • serial assessment of fetus (risk of IUGR).
• All women will be on immunosuppressive therapy, which must be continued; commonly used are prednisolone, azathioprine, and tacrolimus.
• Aim for vaginal delivery with continuous fetal monitoring (parenteral steroids are necessary to cover labour, due to adrenal suppression).
• Prophylactic antibiotics are recommended for obstetric procedures.
• A transplanted kidney does not obstruct labour; CS should be for obstetric reasons—the current rate is 40% (patients with pelvic osteodystrophy may need elective CS).

⚠ Mycophenalate mofetil is associated with congenital abnormalities and should be stopped before conception.

Risk factors

Maternal risks

- *Increased risk of ectopic pregnancy:* as a result of pelvic adhesions 2°
  to surgery, peritoneal dialysis, and pelvic infection.
- 15% develop significant deterioration in renal function, which may be
  permanent.
- In most cases pregnancy has no effect on graft survival or function.
- *Graft rejection ~5%:* same as in non-pregnant women.
- *Hypertension, proteinuria, and pre-eclampsia:* 30–40%.
- *Infections, especially urinary tract:* up to 40%.

Fetal risks

- Miscarriage and congenital anomaly rates are unchanged.
- *IUGR 30%,* higher if the mother is on ciclosporin.
- *Preterm delivery 45–60%:* may be iatrogenic, spontaneous, or 2° to
  preterm rupture of membranes.

⚠ If maternal complications occur before 28wks the chance of a successful pregnancy outcome falls from 95% to 75%.

Investigations in pregnancy following renal transplantation

At each visit

- FBC, U&E, urate.
- MSU.
- PCR.

Every 2–4wks

- USS for fetal growth and Doppler studies.

Every 4wks

- Drug levels of ciclosporin and tacrolimus.

Every 6wks

- Calcium, phosphate, albumin, and LFTs.
- 24h urine for creatinine clearance and protein.

Graft rejection

Consider the diagnosis if there is deteriorating renal function with:

- Fever.
- Oliguria.
- Renal enlargement and tenderness.

▶ It can be difficult to diagnose and a renal biopsy may be required.

⚠ Blood transfusion should be avoided if possible as it increases likelihood of sensitization making graft rejection more of a problem.

Acute renal failure

Characterized by oliguria (<400mL/day), ↑ urea and creatinine, hyperka-laemia, and metabolic acidosis. Rare in pregnancy, typically complicating the post-partum period. There are three phases:

- *Oliguria:* few days to several weeks.
- *Polyuria:* 2 days to 2wks, dilute urine is produced, and as waste products are still not excreted, renal function still deteriorates.
- *Recovery:* urine volume returns to normal with a gradual improvement in renal function.

Management of acute renal failure

- Seek advice from a physician or nephrologist.
- Most cases are reversible with appropriate management (permanent problems more likely with pre-existing renal disease).
- Assessment should include the following investigations:
  - FBC, coagulation, U&E, plasma osmolality, glucose, albumin
  - blood cultures, MSU, HVS
  - urinalysis and urine osmolality and electrolytes
  - ECG (looking for changes due to ↑ K⁺) and arterial blood gases (ABG)
  - fetal assessment with CTG and USS
  - renal USS if obstruction suspected.
- Interventions should include catheterization, central venous line, and renal biopsy if improvement is delayed; only a minority require dialysis.
- Replace fluid/blood loss but avoid fluid overload as there is a significant risk of pulmonary oedema (accurate documentation of input/output, daily weight, and central venous pressure monitoring).
- Maintain BP at levels that allow adequate renal perfusion.
- Review medication and stop nephrotoxic drugs.
- Correct hyperkalaemia, coagulopathy, and give antibiotics if infection suspected.
- Dialysis is required for persistent hyperkalaemia, acidosis, pulmonary oedema, or uraemia.

Some causes of renal failure in pregnancy

Pre-renal (hypovolaemic)
- Haemorrhage:
  - antepartum (abruption, placenta praevia, etc.)
  - post-partum (uterine atony, genital tract trauma, etc.)
- Hyperemesis.
- Septic shock.
- Acute fatty liver of pregnancy.

Intrinsic
- Pre-eclampsia.
- HELLP syndrome.
- Sepsis (Gram −ve, etc.).
- Drug reaction.
- Amniotic fluid embolus.

Post-renal
Obstruction
- Ureteric damage.
- Pelvic or broad ligament haematoma.

⚠ Non-pregnancy-related problems may also be the cause.

Treatment of hyperkalaemia
- 10mL calcium gluconate (10%) IV slowly, for cardioprotection.
- 15U soluble insulin with 50g of glucose 50% IV over 20min.
- Consider use of Calcium Resonium®.

◆ These are only temporary measures; dialysis may be required.

Systemic lupus erythematosus

More common in women than men (9:1) with a higher prevalence in the Afro-Caribbean population than in whites (5:1). The incidence is 1:1000 and onset during the reproductive age is common. It is a connective tissue disease of relapses (flares) and remissions. Diagnosis is based on the four features from the American Rheumatism Society Criteria present either consecutively or concurrently.

Monitoring disease severity in pregnancy

- Flare-ups can be difficult to diagnose as similar symptoms occur in normal pregnancy, e.g. fatigue, hair loss, joint aches, anaemia.
  - ESR is raised in normal pregnancy and CRP is not a marker of disease activity
  - C3(↓) or anti-DNA levels (↑) are an objective index of disease activity.
- Renal disease can also be difficult to distinguish from pre-eclampsia, as hypertension, proteinuria, and thrombocytopaenia are common to both conditions:
  - raised urate and liver transaminases are not features of systemic lupus erythematosus (SLE)
  - falling C3 and rising anti-DNA levels suggest lupus nephritis
  - renal biopsy is diagnostic, but rarely performed in pregnancy.

Maternal risks

- Long-term prognosis is not affected by pregnancy.
- There is increased risk of flare-up, especially in the puerperium.
- Hypertension, pre-eclampsia, and placental abruption are more common.

⚠ Do not stop hydroxychloroquine as this may precipitate a flare.

Fetal risks

- Increased risk of miscarriage, preterm delivery, preterm rupture of membranes, IUGR, and *in utero* fetal death.
- These risks are due to anticardiolipin antibodies, lupus anticoagulant, renal impairment, or hypertension. Risk is low if all these are absent.
- Congenital heart block may occur in women with anti-Ro (or La) antibodies, which cross the placenta (risk of occurrence if anti-Ro +ve is 2–3%, increasing to 25% if previously affected child).
- Transient skin lesions similar to cutaneous lupus can occur in neonates (usually in first 2wks of life).

Management

- Multidisciplinary team management.
- Prepregnancy counselling of maternal and fetal risks based on BP, renal function, anti-Ro, and antiphospholipid antibody status.
- Treat hypertension and modify medication if necessary (see 🕮 Blood pressure in pregnancy: hypertension, p. 62).
- Advise conception during periods of disease remission: less risk of flare.
- Obtain objective evidence of flare-up.
- Flare-ups should be treated by starting or ↑ dose, or steroids.
- Assess fetal growth and well-being (uterine artery Doppler at 24wks is a useful screening test).

Diagnosis of SLE: American Rheumatism Association criteria

Diagnosis requires four of the following features, either simultaneously or following each other:

- Facial butterfly rash.
- Discoid lupus.
- Photosensitivity of skin rash.
- Oral or nasopharyngeal ulceration.
- Arthritis: non-erosive, migratory of two or more peripheral joints.
- Serositis: pleurisy or pericarditis.
- Renal problems: proteinuria >500mg/day or cellular casts.
- Neurological problem: psychosis or convulsions.
- Haemotological problem: haemolytic anaemia, leucopaenia ($<4 \times 10^9$/L), lymphopaenia ($<1.5 \times 10^9$/L) or thrombocytopaenia ($<100 \times 10^9$/L).
- Anti-DNA, antinuclear antibodies (ANAs), chronic false +ve syphilis serology for >6mths, or +ve lupus erythematosus (LE) cell preparation.

Antiphospholipid antibody syndrome

This condition is diagnosed on the basis of the presence of one or more clinical features and one or more positive laboratory findings. The condition may be complicated by hypertension, pulmonary hypertension, epilepsy, thrombocytopaenia, leg ulcers, and valvular problems. It is called 1° if features of connective tissue disease are absent or it can occur 2° to established connective tissue disease. Lupus anticoagulant is an inhibitor of the coagulation pathway, and anticardiolipins are antibodies against the phospholipid components of cell walls.

Diagnostic criteria

Clinical criteria
- *Vascular thrombosis:* arterial or venous.
- Three or more consecutive miscarriages (<10wks).
- One or more fetal death >10wks.
- One or more preterm delivery (<34wks) due to pre-eclampsia or placental insufficiency.

Laboratory criteria
- Anticardiolipin antibody (IgG or IgM) in medium or high titre on at least two occasions >6wks apart.
- Lupus anticoagulant present on at least two occasions >6wks apart.

Maternal risks
- These include placental abruption and pre-eclampsia.
- Previous poor obstetric history is an important predictor of outcome (the risk is less with just recurrent miscarriages).

Fetal risks
- Risks include early and late miscarriage, *in utero* death, IUGR.
- Fetal outcome may be improved by multidisciplinary management, fetal monitoring (including growth, umbilical and uterine artery Dopplers), appropriate drug therapy, and timely delivery.
- Anticardiolipin antibody is the best predictor of fetal outcome: the higher the titre, the greater the fetal risk, but quantifying risk is difficult.
- Possible mechanisms of fetal injury are recurrent placental infarction and direct cellular injury.
- Liaise with anaesthetist if the woman is on LMWH (regional anaesthesia is contraindicated within 12h of a prophylactic dose of heparin and 24h of therapeutic dose).

Antiphospholipid antibody syndrome: recommendations
- No thrombosis or pregnancy loss: no treatment or aspirin 75mg.
- Previous thrombosis: aspirin + LMWH.
- Previous recurrent 1st-trimester miscarriages: aspirin +/– LMWH.
- Previous IUD or IUGR or severe pre-eclampsia: aspirin + LMWH.

Start aspirin when pregnancy confirmed; LMWH when fetal heart seen.

🖙 Take home baby rate: 40% aspirin alone; 70% aspirin and LMWH.

🖙 Some studies have disputed improved pregnancy outcomes with LMWH compared with aspirin alone.

Consider stopping heparin if 24wk uterine artery Doppler is normal. The improved live birth rate is due to ↓ miscarriages.

⚠ Steroids are not recommended → less success and more side effects.

Rheumatoid arthritis

This is more common in women than men, with an incidence of 1:1000–2000 pregnancies. Characterized by symmetrical chronic inflammation and destruction of synovial joints. Autoantibodies are formed to immunoglobulins, which are deposited as immune complexes in the synovial fluid and elsewhere. 80–90% have rheumatoid factor and 20–30% are ANA +ve. It is a multisystem disorder with extra-articular features including anaemia, nodules, carpal tunnel syndrome, and eye and lung involvement.

Maternal risks

- The condition improves in pregnancy in 75% of cases, but flare-up is common in the puerperium.
- At this age atlantoaxial subluxation rarely causes problems during intubation.

Fetal risks

There is usually no adverse effect on pregnancy unless the woman is anti-Ro +ve or has antiphosphlipid antibodies (5–10%).

Drugs used in the treatment of autoimmune diseases

Safe to continue in pregnancy
- Paracetamol.
- Steroids.
- Hydroxychloroquine.
- Sulfasalazine (in conjunction with 5mg folic acid).
- Azathioprine.
- Biological agents, such as infliximab (until 3rd trimester as effect on neonatal immune system is unknown).

Discontinue/avoid in pregnancy
- *NSAIDs:* oligohydramnios, premature closure of ductus arteriosus and neonatal haemorrhage especially with 3rd-trimester use.
- *Gold:* teratogenic effect seen in animals only.
- *Penicillamine:* connective tissue abnormalities only in high doses.
- *Cyclophosphamide (alkylating agent):* risk of leukaemia.
- *Methotrexate (folate antagonist):* causes miscarriage and congenital anomalies.

Myasthenia gravis

Uncommon condition; highest incidence in women of childbearing age. It is caused by autoimmune disruption of nicotinic acetylcholine receptors at the skeletal muscle motor end plate, leading to muscle weakness and fatigue. 90% have acetylcholine receptor antibodies. Muscles affected include eyes (ptosis, diplopia), face, neck, limbs, and trunk. Diagnosis confirmed by prompt, transient improvement in muscle strength with Tensilon test. Condition can be worsened by infection, hypokalaemia, exercise, emotion, and drugs (aminoglycosides, $MgSO_4$, local anaesthetic, β-blockers, β-agonists, narcotics, and neuromuscular blocking drugs).

Effect of pregnancy on myasthenia

- No change 60%, improvement 20%, deterioration 20%.
- There is no consistent effect between pregnancies.
- Symptoms commonly worsen post-partum.
- Previous thymectomy associated with fewer exacerbations in pregnancy.
- Hyperemesis, delayed gastric emptying, ↑ volume of distribution of drugs, ↑ renal clearance can lead to subtherapeutic drug levels.
- Increased doses of anticholinesterases may be required as pregnancy advances; this is best achieved by decreasing dose intervals.
- Parenteral anticholinesterases should be given in labour to avoid absorption problems.

Effect of myasthenia on pregnancy

- Preterm delivery, polyhydramnios, and IUGR are all increased.
- The 1st stage of labour is not prolonged (the smooth muscle of the myometrium is not affected by the condition).
- In the 2nd stage there can be skeletal muscle fatigue; instrumental delivery may be required to prevent maternal exhaustion.
- Neonatal myasthenia can occur following delivery in 10–20% of babies:
  - it results from transplacental passage of maternal antibodies
  - there is poor correlation between the condition and maternal disease activity or antibody levels
  - presentation is with generalized hypotonia, poor sucking/feeding, and a weak cry
  - onset is within 24h and the condition resolves by 2mths
  - treatment is with anticholinesterases.

⚠ $MgSO_4$ is contraindicated for treatment of eclampsia in myasthenia.

Management

- Inform neurologist, paediatrician, and anaesthetist of pregnancy.
- The usual treatment options have all been used in pregnancy:
  - long-acting anticholinesterases (e.g. pyridostigmine)
  - immunosuppression: steroids, azathioprine
  - plasmapheresis
  - thymectomy.

Diabetes: established disease in pregnancy

- Established diabetes affects 1–2% of pregnancies.
- Without good glycaemic control there is increased fetal and neonatal morbidity and mortality.
- Management should be by a multidisciplinary team including:
  - obstetrician
  - physician/diabetologist
  - diabetic specialist nurse/midwife
  - dietitian.
- Glucose metabolism is altered by pregnancy.
- Many pregnancy hormones are diabetogenic (human placental lactogen, cortisol, glucagon, oestrogen, and progesterone).
- Insulin requirements ↑ throughout and are maximal at term.

Effect of diabetes on pregnancy

- *Maternal hyperglycaemia:* leads to fetal hyperglycaemia.
- *Fetal hyperglycaemia:* leads to hyperinsulinaemia (through β-cell hyperplasia in fetal pancreatic cells). Insulin acts as a growth promoter:
  - macrosomia
  - organomegaly
  - ↑ erythropoiesis
  - fetal polyuria (polyhydramnios).
- *Neonatal hypoglycaemia:* caused by the removal of maternal glucose supply at birth from a hyperinsulinaemic fetus.
- *Respiratory distress syndrome:* more common in babies born to diabetic mothers due to surfactant deficiency occurring through reduced production of pulmonary phospholipids.

Effect of pregnancy on diabetes

- *Ketoacidosis:* rare, but may be associated with hyperemesis, infection, tocolysis (β-sympathomimetics), or steroid therapy.
- *Retinopathy:* there is a two-fold increased risk of development or progression of existing disease. Rapid improvement in glycaemic control leads to increased retinal blood flow, which can cause retinopathy. All diabetic women should have assessment for retinopathy in pregnancy, and proliferative retinopathy requires treatment. Early changes usually revert after delivery.
- *Nephropathy:* affects 5–10% of women. Renal function and proteinuria may worsen during pregnancy. This is usually temporary. There is increased maternal risk of pre-eclampsia and fetal risk of IUGR in this population and increased surveillance is required.
- *Ischaemic heart disease:* pregnancy increases cardiac workload. Women with symptoms should be assessed by a cardiologist before conception.

Complications of diabetes in pregnancy

Maternal
- UTI.
- Recurrent vulvovaginal candidiasis.
- Pregnancy-induced hypertension/pre-eclampsia.
- Obstructed labour.
- Operative deliveries: CS and assisted vaginal deliveries.
- ↑ Retinopathy (15%).
- ↑ Nephropathy.
- Cardiac disease.

Fetal
- Miscarriage*
- *Congenital abnormalities:**
  - neural tube defects
  - microcephaly
  - cardiac abnormalities.
  - sacral agenesis
  - renal abnormalities.
- Preterm labour.
- Polyhydramnios (25%).
- Macrosomia (25–40%).
- IUGR.
- Unexplained IUD.

Neonatal
- Polycythaemia.
- Jaundice.
- Hypoglycaemia.
- Hypocalcaemia.
- Hypomagnesaemia.
- Hypothermia.
- Cardiomegaly.
- Birth trauma: shoulder dystocia, fractures, Erb's palsy, asphyxia.
- Respiratory distress syndrome.

* In diabetics with poor control.

Diabetes: antenatal management

Prepregnancy counselling

Offer to all diabetic women of reproductive age; include:

- *Achievement of optimal control:* keep fasting blood glucose between 3.5 and 5.9mmol/L and 1h post-prandial <7.8mmol/L (↑ risk of miscarriage and congenital abnormalities with poor control).
- *Assessment of severity of diabetes:* check for hypertension, retinopathy (fundoscopy, ophthalmology assessment), nephropathy (U&E, urinalysis, urinary protein:creatinine ratio, 24h urine for protein, creatinine clearance), neuropathy (clinical assessment), and cardiac disease.
- *Education:* ensure understanding of effects of hyperglycaemia on fetus and need for tight control—instruct to inform doctor as soon as pregnancy confirmed; some drugs may need stopping (ACEIs).
- *General health:* stop smoking, optimize weight (aim for a normal BMI), minimize alcohol (max 1–2U bd/wk).
- *Folic acid:* ↑ risk of neural tube defects, so start on 5mg folic acid.
- *Rubella status:* offer vaccination if not rubella immune.
- *Contraception:* ensure effective contraception until good control achieved and pregnancy desired.

Antenatal care

Manage by a multidisciplinary team with a diabetologist.

- *Control:* as for prepregnancy, aim for normoglycaemia. Monitor glucose at least 4 times/day, usually before meals, but post-meal glucose may give tighter control. Women can alter their own insulin based on their glucose. Insulin can be given as SC injections 2 or 4 times/day or as a continuous infusion. The latter is no better than injections.
- *HbA1c every month:* this gives an objective measurement of control over the preceding 2mths.
- *Dietitian review:* low sugar, low fat, high fibre diet—low glycaemic index.
- *Dating ultrasound:* to confirm viability and gestation.

● Down's syndrome screening: consider nuchal translucency or invasive testing. Serum screening is affected by diabetes (↓ AFP); therefore, less accurate unless appropriate normograms used.

- *Anomaly scan:* 5–10-fold ↑ risk of congenital anomalies. Risk depends on glycaemic control prior to conception and early pregnancy.
- *Fetal echocardiography:* at 20–24wks.
- *Antenatal surveillance:* individualize care. Serial USS every 2–4wks to detect polyhydramnios, macrosomia, or IUGR. Increased surveillance if problems detected. The use of umbilical artery Doppler should be restricted to cases of IUGR; it is not of value as a screening test.
- *Hypoglycaemia:* awareness of hypoglycaemia may be lost. Educate patient and family and supply with glucagon.

Diabetes: labour and post-partum care

Timing and mode of delivery should be individualized and based on EFW and obstetric factors (previous mode of delivery, gestation, glycaemic control, and antenatal complications).

Timing of delivery

☙ Some obstetricians advise elective delivery by induction of labour at 38–39wks if there are no maternal or fetal complications and good glycaemic control. Outcomes may not be better than awaiting spontaneous labour. Delivery should be expedited if complications occur.

Mode of delivery

Vaginal delivery is preferred. Continuous electronic fetal monitoring is advised in labour. Consider elective CS if EFW is >4.5kg. If EFW is 4–4.5kg use obstetric factors to influence decision. CS rates are high: 50–60%. Give antibiotic and thromboprophylaxis if CS is carried out.

☙ Shoulder dystocia is more common at all birth weights than in the non-diabetic population. Experienced obstetricians should perform instrumental deliveries because this is an independent risk factor.

Glycaemic control

- *Diet controlled:* check blood glucose hourly. If glucose >6.0mmol/L, start sliding scale.
- *Insulin dependent:* continue SC insulin until in established labour, then convert to insulin sliding scale (Table 5.1). If induction of labour or CS, continue normal insulin until day of procedure, then start sliding scale in early morning.

⚠ Avoid maternal hyperglycaemia → causes fetal hypoglycaemia.

⚠ If steroids are given for threatened preterm labour, monitor glucose closely—hyperglycaemia should be anticipated.

Post-partum care

- Encourage breast-feeding. ☙ Avoid oral hypoglycaemic drugs if breast-feeding—metformin and insulin are safe.
- Baby needs early feeding and glucose monitoring.

Contraception

- Avoid the COCP if breast-feeding or vascular complications. Progesterone-based contraception is safe and there are no contra-indications to an IUCD. This should be fitted from 6wks post-partum onwards. Sterilization or vasectomy should be considered if the family is complete.
- Review sliding scale regularly.
- Renew insulin syringe every 24h.
- IV fluids should always be given with the sliding scale:
  - stable situations—5% glucose
  - high blood glucose—normal saline.

Table 5.1 Insulin: IV sliding scale

Blood glucose (mmol/L)	Insulin rate (mL/h)
<3.0	0
3.1–4	0.5
4.1–6	1.0
6.1–8	1.5
8.1–11	2.0
11.1–15	3.0
>15.1	Call doctor

Prescription: 50U human actrapid in 50mL normal saline (sodium chloride 0.9%), via a continuous infusion pump.

Post-partum insulin requirements

Insulin requirements fall dramatically after delivery of the placenta. Halve the sliding scale initially. Change back to SC insulin when eating and drinking. Start with the prepregnancy dose of SC insulin. If this is not known, it is roughly half the last dose. The dose may need to be further reduced if breast-feeding. Stop the sliding scale 1h after giving the SC dose.

▶ Aim for blood sugar monitoring (BM) 4–9mmol/L in the post-partum period.

Gestational diabetes

The World Health Organization (WHO) now includes gestational impaired glucose tolerance (IGT) with gestational diabetes. A proportion of women diagnosed in pregnancy will actually have previously unrecognized type 1 or 2 diabetes (20–30%). WHO does not advocate universal screening. Selective screening should be based on risk factors.

Risk factors for gestational diabetes
- BMI above 30kg/m².
- Previous macrosomic baby weighing 4.5kg or above.
- Previous gestational diabetes.
- First-degree relative with diabetes.
- Family origin with a high prevalence of diabetes (South Asian, black Caribbean, and Middle Eastern).

The diagnosis is based on an oral glucose tolerance test (OGTT) (Box 5.4), usually undertaken at 26–28wks gestation. A normal result in early pregnancy does not mean that gestational diabetes will not develop, and an OGTT should be repeated at 34wks if there are concerns.

Management
- Management by a multidisciplinary team.
- Measure glucose 4–6 times/day (1h post-prandial measurements may be more effective in preventing macrosomia than pre-meal glucose).
- *Diet should be first-line treatment:*
  - aim for normoglycaemia and avoid ketosis.
  - weight should remain steady if diet followed
  - compliance is often poor—dietitian input may help.
- *Start insulin if:*
  - pre-meal glucose >6.0mmol/L.
  - 1h post-prandial glucose >7.5mmol/L.
  - AC >95th centile despite apparent good control.
- There is no increased risk of miscarriage or congenital anomalies; other fetal and neonatal risks are similar to established diabetes (IUGR is less likely).
- Antenatal and intrapartum care as for established diabetes.
- *Post-partum:*
  - stop insulin and glucose infusions
  - check glucose prior to discharge to ensure normal (risk of previously undiagnosed type 2 diabetes)
  - arrange OGTT at 6wks post-partum
  - *education*—50% risk of developing type 2 diabetes mellitus over next 25yrs (this risk can be reduced by maintaining physical activity and avoiding obesity).

Box 5.4 Oral glucose tolerance test
- Overnight fasting (8h minimum):
  - water only may be consumed during this time
  - no smoking.
- 75g Glucose load in 250–300mL water.
- Plasma glucose measured fasting and at 2h.

Results
- Diabetes:
  - fasting glucose >6.0mmol/L but <7.0mmol/L
  - 2h glucose ≥11.1mmol/L.
- IGT:
  - fasting glucose >6.0mmol/L but <7.0mmol/L
  - 2h ≥7.8 <11.0mmol/L.

⚠ Only one value needs to be abnormal to make the diagnosis.

Thyrotoxicosis

Thyrotoxicosis occurs in 1:500 pregnancies. The most common cause is Graves' disease (95%). This is an autoimmune disease characterized by the production of TSH receptor stimulating antibodies. Most women have been diagnosed before pregnancy and may be on treatment. Many symptoms and signs occur in normal pregnancy. The most discriminatory features are weight loss, tremor, persistent tachycardia, and eye signs. Diagnosis is made by a low TSH and high free T_4 or free T_3 levels.

▶ Use pregnancy-specific reference ranges for each trimester. See Table 5.2.

Effect of pregnancy on thyrotoxicosis

- Usually improves in the 2nd and 3rd trimester.
- Pregnancy is a state of relative immunodeficiency, but with return of normal immunity in the puerperium it is likely to deteriorate.

Effect of thyrotoxicosis on pregnancy

- Maternal and fetal outcome usually good if disease is controlled.
- Untreated or poorly controlled thyrotoxicosis is associated with sub-fertility (amenorrhoea due to weight loss), ↑ risk of miscarriage, IUGR, and premature delivery.

⚠ With the stress of infection, labour, or operative delivery a 'thyroid storm' can occur in poorly controlled patients. This is a medical emergency, characterized by pyrexia, confusion, and cardiac failure. Neonatal/fetal thyrotoxicosis occurs in up to 10% of babies born to women with current or past history of Graves' disease (transplacental passage of thyroid receptor stimulating antibodies).

▶ Check antibody levels in all women with a history of Graves' disease.
- If antibodies are present, monitor by fetal heart rate, and serial USS for growth and fetal goitre (treatments include antithyroid drugs titrated to fetal heart rate, or delivery).
- Antibodies have a half-life of around 3wks, therefore transient neonatal hyperthyroidism may occur.

Treatment

- *Antithyroid drugs:* carbimazole and propylthiouracil (PTU) are the two drugs used. The aim of treatment is to achieve clinical euthyroid with T_4 at the upper limit of normal. Use the lowest dose of drug to achieve this. Both drugs cross the placenta and may cause fetal hypothyroidism in high doses. PTU is preferred for new cases as there is less transfer across the placenta and into breastmilk. β-Blockers may safely be used for symptom relief in new cases for a short period of time.
- Surgery: thyroidectomy can be safely done in pregnancy. Indications include dysphagia, stridor, suspected carcinoma, and allergies to both antithyroid drugs.

☛ Radioactive iodine is contraindicated in pregnancy and breast-feeding.

Causes of thyrotoxicosis

- Graves' disease.
- Toxic multinodular goitre.
- Toxic adenoma.
- Carcinoma.
- Subacute thyroiditis.
- Amiodarone.
- Lithium.

⚠ Women with hyperemesis or a molar pregnancy may mimic biochemical hyperthyroidism as hCG, at high levels, can stimulate TSH receptors. They usually have no clinical signs of thyrotoxicosis and should not be treated.

Management

- Graves' disease often improves in pregnancy, but relapses postpartum.
- With treatment the outlook is good for mother and baby.
- Untreated thyrotoxicosis is dangerous for mother and baby.
- PTU and carbimazole may be used as treatment; both cross the placenta.
- Avoid radioactive iodine.
- Check for TSH receptor stimulating antibodies.
- Monitor thyroid function every 4–6wks in new cases, less frequently in stable cases.
- Monitor fetus by fetal heart rate and serial USS for growth and presence of goitre.
- Breast-feeding is safe with doses of PTU <150mg/day and carbimazole <15mg/day. Monitor TFTs in baby at higher doses.

Table 5.2 Reference ranges for TFTs by trimester

	Non-pregnant	1st trimester	2nd trimester	3rd trimester
TSH (µ/l)	0.3–4.2	0–5.5	0.5–3.5	0.5–4
Free T$_4$ (pmol/L)	9–26	10–16	9–15.5	8–14.5
Free T$_3$ (pmol/L)	2.6–5.7	3–7	3–5.5	2.5–5.5

Hypothyroidism

Hypothyroidism complicates around 1% of pregnancies. Most cases have been diagnosed previously and patients are on replacement therapy. New diagnosis in pregnancy is rare. The commonest cause is autoimmune and may be associated with other autoimmune conditions.

- Classical symptoms and signs may be seen in normal pregnancy. The most discriminatory features are cold intolerance, bradycardia, and slow relaxation of tendon reflexes.
- The diagnosis is made by a low free T_4. TSH is also raised, but in isolation is not diagnostic.

▶ Use pregnancy-specific reference ranges for each trimester (Table 5.2). Free T_4 levels are normally lower in the 2nd and 3rd trimester. TSH level is most useful.

Effect of pregnancy on hypothyroidism

No effect usually. Most women do not need to alter their dose of levothyroxine. The most common reason for increasing levothyroxine is an inadequate prepregnancy dose.

Effect of hypothyroidism on pregnancy

- Untreated hypothyroidism is associated with anovulatory infertility.
- Severe or untreated hypothyroidism in pregnancy is associated with increased risk of miscarriage, fetal loss, pre-eclampsia, and low birth weight.
- Hypothyroidism is also associated with gestational diabetes.
- The fetus requires maternal T_4 for normal brain development before 12wks (inadequate replacement may lead to reduced IQ in the offspring); after this time T_3/T_4/TSH do not cross the placenta.

▶ Aim for optimal control before conception.

- Women on adequate replacement therapy are euthyroid at the onset of pregnancy and have good maternal and fetal outcomes.
- Neonatal/fetal hypothyroidism is very rare and caused by the transplacental transfer of TSH receptor blocking antibodies, which may be seen in atrophic thyroiditis.

Treatment

- Most women should continue their maintenance dose of levothyroxine; the dose should only be increased if they are under-replaced (shown by TSH level).
- TSH levels need to be checked before conception and in each trimester, unless there has been a dose adjustment, in which case it should be repeated in 6wks.
- If the diagnosis is made in pregnancy, in the absence of cardiac disease, consider a starting dose of 50 micrograms daily.
- In practice, aim for a TSH level of <2.5μ/L in the first trimester.
- Levothyroxine can be safely taken during breast-feeding.

Causes of hypothyroidism
- Hashimoto's thyroiditis.
- Atrophic thyroiditis.
- Congenital absence of thyroid.
- Iatrogenic:
  - thyroidectomy
  - radioiodine
  - drugs (amiodarone, lithium, iodine, antithyroid drugs).
- Pituitary cause (rare).

Other thyroid diseases

Post-partum thyroiditis

This is an autoimmune condition causing destructive thyroiditis. It presents post-partum due to return to normal immunity after the relative immuno-suppression of pregnancy. Preformed T_4 is released, which may cause transient hyperthyroid symptoms followed by hypothyroidism as the reserve of T_4 is used up.

It can present for up to a year after delivery, but usually occurs 3–4mths post-partum. The incidence varies (5–10%) and it may manifest as transient hypothyroidism (40%), hyperthyroidism (40%), or biphasic with first hyperthyroidism then hypothyroidism (20%). There may be a family history of thyroid disease in 25% of cases. Many women are asymptomatic and often symptoms are vague and may be attributed to the post-partum state. Initiation of treatment should be based on symptoms and not biochemical results. Some women may not require any treatment. Most recover spontaneously. Risk of recurrence in future pregnancy is 70%. Risk of permanent hypothyroidism is 5%/yr for antibody-positive women (90% of patients have thyroid peroxidase antibodies).

- The hyperthyroid phase should be treated with β-blockers (not antithyroid drugs).

⚠ **Differential diagnosis:** Graves' disease.

- The hypothyroid state should be treated with thyroxine; treatment should be withdrawn after 6mths to check for recovery.

⚠ **Differential diagnosis:** Hashimoto's thyroiditis or Sheehan's syndrome.

▶ Long-term follow-up should be with annual TFT.

Thyroid nodules

- Thyroid nodules are common, affecting 5% of women in their reproductive years.

⚠ A small proportion of thyroid nodules are malignant.

- Differential diagnosis is a solitary toxic nodule, subacute (de Quervain's) thyroiditis, or a bleed into a cystic lesion.
- *Investigations:*
  - TFT and thyroid antibodies
  - thyroglobulin level: suggests malignancy if >100 micrograms/L
  - USS—cystic nodules are more likely to be benign than solid nodules
  - fine needle aspiration for cytology (cystic lesion)
  - biopsy (solid lesion).

⚠ Radioiodine is contraindicated in pregnancy.

Malignant lesions can be surgically treated in the 2nd and 3rd trimesters, and postoperatively thyroxine can be safely given to completely suppress TSH in TSH-dependent tumours.

Thyroid nodules: symptoms or signs suggestive of malignancy
- Past history of radiation to neck or chest.
- Fixed lump.
- Lymphadenopathy.
- Rapid growth of painless nodule.
- Voice change.
- Neurological involvement such as Horner's syndrome.

Phaeochromocytoma

This is a tumour of the adrenal medulla that causes excess secretion of catecholamines. They are bilateral in 10% of cases and malignant in 10%. In non-pregnant hypertensive patients the incidence is around 1:1000; it is exceedingly rare in pregnancy. A high index of clinical suspicion is required to make the diagnosis—the condition should be considered in hypertensive pregnant women if there are atypical features. Untreated, mortality is high: maternal mortality ~17% and fetal mortality ~26%. Maternal mortality can be reduced to ~4% with treatment.

Symptoms and signs
- Hypertension.
- Sweating.
- Palpitations.
- Anxiety.
- Headache.
- Vomiting.

⚠ Symptoms may mimic pre-eclampsia and may be paroxysmal.

Investigations
- Raised 24h urinary catecholamines or their metabolites, such as vanillylmandelic acid (VMA) confirm the diagnosis—a level twice normal is highly suggestive and 3 times normal diagnostic (methyldopa and labetalol can interfere with the results).
- Imaging is required to localize the tumour (USS, CT, or MRI are all used but MRI is preferable in pregnancy).

Management
- Multidisciplinary management including endocrine physician and surgeon.
- The main risk from this condition is potentially fatal hypertensive crises that can cause strokes, congestive cardiac failure, and arrhythmias.
- Patients should be commenced on α-blockers (phenoxybenzamine) to control BP, then β-blockers (propranolol) to control tachycardia.

⚠ Do *not* start β-blockers until a few days after α-blockers or a hypertensive crisis may ensue.
- Surgery is the only cure for the condition and should only be undertaken once pharmacological blockade has been achieved (if the diagnosis is made after 24wks, surgery should be delayed until fetal maturity is achieved).
- CS is preferred for delivery as it minimizes potential catecholamine surges (removal of the adrenal tumour can be done at the time of CS or later).
- Anaesthetic experience is vital as the patient may have a catecholamine surge during delivery due to inadequate pharmacological blockade.

Congenital adrenal hyperplasia

This is an autosomal recessive disorder affecting the synthesis of glu-cocorticoids and mineralocorticoids. In response to low levels of these hormones, the pituitary gland produces large amounts of ACTH and this results in excessive production of sex steroids. A number of enzyme deficiencies can lead to this condition: the commonest is 21-hydroxylase deficiency. Many different gene mutations exist, which result in vari-able clinical presentations. Treatment is replacement with corticosteroid +/− fludrocortisone.

Affected individuals present in several ways:
- Salt-losing crisis in neonate.
- Masculinization of female fetus (ambiguous genitalia at birth).
- Precocious puberty in boy.

▶ If a couple has an affected child, risk in subsequent pregnancies is 1:4.

Maternal and fetal risks

Pregnancies in women with congenital adrenal hyperplasia (CAH), diag-nosed in infancy, are uncommon. Many are subfertile due to anovulation; others have psychosexual and emotional difficulties or anatomical prob-lems related to corrective surgery for virilization.
- ↑ Risk of miscarriage, pre-eclampsia, and IUGR.
- ↑ Risk of CS due to android-shaped pelvis.

Management

- Maternal steroid therapy should be continued at same dose throughout pregnancy.
- Genetic counselling should be offered to all couples after the birth of an affected child; antenatal diagnosis can be untaken in subsequent pregnancies, but the female fetus is at risk of virilization before these tests can be undertaken,

▶ Start dexamethasone, 1.5mg/day, as soon as pregnancy confirmed, and before 5wks gestation (dexamethasone crosses placenta and suppresses excessive fetal ACTH production, which prevents masculinization and neuroendocrine effects to female fetus).
- Usually CVS is the preferred method of antenatal diagnosis.
- If the fetus is male, or an unaffected female, stop dexamethasone.
- If the fetus is an affected female options include continuation of dexamethasone throughout pregnancy or termination of pregnancy.

⚠ Mother needs to be monitored for gestational diabetes and ↑ BP.
- If invasive testing is declined, dexamethasone should be given and fetal sex determined by USS.
- Suppression of virilization with dexamethasone is not always successful and parents should be appropriately counselled.
- During labour increase steroid dose—hydrocortisone 100mg IV every 6h.
- Postnatally the child needs to be reviewed by a paediatrician and evidence of virilization sought; replacement glucocorticoid and mineralocorticoid therapy should be continued.

Antenatal diagnosis

- Amniocentesis (≥16wks):
  - Fetal sex.
  - 17-Hydroxyprogesterone and androgen levels in amniotic fluid.
  - Human leucocyte antigen (HLA) typing of amniotic cells.
- Chorionic villus sampling (≥10wks):
  - fetal sex
  - gene probe for specific mutations of 21-hydroxylase.
- PCR of fetal cells in maternal blood may help determine fetal sex.

Addison's, Conn's, and Cushing's syndromes

Addison's disease

Adrenocortical failure with deficiency of glucocorticoids and mineralocorticoids; may be associated with other autoimmune conditions: pernicious anaemia, diabetes, or thyroid disease. Most common cause in the UK is autoimmune destruction of the adrenals. Worldwide, TB is an important cause. It is rare to make a new diagnosis in pregnancy.

- Diagnosis is based on δ cortisol, ↓ ACTH, and poor response to tetracosactide (synthetic ACTH).

▶ Cortisol measurements are normally higher in pregnancy; therefore, care should be taken in interpreting results.

- Pregnancy does not affect the course of Addison's disease and if the condition is treated there are no adverse fetal effects.
- Patients should continue with their usual steroid doses (hydrocortisone 20–30mg/day and fludrocortisone 100 micrograms/day) throughout pregnancy.
- Increased or IV doses of steroids are required to cover periods of stress, such as infection, hyperemesis, labour, or surgery.
- In the puerperium physiological diuresis can cause profound hypotension; therefore tail steroids down to maintenance over several days.
- Breast-feeding is safe.

Conn's syndrome

- This is a rare cause of hypertension in pregnancy. Primary hyperaldosteronism is caused by adrenal aldosterone-secreting adenoma or carcinoma or bilateral adrenal hyperplasia.
- Clinical features are hypokalaemia (K^+ <3.0mmol/L) and hypertension.
- Diagnosis is based on ↓ K^+, ↑ plasma aldosterone, ↓ renin.
- Treat hypertension as usual (but avoid spironolactone which is used outside pregnancy) and give potassium supplements.

Cushing's syndrome

- This is a condition of glucocorticoid excess; very rare in pregnancy as anovulation leads to infertility. Causes in pregnancy are excessive pituitary ACTH secretion (44%), adrenal adenoma (44%), and adrenal carcinoma (12%).
- Diagnosis based on ↑ cortisol, which fails to suppress with high dose dexamethasone suppression test (ACTH levels depend on cause).
- Maternal morbidity and mortality are raised: specific risks include pre-eclampsia, diabetes, and poor wound healing.
- Fetal loss, prematurity, and perinatal mortality are increased and adrenal insufficiency can occur in the neonate.
- Surgery is the treatment of choice for adrenal and pituitary causes, and it may be successfully performed in pregnancy.
- Limited knowledge of use of drugs in pregnancy. Medical treatment include drugs that suppress cortisol production (metyrapone) or ACTH activity (cyproheptadine).
- Avoid breast-feeding.

Clinical features of Addison's disease
- Weight loss.
- Vomiting.
- Postural hypotension and syncope.
- Weakness.
- Hyperpigmentation (skin folds, scars, mouth).

Clinical features of Cushing's syndrome
- Bruising.
- Myopathy.
- Hypertension.
- Excessive weight gain/oedema.
- Hirsutism.
- Excessive striae.
- Headaches.
- Acne.
- Obesity.
- Impaired glucose tolerance/diabetes.

Hyperprolactinaemia

Prolactinomas are the commonest pituitary tumours seen in pregnancy. They can be classified according to their size into microprolactinoma (<1cm) and macroprolactinoma (>1cm). Outside pregnancy, diagnosis is based on a raised serum prolactin level in conjunction with imaging of the pituitary fossa by CT or MRI. In pregnancy, there is a 10-fold physiological rise in prolactin levels, so prolactin level is not a useful test in diagnosis or follow-up.

Clinical features of prolactinoma
- Amenorrhoea.
- Galactorrhoea.
- Headache.
- Visual field defects (bitemporal hemianopia).
- Diabetes insipidus.

Effect of pregnancy on prolactinoma
There is a possibility that prolactinomas will increase in size in pregnancy and cause symptoms. The highest risk (15%) is in the 3rd trimester with macroprolactinomas. Pregnancy should be delayed until tumour shrinkage has occurred with drug therapy. This reduces the risk of symptomatic tumour expansion to 4%. The risk is small for microprolactinomas (1.6%).

Effect of prolactinoma on pregnancy
Untreated, high prolactin levels lead to infertility. With preconception treatment fertility can be restored. Most cases have no complications in pregnancy. Breast-feeding is not contraindicated.

Management
- Outside pregnancy dopamine receptor agonists (cabergoline and bromocriptine) reduce prolactin levels; these should be stopped upon confirmation of pregnancy.
- The patient should report symptoms that might suggest tumour expansion—headache, visual disturbance, thirst, and polyuria; this should then be investigated by CT or, preferably, MRI of the pituitary.
- Formal visual field testing is recommended in pregnancy for symptomatic and asymptomatic patients with macroprolactinomas.
- Bromocriptine can safely be restarted if there is concern regarding tumour expansion and can be continued during breast-feeding, but may suppress milk production.
- Surgery is reserved for macroprolactinomas that fail to shrink despite drug therapy, but is usually delayed until after delivery.

Causes of hyperprolactinaemia
- Normal pregnancy and breast-feeding.
- Pituitary adenomas.
- Hypothalamus or pituitary stalk lesions.
- Empty sella syndrome.
- Hypothyroidism.
- Chronic renal failure.
- Drugs: phenothiazines, metoclopramide, methyldopa.

Hypopituitarism

This is anterior pituitary failure. Diagnosis is based on reduced levels of anterior pituitary and target organ hormone levels: thyroxine, TSH, cortisol, ACTH, follicle-stimulating hormone (FSH), luteinizing hormone (LH), and growth hormone. There is also a failed response to an insulin stress test with lack of increase in growth hormone, ACTH, and prolactin levels.

Causes of hypopituitarism
- Pituitary surgery.
- Radiotherapy.
- Pituitary or hypothalamic tumours.
- Post-partum pituitary infarction (Sheehan's syndrome).
- Autoimmune lymphocytic hypophysitis.

⚠ Imaging of the pituitary area, by MRI or CT, should be undertaken to exclude a space-occupying lesion.
- Pregnancy is possible, but may require ovulation induction with gonadotrophins.
- Once pregnancy is achieved the feto-placental unit can sustain pregnancy by sufficient production of oestradiol and progesterone.
- Maternal and fetal outcome is normal if the condition is adequately treated.
- Inadequately treated cases are at increased risk of adverse outcomes including maternal hypotension, hypoglycaemia, and mortality, miscarriage, and stillbirth.
- Treatment involves replacement therapy with levothyroxine and hydrocortisone (additional IV hydrocortisone is required in labour).
- Milk production may be impaired because of prolactin deficiency.

Sheehan's syndrome
- This is caused by avascular necrosis of the pituitary, as a result of hypotension usually secondary to a post-partum haemorrhage. The pituitary is particularly vulnerable in pregnancy due to its 2–3-fold increase in size. Partial or complete pituitary failure can occur. The posterior pituitary is unaffected as it has a different blood supply. Treatment is as above. Pregnancies have been reported following this diagnosis.

Clinical features of Sheehan's syndrome
- Failure of lactation.
- Persistent amenorrhoea.
- Loss of pubic and axillary hair.
- Hypothyroidism.
- Adrenal insufficiency (vomiting, hypotension, hypoglycaemia).

Diabetes insipidus

- Incidence 1:15 000 pregnancies.
- Caused by a lack of antidiuretic hormone (ADH).
- *Four types:*
  - *central*—lack of ADH production by the posterior pituitary caused by expanding tumours
  - *nephrogenic*—ADH resistance in the kidney
  - *transient*—production of an enzyme by the placenta that results in increased breakdown of ADH, occurs in association with pre-eclampsia or acute fatty liver of pregnancy
  - *psychogenic*—compulsive water drinking.
- *Clinical features:* excessive thirst and polyuria.
- Pregnancy may unmask the condition or make it worse (60%).
- Treatment is with desmopressin intranasally.

Obesity in pregnancy: maternal risks

- Obesity is an increasing problem in the developed world.
- The WHO definition of normal weight is a BMI between 18.5 and 24.9:
  - overweight is BMI between 25.0 and 29.9
  - obese is BMI ≥30.
- 1 in 5 pregnant women in the UK are now obese.
- The 2006–8 Confidential Enquiry unit Maternal and Child Health (CEMACH) report identified that obesity carries a greater risk of maternal death.

Maternal risks associated with obesity

Hypertension and pre-eclampsia

- Over twice as likely to develop gestational hypertension.
- Women with a BMI >30 have a significantly ↑ risk of pre-eclampsia.
- Excessive weight gain in pregnancy is associated with higher rates of pre-eclampsia in already overweight women.

Gestational diabetes

Over 3 times more likely to develop gestational diabetes compared with women with a normal BMI.

Thromboembolism

The incidence of thromboembolic disease in pregnancy is doubled in obese women.

Antenatal requirements for obese women

- 5mg folic acid pre-conception and until 12wks.
- 400 micrograms vitamin D.
- VTE risk assessment.
- Referral for consultant care.
- Anaesthetic referral.
- GTT at 24–28wks.

It may be difficult to palpate the uterus in obese women, leading to:

- Missed diagnosis of breech presentation.
- Missed diagnosis of IUGR or macrosomia.
- Unsuccessful ECV attempts.

⚠ USS is also technically difficult and may be inaccurate.

Postnatal complications associated with obesity

- Increased rates of postoperative complications also occur, including:
  - wound infection and endometritis
  - lower respiratory tract infection
  - PPH.
- Also associated with a reduction in breast-feeding frequency.

Peripartum risks of obesity

- Difficulty in siting regional anaesthesia due to body habitus.
- If a general anaesthesia (GA) is needed:
  - intubation is technically more difficult
  - ↑ risk of aspiration.
- Difficulty monitoring both the fetus and uterine contractions.
- Higher rate of:
  - induction of labour
  - failed induction
  - CS.
- If vaginal delivery, there is an ↑ rate of:
  - instrumental deliveries
  - shoulder dystocia
  - 3rd and 4th degree perineal tears.
- High prepregnancy BMI and weight gain in the interpregnancy interval has been shown to ↓ the success of VBAC by 50%.

Strategies for managing pregnancy in obese women

- Counselling regarding weight loss and lifestyle changes prepregnancy would be ideal.
- Increased vigilance for pre-eclampsia:
  - regular antenatal checks with urine dipstick analysis (low threshold for quantifying proteinuria with a 24h collection)
  - measure arm circumference to ensure the correct size BP cuff.
- Increased vigilance for diabetes:
  - consider random blood sugar at booking
  - urine dipstick analysis at each visit for glycosuria
  - GTT at 24–28wks (NICE).
- Increased vigilance for both macrosomia and IUGR: may need serial USS to monitor growth as SFH measurement may not be accurate.
- May require USS at 36wks gestation for presentation (to prevent an undiagnosed breech) if unable to palpate the fetus accurately.
- Further weight gain during the pregnancy should be discouraged.

Obesity in pregnancy: fetal risks

Miscarriage

Overweight women have a significantly ↑ rate of early miscarriage (both spontaneous and IVF pregnancies); this is thought to be related to ↓ insulin sensitivity.

Congenital abnormalities

✿ There is conflicting evidence regarding obesity and congenital abnormalities.

Some groups have reported an ↑ rate of neural tube defects, heart, and intestinal abnormalities, with increased serum insulin, triglycerides, uric acid, and oestrogens; in addition to increased insulin resistance, hypoxia and hypercapnia have been proposed as mechanisms for these effects.

Stillbirth

Significant risk factor for antepartum stillbirth:
- Risk of stillbirth ↑ consistently with ↑ prepregnancy BMI.
- Morbidly obese women are 3 times more likely to have a stillbirth than women with normal BMI.

Macrosomia

Well-recognized risk factor for fetal macrosomia (independent of maternal diabetes) which carries ↑ risk of:
- Instrumental delivery.
- CS.
- 3rd degree perineal tears.
- PPH.

Long-term risks for fetus
- Maternal weight is an independent determinant of childhood obesity.
- Macrosomic fetuses have an ↑ risk of adolescent and adult obesity related to an ↑ incidence of the metabolic syndrome.

Summary of risks relating to obesity in pregnancy
For the mother
- Maternal death or severe morbidity.
- Cardiac disease.
- Spontaneous 1st trimester or recurrent miscarriage.
- Pre-eclampsia.
- Gestational diabetes.
- Thromboembolism.
- Post-CS wound infection.
- Infection from other causes.
- PPH.
- Low breast-feeding rates.

For the baby
- Stillbirth and neonatal death.
- Congenital abnormalities.
- Prematurity.

Drugs in pregnancy

Prescribing in pregnancy requires the clinician to walk a delicate line between benefit (usually for the mother) and potential harm (usually to the fetus). This tends to generate anxiety and at its worst may lead to the omission of necessary treatment with significant adverse effects.

Most drugs cross the placenta to a certain extent and therefore are potentially teratogenic or fetotoxic. The exception is very large molecules, such as heparin and insulin. As women delay becoming pregnant until later life, more and more will become pregnant whilst taking medication for common conditions such as essential hypertension. Similarly, some women with conditions that were once thought incompatible with pregnancy are now becoming pregnant due to improved medication (e.g. women with CF, transplant recipients).

Timing of exposure

Drugs can cause teratogenesis in the fetus. This is defined as dysgenesis of fetal organs in terms of either structure or function. Other manifestations include IUGR and fetal death.

The timing of exposure is critical. There are three main phases of human development:

- *Pre-embryonic:*
  - conception to 17 days after (implantation and blastocyst formation)
  - adverse effects usually result in miscarriage.
- *Embryonic:*
  - day 17 to day 55 after conception (organogenesis)
  - congenital malformations likely due to the rapidly dividing tissues
  - the earlier the timing of the insult, the greater the damage.
- *Fetal phase:*
  - from 8wks after conception to term
  - any effects of drugs impact on fetal growth and function of organs.

General principles for using

- The benefits from continuing medication in pregnancy and when breast-feeding often outweigh the potential risks.
- Prepregnancy assessment should be offered to all women of childbearing age on regular medication with the option to change to alternative medication where possible.
- Try to avoid 1st trimester use if possible.
- Use drugs already used in pregnancy rather than new ones.
- Use the minimum dose to achieve the desired effect.
- The latest information on specific medications should be sought to enable the clinician to adequately assess the risks involved and allow the woman to make an informed choice.

▶ Help can be obtained from the Organization of Teratology Information Specialists (OTIS). This is funded by the Health Protection Agency to provide a 24h service on all aspects of toxicity of drugs and chemicals in pregnancy throughout the UK.

📖 http://www.otispregnancy.org/

📖 www.nyrdtc.nhs.uk/Services/teratology/teratology.html

Labour and delivery

Labour: overview

Labour is the process by which the fetus is delivered after the 24th week of gestation. The onset of labour is defined as the point when uterine contractions become regular and cervical effacement and dilatation becomes progressive. Hence, it is difficult to define the precise time of the onset. For clinical management the duration of observed labour is considered and not the duration the mother had painful contractions at home. Show and rupture of membranes may or may not be associated with labour, and these characteristics in themselves do not suggest onset of labour. In most cases, labour is characterized by:

- Onset of uterine contractions, which ↑ in frequency, duration, and strength over time.
- Cervical effacement and dilatation.
- Rupture of membranes with leakage of amniotic fluid.
- Descent of the presenting part through the birth canal.
- Birth of the baby.
- Delivery of the placenta and membranes.

The mechanism of labour

The head usually engages in the transverse position and the passage of the head and body follows a well-defined pattern through the pelvis (Fig. 6.1). Not all the diameters of the fetal head can pass through a normal pelvis (see 📖 Diameters of the female pelvis, p. 12). The process of labour therefore involves the adaptation of the fetal head to the various segments of the pelvis.

Sequence for the passage through the pelvis for a normal vertex delivery

- *Engagement and descent:* the head enters the pelvis in the occipitotransverse position with flexion ↑ as it descends.
- *Internal rotation to occipitoanterior:* occurs at the level of the ischial spines due to the forward and downward sloping of the levator ani muscles.
- *Crowning:* the head extends, distending the perineum until it is delivered.
- *Restitution:* the head rotates so that the occiput is in line with the fetal spine.
- *External rotation:* the shoulders rotate when they reach the levator muscles until the biacromial diameter is anteroposterior (the head externally rotates by the same amount).
- *Delivery of the anterior shoulder:* occurs by lateral flexion of the trunk posteriorly.
- *Delivery of the posterior shoulder:* occurs by lateral flexion of the trunk anteriorly and the rest of the body follows.

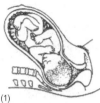

(1)
First stage of labour. The cervix
dilates. After full dilation
the head flexes futher and
descends further into the pelvis.

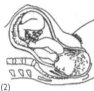

(2)
During the early second
stage the head rotates at
the levels of the ischial spine
so the occiput lies in the
anterior part of the pelvis.
In late second stage the
head broaches the vulval ring
(crowning) and the perineum
stretches over the head.

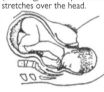

(3)
The head is born. The shoulders still lie
transversely in the midpelvis.

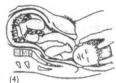

(4)
Birth of the anterior shoulder.
The shoulders rotate to lie in the
anteroposterior diameter of the
pelvic outlet. The head rotates
externally, 'restitutes', to its
direction at onset of labour.
Downward and backward traction
of the head by the birth attendant
aids delivery of the anterior shoulder.

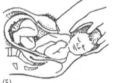

(5)
Birth of the posterior
shoulder is aided by lifting
the head upwards whilst
maintaining traction.

Fig. 6.1 Mechanism of labour and delivery. Reproduced from Collier J, Longmore
M, Brinsden M. (2003). *Oxford Handbook of Clinical Specialties*, 6th edn. Oxford:
OUP. By permission of Oxford University Press.

Labour: 1st stage

The 1st stage is divided into two phases:
- *Latent phase:* the period taken for the cervix to completely efface and dilate up to 3cm.
- *Active phase:* from 3cm to full dilatation (10cm).

Braxton Hicks contractions are mild, often irregular, non-progressive contractions that may occur from 30wks gestation (more common after 36wks) and may often be confused with labour. However, contractions in labour are painful, with a gradual increase in frequency, amplitude, and duration.

Failure to progress is suspected if:
- There is <2cm dilatation in 4h (on a 4hr action line partogram the plotted progress falls to the right).
- Slowing in progress in parous women.

▶ Consideration should also be given to effacement of cervix and descent of the head.
- If labour is slow from onset, it is 1° *dysfunctional labour.*
- If there was previous adequate progress then it is 2° *arrest.*

Some causes of poor progress in the 1st stage

- Inefficient uterine activity (*power*—commonest cause).
- Malpositions, malpresentation, or large baby (*passenger*).
- Inadequate pelvis (*passage*).
- A combination of two or more of the above.

Poor progress in the 1st stage

Assessment
- Review the history.
- Abdominal palpation, frequency, and duration of contractions.
- Review fetal condition; fetal heart rate and colour/quantity of amniotic fluid.
- Review maternal condition including hydration and analgesia.
- Vaginal assessment; cervical effacement, dilatation, caput, moulding, position, and station of the head.

Management
- Amniotomy (artifical rupture of membranes (ARM)) and reassess in 2h.
- Amniotomy + oxytocin infusion and reassess in 2h: this should always be considered in nulliparous women.
- Lower segment CS (if there is fetal distress).

⚠ For multiparous women and those with a previous CS an experienced obstetrician should review before starting oxytocin.

NICE. (2007). *Intrapartum care: management and delivery of care to women in labour.* NICE guideline CG55. ℘ http://guidance.nice.org.uk/CG55

Monitoring in labour (recorded on the partogram (Fig. 6.2))
- The FHR should be monitored every 15min (or continuously with a CTG).
- The contractions should be assessed every 30min.
- Maternal pulse should be checked hourly.
- BP and temperature should be checked 4-hourly.
- VE should be offered every 4h to assess progress.
- Maternal urine is tested 4-hourly or when passed for ketones and protein.

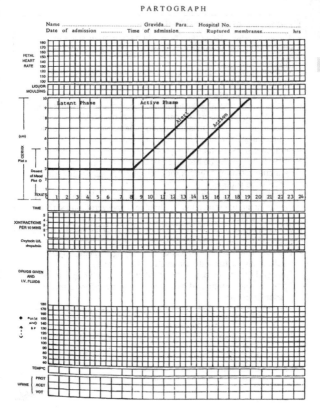

Fig. 6.2 Partogram.

Labour: 2nd stage

The 2nd stage is the time from full cervical dilatation until the baby is born.

▶ If the woman has an epidural and the CTG is reassuring, 1h is usually allowed for passive descent before active pushing is commenced.
   During this hour it is important to ensure that good contractions are maintained and oxytocin may be commenced.

▶ Birth should take place within 3h of the start of 2nd stage for nulliparous women and within 2h for multiparous women.

Description of a normal 2nd stage

- The active 2nd stage commences when the mother starts expulsive efforts using her abdominal muscles with the Valsalva manoeuvre to 'bear down'.
- Women may choose many different positions to deliver in: squatting, standing, on all fours, or supine: lithotomy is required for instrumental deliveries.
- As the head comes down, it distends the perineum and anus: a pad may be used to support the perineum and cover the anus, while the other hand is used to maintain flexion and prevent sudden deflexion and to control the rate of delivery of the head (this attempts to slow perineal distension, minimizing tears by preventing rapid delivery).
- An episiotomy may be performed if there is concern that the perineum is tearing towards the anal sphincter: episiotomy should not be used routinely.
- With the next contraction gentle traction guides the head towards the perineum until the anterior shoulder is delivered under the subpubic arch.
- Gentle traction upwards and anteriorly helps to deliver the posterior shoulder and the remainder of the trunk.
- The cord is double-clamped and cut: delaying clamping for 2–3min results in higher haematocrit levels in the neonate.
- The condition of the baby is assessed at 1, 5, and 10min using the Apgar scoring system, and if all is well, baby is handed to the mother as soon as possible.

Delay in the 2nd stage of labour

Nulliparous women

- Suspected if delivery is not imminent after 1h of active pushing: VE should be offered and amniotomy recommended.
- If not delivered in 2h: requires review by obstetrician to consider instrumental delivery or CS.

Multiparous women

- If delivery is not imminent after 1h of active pushing: requires review by obstetrician to consider instrumental delivery or CS.

⚠ Delay in the 2nd stage in a multiparous woman must always raise suspicions of malposition or disproportion.

Labour: 3rd stage

The 3rd stage is the duration from delivery of the baby to delivery of the placenta and membranes.

Active management of the 3rd stage
Consists of:
- Use of uterotonics.
- Clamping and cutting of the cord.
- Controlled cord traction.

Benefits
- ↓ Rates of PPH >1000mL.
- ↓ Mean blood loss and postnatal anaemia.
- ↓ Length of the 3rd stage.
- ↓ The need for blood transfusions.

Adverse effects
- Nausea and vomiting.
- Headache.

Physiological management of the 3rd stage
Consists of:
- No Syntometrine® or oxytocin is given.
- Cord is allowed to stop pulsating before it is clamped and cut.
- The placenta is delivered by maternal effort alone.

⚠ The cord must not be pulled and the uterus not pushed on in any direction to help to expel the placenta.

A planned physiological 3rd stage should be changed to active management in the event of:
- Haemorrhage.
- Failure to deliver the placenta within 1h.
- Maternal desire to shorten the 3rd stage.

Description of an actively managed 3rd stage

- Syntometrine® IM (ergometrine 0.5mg + oxytocin 5IU) or oxytocin 10IU IM is given as the anterior shoulder of the baby is born.
- A dish is placed at the introitus to collect the placenta and any blood loss, and the left hand is placed on the abdomen over the uterine fundus.
- As the uterus contracts to 20-wk size, the placenta separates from the uterus through the spongy layer of the decidua basalis.
- The uterus will then feel firmer, the cord will lengthen, and there is often a trickle of fresh blood (separation bleeding).
- Controlled cord traction (CCT) is applied with the right hand, whilst supporting the fundus with the left hand (Brandt–Andrew's technique).

⚠ Multiple pregnancy must be excluded before uterotonics are given.

▶ NICE recommends the use of oxytocin 10IU rather than Syntometrine® as it appears to have similar efficacy but with fewer side effects.

Care immediately after delivery

- Most complications occur in the first 2h after delivery, including;
  - PPH
  - uterine inversion
  - haematoma formation.
- Usually women are kept in the delivery unit during this time to observe: pulse, BP, temperature, uterine size and contractions, fresh bleeding per vaginum, or painful swelling of the vulva, vagina, or perineum.
- Where there is an increased risk of PPH (e.g. in multiple pregnancy), an oxytocin infusion (40U in 500mL saline) should be given prophylactically for 3–4h.
- Encouragement should be given for skin-to-skin contact as soon as possible and the mother and baby should not be separated for the 1st hour.
- Support should be provided for breast-feeding, which should be initiated in the 1st hour.
- If there are no complications during these 2h, the mother may then be transferred to the postnatal ward: some women may then go home after a further 3–4h of observation.

Induction of labour: indications

- 10–20% of all pregnancies are induced.
- Overall success rate is about 60–80% at term.
- Chance of achieving vaginal birth after IOL <34wks is <35%.
- The indication may be obstetric or medical.
- IOL on maternal request should be avoided as it is associated with risks for both mother and fetus.

Obstetric indications

- Uteroplacental insufficiency (one of the most common indications).
- Prolonged pregnancy (41–42wks).
- IUGR.
- Oligo- or anhydramnios.
- Abnormal uterine or umbilical artery Dopplers.
- Non-reassuring CTG.
- PROM.
- Severe pre-eclampsia or eclampsia after maternal stabilization.
- Intrauterine death of the fetus (IUD).
- Unexplained antepartum haemorrhage at term.
- Chorioamnionitis.

♦ There is inadequate evidence for induction for suspected fetal macrosomia. Some advocate IOL around 40–41wks with an aim of preventing further intrauterine growth and associated risks like shoulder dystocia and birth trauma.

Medical indications

With underlying maternal medical conditions, planned early IOL may potentially limit the maternal risks associated with pregnancy. Careful timing is required to balance the best interests of the mother with any potential risks of prematurity.

Such situations may include:
- Severe hypertension.
- Uncontrolled diabetes mellitus.
- Renal disease with deteriorating renal function.
- Malignancies (to facilitate definitive therapy).

Cervical ripening

Predictors for successful induction of labour

Strong predictors for a successful IOL are:
- Gestational age at induction.
- Parity.
- Modified Bishop's score of the cervix (Table 6.1): overview of the 'ripeness' of the cervix (↑ score, ↑ success).

Mechanical methods of cervical ripening

Separation of the membranes from the cervix leads to the local release of prostaglandins.
- A common method is artificial separation ('stretch and sweep').
- This requires that the cervical os admits a finger, and involves digitally separating the membranes from the cervix.
- It is uncomfortable and may lead to some bleeding.
- 30% will go into spontaneous labour in <7 days.
- In the majority it results in a more favourable cervix.

Pharmacological methods

Prostaglandins (PGE2 = dinoprostone)
- Preferred agents for cervical ripening.
- Usually given intravaginally into the posterior fornix.
- The gel form is absorbed well.
- Tablet forms are easier to remove if hyperstimulation occurs (5–7%).
- Vaginal prostaglandins (3mg tablets, 2mg gel) increase vaginal delivery rates within 24h with no increase in operative delivery rates.

Oxytocin infusion
- Has been shown to increase cervical prostaglandin levels.
- As most receptors are located in the myometrium, it is more suitable for initiating uterine contractions.
- Best used where membranes have ruptured, whether spontaneously or after amniotomy.

▶ Other agents have been tried but there is limited evidence for their safety and efficacy.

Other methods

There is no evidence to suggest that the following are effective in cervical ripening or IOL:
- Sexual intercourse.
- Herbal remedies (raspberry leaf tea).
- Nipple stimulation.
- Acupuncture.
- Castor oil.

Table 6.1 Modified Bishop's score: to assess the favourability for induction of labour. A total score of >8 indicates a favourable cervix

Score	0	1	2
Position of cervix	Posterior	Axial	Anterior
Length of cervix	2cm	1cm	<0.5cm
Consistency of cervix	Firm	Soft	Soft and stretchy
Dilatation of cervix	0	1cm	>2cm
Station of the presenting part (distance in cm in relation to the ischial spines)	−2	−1	0

Data from Kennedy *et al.*, 1982.

Induction of labour: methods

Amniotomy
- ARM or amniotomy releases local prostaglandins causing cervical ripening and myometrial contractions.
- If regular, painful uterine contractions are not initiated or there are no cervical changes after 2h, then oxytocin infusion should be commenced.
- Starting oxytocin at the time of amniotomy has been shown to decrease the induction–delivery interval, thereby decreasing both the fetal and maternal risk of sepsis.
- ARM alone is not recommended for IOL.

Prostaglandins for induction of labour
- A CTG should be performed 30min before, as well as after insertion of prostaglandins to confirm fetal well-being and to detect possible hyperstimulation.
- VE after 6h: if the cervix is not favourable, another dose may be administered (>2 doses need to be reviewed by a consultant; multiparous women seldom require more than 1 dose).
- Oxytocin should not be started for 6h to avoid the risk of uterine hyperstimulation.

Synthetic oxytocin for induction or augmentation of labour
- It should be started on a low dose (1–4mU/min).
- It is increased (usually doubled) every 30min to achieve optimal contractions (3–4 every 10min, each lasting 40–60s).
- Continuous CTG monitoring should be used:
  - the sensitivity of the myometrium to oxytocin ↑ during labour and it may be necessary to ↓ the rate of infusion as labour advances
  - infusion pumps should be used to carefully control the amount given and avoid the risk of uterine hyperstimulation.

✒ Women should be advised that the use of oxytocin will reduce the length of labour and may reduce the operative births due to dystocia without any major impact on neonatal outcomes (Cochrane review).

Risks and complications of IOL

- *Prematurity:*
  - may be iatrogenic (severe pre-eclampsia)
  - unintentional (failure to correctly assess the gestational age).
- Cord prolapse with rupture of membranes if the presenting part is not engaged.
- *Side effects of pharmacological agents used:*
  - pain or discomfort
  - uterine hyperstimulation
  - fetal distress
  - uterine rupture (rare but ↑ in grand multipara or a scarred uterus).
- Prostaglandins rarely cause non-selective stimulation of other smooth muscle leading to:
  - nausea and vomiting
  - diarrhoea
  - bronchoconstriction (caution in asthmatics)
  - maternal pyrexia may result due to the effect on thermoregulation in the hypothalamus.
- CS due to failed induction.
- Atonic post-partum haemorrhage.
- Intrauterine infection with prolonged induction.

⚠ Oxytocin has the properties of ADH, and U&E should be checked if it has been used for >12h as it may very rarely cause dilutional hyponatraemia.

Induction of labour: special circumstances

Prelabour rupture of membranes

Prostaglandins should be used before starting syntocinon for IOL if the cervix is unfavourable.

Stabilizing induction

This is carried out when the presenting part is not engaged or when there is an unstable lie, to avoid the risk of cord prolapse.
- The head is 'stabilized' by an assistant holding it suprapubically and if possible by pushing the head into the pelvic brim.
- Amniotomy is performed.
- Once cord prolapse is excluded, oxytocin infusion is started.

▶ This is usually performed in the delivery unit with the theatre and team available should an emergency of cord prolapse occur. It is good to have an epidural that could be topped up sufficiently to allow an emergency CS.

Grand multipara (≥ para 5)

⚠ The risk of uterine rupture is higher and hence caution should be exercised.

- Prostaglandin gel should only be used in exceptional circumstances.
- Onset of labour is awaited for up to 4h after ARM.
- In the absence of contractions oxytocin infusion can be started and titrated to get 3–4 every 10min, each lasting >40s.
- Once contractions are established it should be possible to stop the oxytocin as most will continue to labour and deliver normally.

⚠ Malpresentation (obstructed labour) must be excluded before starting oxytocin.

Induction for intrauterine death at term

The WHO and RCOG Guidelines recommend misoprostol 25 micrograms every 2–4h.
- As this strength is not available in the UK 200 microgram tablets can be dissolved in 40mL water and 5mL aliquots administered.
- Although uniformity of strength cannot be guaranteed it is potentially safer than administering a higher dose.

IOL with previous CS

⚠ The risk of scar dehiscence with previous uterine surgery is:
- 5:1000 with spontaneous labour.
- 8:1000 with use of oxytocin.
- 24:1000 with prostaglandins.

▶ Women should be counselled regarding these risks and have continuous CTG monitoring throughout the whole of the induction process when contractions are present.

▶ Facilities should be available for immediate CS should there be a scar rupture and fetal bradycardia.

Further reading

Kennedy JH, Stewart P, Barlow DH, *et al.* (1982). Induction of labour: a comparison of a single prostaglandin E2 vaginal tablet with amniotomy and intravenous oxytocin. *Br J Obstet Gynaecol* **89**:704–7.

NICE. (2011). *Induction of labour*, NICE guideline CG70. ✎ http://www.nice.org.uk/CG70

RCOG. (2011). Green-top guidelines. *Induction of labour for intrauterine death at term*. ✎ www.rcog.org.uk

WHO. (2011). Recommendations on induction of labour. ✎ http://whqlibdoc.who.int/publications/2011/9789241501156_Eng.pdf

Fetal surveillance in labour: overview

- It is estimated that 10% of CP is due to intrapartum hypoxia (the rest may be attributed to antenatal).
- Blood supply to the placental pool is restricted, with contractions (especially in the 2nd stage) placing a physiological strain on the fetus.
- Ability to withstand the stress is dependent on fetal reserve.
- A fetus that was coping in the antenatal period but has no extra reserve may decompensate in labour.

Intrapartum surveillance

- The options for intrapartum surveillance are:
  - intermittent auscultation (IA)
  - continuous CTG, also known as electronic fetal monitoring (EFM).
- On admission in labour, an assessment should be made to identify fetal and maternal risk factors (see Boxes 6.1 and 6.2).
- If the woman has no risk factors she should be offered intermittent auscultation performed for a full minute after a contraction:
  - at least every 15min in the 1st stage
  - every 5min or after every other contraction in the 2nd stage.

Electronic fetal monitoring

- Results in:
  - ↑ intervention and operative delivery rates
  - no marked ↓ in CP.
- Most likely because:
  - CTG is not specific enough in detecting fetal hypoxia
  - failure to consider the clinical situation
  - poor interpretation
  - delay in taking action
  - intrapartum hypoxia as a cause of CP is rare.
- Additional tests, such as fetal scalp blood sampling in labour, are required to ↑ specificity.

▶ Some centres use fetal ECG ST waveform analysis (STAN) to improve the positive predictive value of the CTG.

▶ Cochrane review suggested that there is reduction of fetal scalp blood sampling and total operative delivery, but not CS and there is no reduction in poor outcome of the neonate.

Box 6.1 Antenatal risk factors that should prompt recommendation of EFM in labour

Maternal
- Previous CS.
- Cardiac problems.
- Pre-eclampsia.
- Prolonged pregnancy (>42wks).
- Prelabour rupture of membranes (>24h).
- Induction of labour.
- Diabetes.
- Antepartum haemorrhage.
- Other significant maternal medical conditions.

Fetal
- IUGR.
- Prematurity.
- Oligohydramnios.
- Abnormal Doppler velocimetry.
- Multiple pregnancy.
- Meconium-stained liquor.
- Breech presentation.

Box 6.2 Intrapartum risks requiring EFM

- Oxytocin augmentation.
- Epidural analgesia.
- Intrapartum vaginal bleeding.
- Pyrexia >37.5°C.
- Fresh meconium staining of liquor.
- Abnormal FHR on intermittent auscultation.
- Prolonged labour.

Further reading

Cochrane review of ST waveform analysis for intrapartum surveillance. www.cochrane.org
NICE. (2007). *Intrapartum care guidelines.* publications.nice.org.uk/intrapartum-care-cg55/guidance#complicated-labour-monitoring-babies-in-labour

Fetal surveillance: cardiotocography

Definitions of terms used in EFM

- *Baseline rate*: mean level of the FHR when this is stable, and after exclusion of accelerations and decelerations.
- *Baseline variability*: degree to which the baseline varies, i.e. bandwidth of baseline after exclusion of accelerations and decelerations. Variability of 5–25 beats/min is defined as normal, 0–5 beats/min as reduced, and >25 beats/min as saltatory.
- *Acceleration*: a transient rise in FHR by at least 15 beats over the baseline lasting for 15s or more (Fig. 6.3).
- *Deceleration*: a reduction in the baseline of 15 beats or more for more than 15s.

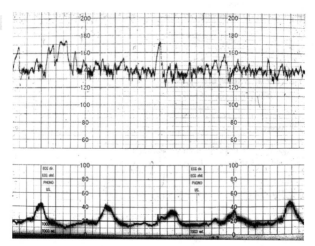

Fig. 6.3 Cardiotocographic trace.

▶ The most useful features in assessing fetal well-being are normal variability and presence of accelerations.

⚠ Always be concerned about a CTG if you cannot identify the baseline rate.

Causes of decreased baseline variability
- Fetal hypoxia.
- Fetal sleep cycle (should be for <40 and maximally 90min).
- Fetal malformation (CNS or cardiac) or arrhythmias.
- Administration of drugs including:
  - methyldopa
  - magnesium sulphate
  - narcotic analgesics
  - tranquillizers
  - barbiturates
  - general anaesthesia.
- Severe prematurity.
- Fetal heart block.
- Fetal anomalies.

Fetal surveillance: cardiotocography abnormalities

Abnormalities in baseline rate

A *bradycardia* is a baseline FHR of less than 110 beats/min.

- 100–110 beats/min is moderate baseline bradycardia and on its own is not considered to be associated with fetal compromise if the baseline variability is normal and accelerations are present.
- A baseline below 100 beats/min should raise the possibility of hypoxia or other pathology.

⚠ Beware of maternal heart rate being recorded as the FHR.

A *tachycardia* is a baseline FHR >160 beats/min and is associated with maternal pyrexia and tachycardia, prematurity, and fetal acidosis.

- 160–180 beats/min is moderate baseline tachycardia and on its own is probably not indicative of hypoxia if the baseline variability is normal and accelerations are present.
- A baseline >180 beats/min should always raise suspicion of underlying pathology.

Decelerations

- *Early decelerations:* the peak of the deceleration coincides with the peak of the contraction (Fig. 6.4). This is related to head compression and, therefore, should only be seen in active second stage of labour.
- *Late decelerations:* have at least a 15s time lag between the peak of the contraction and the nadir of the deceleration (Fig. 6.5).

⚠ They may be suggestive of acidosis, especially if accompanied with tachycardia and reduced baseline variability.

⚠ Shallow, late decelerations in the presence of reduced baseline variability on a non-reactive trace should be of particular concern and may even be pre-terminal, especially if there are associated clinical risks including IUGR, absent FM, bleeding, infection, prolonged pregnancy, or severe pre-eclampsia.

- *Variable decelerations:* have variable pattern in timing, size, and shape and are associated with cord compression (Fig. 6.6).
  - *typical* variables are U or V shaped, quick to drop and to recover, and often have 'shouldering' (not usually associated with hypoxia)
  - *atypical* variables have a duration of >60s, a loss >60 beats from the baseline, slow recovery, a combined variable, and a late deceleration component
  - with progressive hypoxia the decelerations become deeper and wider with rising baseline rate. Subsequent reduction of baseline variability suggests possible fetal acidosis.

Other abnormalities *Sinusoidal pattern:* a rare undulating pattern (sine wave) with little, or no, variability. Can indicate significant fetal anaemia, but in short spells (<10min) may be a result of fetal behaviour (thumb-sucking).

⚠ A sinusoidal pattern should always be taken seriously. Blood group antibodies, Kleihauer test, and a scan for middle cerebral artery velocity to detect fetal anaemia may be indicated.

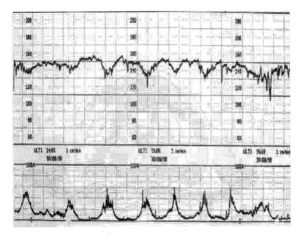

Fig. 6.4 Cardiotocograph trace with early decelerations.

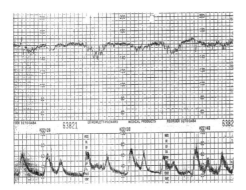

Fig. 6.5 Cardiotocograph trace with late decelerations.

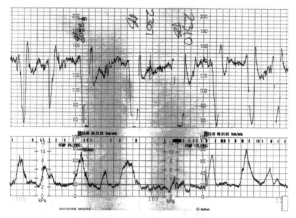

Fig. 6.6 Cardiotocograph trace with variable decelerations.

Fetal surveillance: cardiotocography classification

In order to help with the difficulties encountered when assessing a CTG a classification scheme was introduced that can be used to define a CTG as normal, suspicious, or pathological (Table 6.2).

Table 6.2 Fetal heart-rate feature classification

	Baseline (beats/min)	Variability (beats/min)	Decelerations	Accelerations
Reassuring	110–160	≥5	None	Present
Non-reassuring	100–109 161–180	<5 for ≥40 but <90min	Early decelerations Variable decelerations being present for 50% of contractions for ≥90min Single prolonged deceleration up to 3min	The absence of accelerations in an otherwise normal CTG is of uncertain significance
Abnormal	<100 >180 Sinusoidal pattern for ≥10min	<5 for ≥90min	Atypical variable decelerations Late decelerations being present for >50% of contractions for ≥30min Single prolonged deceleration >3min	

NICE. (2011). *Intrapartum care: management and delivery of care to women in labour.* CG55. http://www.nice.org.uk

CTG classification using Table 6.2

• *Normal:* all four features are in the reassuring category.
• *Suspicious:* no more than one non-reassuring feature when analysing the CTG.
• *Pathological:* two or more non-reassuring features or one or more abnormal features.

Maternal factors that may contribute to an abnormal CTG

• The woman's position: advise her to adopt left lateral.
• Hypotension.
• Vaginal examination.
• Emptying bladder or bowels.
• Vomiting.
• Vasovagal episodes.
• Siting and topping-up of regional anaesthesia.

Fetal blood sampling

• This is used to improve the specificity of CTG in the detection of fetal hypoxia.
• It should be obtained if the trace is pathological, unless obvious immediate delivery may be required (e.g. bradycardia of <80 beats/min for >3min).
• The woman should be in left lateral.

Interpretation of the FBS results

• *Normal (pH ≥7.25):* repeat FBS within 1h if CTG remains pathological.
• *Borderline (pH 7.21–7.24):* repeat FBS within 30min if CTG remains pathological.
• *Abnormal (pH ≤7.20):* immediate delivery.

Meconium-stained liquor

Meconium is made up of water, bile pigment, mucus, and amniotic fluid debris. Detection in amniotic fluid causes anxiety as it is associated with ↑ perinatal morbidity and mortality; it may be aspirated by fetus.

- Meconium-stained amniotic fluid (MSAF) is rare in preterm infants (<5%) and is associated with infection and chorioamnionitis.
- Incidence of MSAF gradually increases from 36 to 42wks.
- Passage of meconium signifies the maturation of central nervous and gastrointestinal systems. Sometimes hypoxia causes peristalsis of the bowel and relaxation of anal sphincters resulting in MSAF.

Meconium aspiration syndrome

- Occurs in 1:1000 births in Europe.
- May happen *in utero* when fetal breathing movements draw amniotic fluid into the airway. Fetal gasping *in utero* is thought to be associated with prolonged decelerations that cause transient hypoxia, as 50% of meconium aspiration syndrome (MAS) occur in fetuses that were not acidotic in labour.
- Meconium:
  - causes mechanical blockage of the airway
  - acts as a chemical irritant, causing pneumonitis and alveolar collapse
  - predisposes to secondary bacterial infection.

⚠ Suction of the mouth and upper airway immediately after delivery is not currently recommended if the baby is active and crying.

⚠ If the newborn has respiratory difficulty, meconium should be cleared from the oro- and nasopharynx and, if needed, from the trachea by using a laryngoscopy.

▶ This will not help with pre-existing *in utero* aspiration.

Classification of MSAF

- *Grade 1 (light):* meconium lightly stains the amniotic fluid that is usually copious.
- *Grade 2 (moderate):* dark green staining of amniotic fluid that appears opalescent.
- *Grade 3 (thick):* thick, opaque meconium in scanty amniotic fluid ('pea soup meconium').

Management of meconium-stained liquor

- Recommend immediate induction of labour if prelabour rupture of membranes.
- Advise continuous fetal monitoring.
- Advise delivery in a unit able to provide fetal blood sampling and advanced neonatal life support at birth:
  - if the baby is born with depressed vital signs it will require laryngoscopy and suction by a healthcare professional trained in advanced neonatal life support
  - if the baby is born in good condition it will still require close monitoring for 12h.

Operative vaginal delivery: overview

CS in the 2nd stage of labour is associated with increased morbidity to the mother. Instrumental vaginal delivery helps to avoid maternal and perinatal morbidity and mortality and an emergency CS.

In the UK, the operative vaginal delivery rate is stable at between 10 and 15%. Important to appreciate that forceps and ventouse are complementary to each other and that operator's skill and experience, as well as clinical findings, should decide which one to use.

▶ If in doubt, senior help must be called.

Indications for instrumental delivery

Maternal
- Exhaustion.
- Prolonged 2nd stage:
  - >1h of active pushing in multiparous women
  - >2h in primiparous women.
- Medical indications for avoiding Valsalva manouevre, such as:
  - severe cardiac disease
  - hypertensive crisis
  - uncorrected cerebral vascular malformations.
- Pushing is not possible (paraplegia or tetraplegia).

Fetal
- Fetal compromise.
- To control the after-coming head of breech (forceps).

▶ It is important to discuss with the woman why an operative delivery is indicated, the instrument chosen, the likelihood of success, and the alternatives available (emergency CS).

⚠ Consent (verbal or written) must be obtained by explaining the indication and it should be recorded.

Complications of operative vaginal delivery

- Forceps are associated with increased maternal trauma (including anal sphincter trauma).
- Rotational forceps may cause spiral tears of the vagina.
- Fetal injuries with forceps are rare but may occur (mostly due to incorrect application of the blades) including:
  - facial nerve palsy
  - skull fractures
  - orbital injury
  - intracranial haemorrhage.
- Ventouse is associated with fetal injuries including:
  - scalp lacerations and avulsions (rarely, alopecia in the long term)
  - cephalohaematoma
  - retinal haemorrhage
  - rarely, subgaleal haemorrhage and/or intracranial haemorrhage.

⚠ The use of sequential instruments (usually forceps after a failed ventouse) is associated with an increased risk of fetal trauma when attempted with no significant descent.

▶ It is not uncommon for ventouse to slip when the head is at the introitus, then delivery is completed by a lift-out forceps—hence, the discrepancy in the Cochrane review of more failed ventouse deliveries, but a lower CS rate compared with forceps deliveries.

Operative vaginal delivery: instruments

Forceps

These consist of curved blades that sit around the fetal head and allow traction to be applied along the 'flexion point' of the head (3cm in front of the occiput). This is usually to speed up delivery, but may be used to slow rate of the head in a breech delivery (see Fig. 6.7).

Low cavity forceps (Wrigley's)
- Short and light.
- These are also the forceps used at CS.

Mid-cavity non-rotational forceps (Neville-Barnes', Haig Ferguson, Simpson's)
- Used when the sagittal suture is in the direct anteroposterior position (usually direct occipito-anterior (DOA)).
- Malposition (direct occipito-posterior (DOP) or direct occipito-lateral (DOL)) can be corrected manually between contractions and the blades applied once the head is in the DOA position.

Mid-cavity rotational forceps (Keilland's)
- Reduced pelvic curve on the blades of the forceps allows rotation about the axis of the handle.
- Helps to correct asynclitism and malposition.
- Must only be attempted by an experienced operator.

Vacuum extraction (ventouse)

Works on the principle of creating 'negative pressure' to allow scalp tissues to be sucked into the cup. This creates artificial caput called a 'chignon'. The cup is held in place by the atmospheric pressure on the cup against the negative pressure created.

⚠ It should not be used at <34wks gestation (see Fig. 6.7).

Metal cup
- Available with 60, 50, or 40mm standard anterior (for positions) or posterior cup (for occipito-lateral (OL) or occipito-posterior (OP) positions).
- Pressure is created by a suction pump.
- Excessive traction is likely to cause fetal trauma.

Soft cup
- Soft and easier to apply (important in women without epidural) for OA positions.
- Moulds around the fetal head covering a greater surface area.
- Causes fewer scalp abrasions.

Kiwi Omni Cup™
- Single-use cup.
- Pressure created with hand pump (quick in an emergency).
- Allows application to flexion point in OL and OP position.

Comparison of forceps and vacuum extractor

- Ventouse is more likely to fail.
- Ventouse is more likely to cause fetal trauma such as:
  - cephalohaematoma
  - retinal haemorrhage.
- Ventouse is more likely to be associated with maternal concerns about the baby.
- Forceps are more likely to cause significant maternal genital tract trauma.
- There is:
  - slightly less CS delivery with ventouse delivery
  - no difference in low 5min Apgar scores
  - no difference in need for neonatal phototherapy.

▶ Bottom line—ventouse appears safer for mother but forceps may be safer for baby.

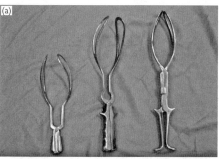

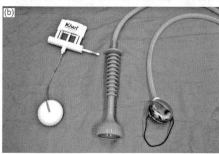

Fig. 6.7 (a) Forceps (Wrigley's, Neville-Barnes', Keilland's). (b) Ventouse cups (Kiwi Omni Cup™, silc cup, Bird's cup). With permission of Clinical Innovations Europe Ltd, 2008, and Menox AB, Goteborg, Sweden, 2008.

Operative vaginal delivery: criteria

▶ The techniques involved with both ventouse and forceps can only be learned under direct supervision from an experienced operator and are therefore not described in the book.

The following criteria should be satisfied before attempting an operative vaginal delivery. This may be best remembered as *'FORCEPS'*.

- F **F**ully dilated cervix (i.e. confirm 2nd stage).
- O **O**bstruction should be excluded (head ≤1/5 palpable abdominally).
- R **R**uptured membranes.
  Review the procedure (if forceps blades don't lock, or lack of rotation or descent despite three attempts at traction).
- C **C**onsent.
  Catheterize bladder ('in and out' technique, indwelling catheters must be removed).
  Check instrument prior to application.
- E **E**xplain the procedure to the patient.
  Epidural (or pudendal) analgesia.
  Examine the genital tract to exclude genital tract trauma.
- P **C**heck **P**resentation and **P**osition of the head (must be sure before applying any instrument).
  Power: are the contractions effective? Correct with syntocinon—(propulsion is better than extraction).
  Correct **P**lacement of forceps blades or ventouse cup (ensure no maternal tissues are caught).
- S **S**tation of the presenting part (not above ischial spines).
  Senior help should be called if needed.

See Fig. 6.8.

Further reading

RCOG. (2011). *Green-top guideline 26: Operative vaginal delivery.* ✍ http://www.rcog.org.uk/womens-health/clinical-guidance/operative-vaginal-delivery-green-top-26

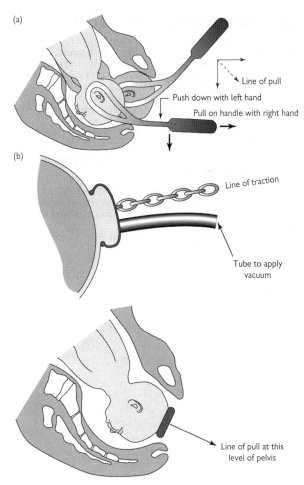

(a)

Line of pull

Push down with left hand

Pull on handle with right hand

(b)

Line of traction

Tube to apply vacuum

Line of pull at this level of pelvis

Fig. 6.8 Assisted delivery techniques: (a) forceps delivery; (b) ventouse delivery. Reproduced from Chamberlain G, Steer P. (1999). ABC of labour care: operative delivery. *Br Med J* **318**: 1260–4. With permission. © BMJ Publishing Group Ltd 1999.

Operative vaginal delivery: trial

This term is used when it is not possible to determine with sufficient confidence that an instrumental delivery will be successful. It should, therefore, take place in theatre, where it is possible to move to an immediate CS, avoiding failed delivery in delivery room and subsequent delay in performing CS, which may compromise fetal well-being.

• The woman should be fully informed of the likely success and sign a consent form for 'Trial of instrumental vaginal delivery +/– emergency CS'.

• If procedure is abandoned, assistance may be required to 'push head up' from vagina during CS as head may be impacted in pelvis.

⚠ Senior obstetric input is recommended in 2nd stage CS, especially after a failed trial of instrumental delivery.

When to abandon and deliver by emergency Caesarean

• No evidence of progressive descent with each pull (care must be taken with the ventouse to not interpret increasing caput as descent of the head).

• Where delivery is not imminent following three pulls of a correctly applied instrument by an experienced operator.

Risk factors for failed operative vaginal delivery

• BMI >30.
• EFW >4000g or clinically big baby.
• OP position.
• Mid-cavity delivery or if head is >1/5 palpable abdominally.

Episiotomy

More than 85% of women delivering vaginally in the UK will sustain some degree of perineal trauma. Episiotomy is a surgical incision to enlarge the vaginal introitus. The decision to perform an episiotomy is made by the birth attendant. The worldwide rates of episiotomy vary dramatically (14% in England, 8% in the Netherlands, 50% in the USA). There is clear evidence to recommend a *restricted* use of episiotomy.

WHO recommends that episiotomy should be considered in the following circumstances:
- Complicated vaginal delivery:
  - breech
  - shoulder dystocia
  - forceps
  - ventouse.
- If there is extensive lower genital tract scarring:
  - female genital mutilation
  - poorly healed 3rd or 4th degree tears.
- When there is fetal distress.

▶ It is also often recommended if there is an indication that there may be extensive perineal trauma such as the appearance of multiple vaginal/perineal tears or perineal button-holing.

Types of episiotomy
- Mediolateral episiotomy extends from the fourchette laterally (thus reducing the risk of anal sphincter injury).
- Midline episiotomy extends from the fourchette towards the anus (common in the USA, but not recommended in the UK).

How to perform an episiotomy (see Fig. 6.9)
- If the woman does not have a working regional block (epidural) then the perineum should be infiltrated with lidocaine (lignocaine).
- Two fingers should be placed between the baby's head and the perineum (to protect the baby).
- Sharp scissors are used to make a single cut in the perineum about 3–4cm long (ideally this should be at the height of the contraction when the perineum is at its thinnest).

▶ Every effort should be made to anaesthetize the perineum early to provide sufficient time for effect.

▶ It will cause bleeding so must not be done too early and should be repaired as soon as possible.

⚠ Always check for any extension or other tears (including a PR examination to ensure no trauma to the anal sphincter).

General complications of perineal trauma including episiotomy
- Bleeding.
- Haematoma.
- Pain.
- Infection.
- Scarring, with potential disruption to the anatomy.
- Dyspareunia.
- Very rarely, fistula formation.

⚠ Women who have undergone female genital mutilation should be seen antenatally and de-infibulation discussed. However, it they present in labour the episiotomy should be anterior and upwards. (See 📖 Female genital mutilation, p. 470).

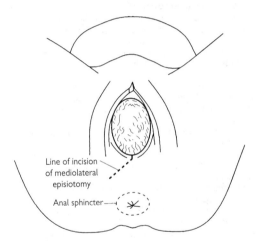

Line of incision of mediolateral episiotomy

Anal sphincter

Fig. 6.9 Performing an episiotomy. Adapted from Wyatt JP, Illingworth RN, Graham CA, et al. (eds) (2006). *Oxford Handbook of Emergency Medicine.* Oxford: OUP. By permission of Oxford University Press.

Perineal tears

Classification of perineal tears
- *1st-degree:* injury to the skin only.
- *2nd-degree:* injury to the perineum involving perineal muscles (includes episiotomy).
- *3rd-degree:* injury to the perineum involving the anal sphincter complex:
  - 3a: <50% of the external anal sphincter (EAS) thickness torn
  - 3b: >50% of the EAS thickness torn
  - 3c: internal anal sphincter (IAS) torn.
- *4th-degree:* injury to perineum involving the anal sphincter complex (EAS and IAS) and the anal/rectal epithelium.

Principles of basic perineal repair (Fig. 6.10)
- Suture as soon as possible to reduce bleeding and infection risk.
- A rectal examination is recommended before starting, to ensure there is no trauma to the anal sphincter complex.
- The attendant should have adequate training for the type of tear: difficult trauma should be repaired in theatre under regional or general anaesthesia by an experienced operator.
- The woman should preferably be in lithotomy position.
- There should be a good light source and adequate analgesia.
- Use of rapid-absorption polyglactin suture material is associated with a significant reduction in pain.
- Apex of the cut should be identified and the suturing started from just above this point.
- A loose, continuous non-locking suturing technique used to appose each layer is associated with less short-term pain than the traditional interrupted method.
- Perineal skin should be sutured with a subcuticular suture as this is associated with less pain.
- Anatomical apposition should be as accurate as possible and consideration given to cosmetic results.
- Rectal examination after completion ensures that no suture has accidentally passed into the rectum or anal canal.

⚠ Needle and swabs must be counted afterwards (lost swabs are a recurring cause of litigation in obstetrics).

Further reading
RCOG. (2007). *Green-top guideline 23: Perineal repair.* ♒ http://www.rcog.or.uk

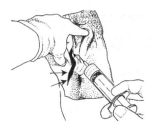

(1)
Swab the vulva towards the perineum. Infiltrate with 1% lignocaine → (arrows).

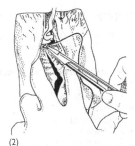

(2)
Place tampon with attached tape in upper vagina. Insert 1st suture above apex of vaginal cut (not too deep as underlying rectal mucosa nearby).

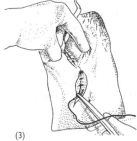

(3)
Bring together vaginal edges with continuous stitches placed 1cm apart. Knot at introitus under the skin. Appose divided levator ani muscles with 2 or 3 interrupted sutures.

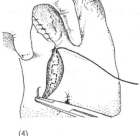

(4)
Close perineal skin (subcuticular) continuous stitch is shown here.

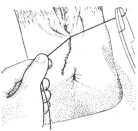

(5)
When stitching finished, remove tampon and examine vagina (to check for retained swabs). Do a PR to check that apical sutures have not penetrated rectum.

Fig. 6.10 Episiotomy repair. Reproduced from Collier J, Longmore M, Brinsden M. (2006). *Oxford Handbook of Clinical Specialties*, 7th edn. Oxford: OUP. By permission of Oxford University Press.

Third- and fourth-degree tears

Approximately 1–3% of vaginal deliveries will result in injury to the anal sphinter. Prediction and prevention are both difficult.

Factors associated with increased risk of anal sphincter trauma

- Forceps delivery.
- Nulliparity.
- Shoulder dystocia.
- 2nd stage >1h.
- Persistent OP position.
- Midline episiotomy.
- Birth weight >4kg.
- Epidural anaesthesia.
- Induction of labour.

Management of 3rd- and 4th-degree tears

- All women sustaining genital tract injury should be carefully examined before suturing is started (including a rectal examination).
- Repair must be carried out by a trained senior clinician in theatre with adequate analgesia.
- The technique used can be end to end or overlapping for the EAS using either polydioxanone suture (PDS) or vicryl suture material.
- The IAS should be repaired with vicryl using interrupted sutures.
- Women must receive broad-spectrum antibiotics and stool softeners.
- They should receive physiotherapy input.
- Ideally, they should be reviewed 6wks later by an obstetrician or gynaecologist.
- Women must be warned of the risk of incontinence of faeces, fluid, and flatus: those experiencing symptoms at 6wks should be referred to a specialist gynaecologist or colorectal surgeon for investigation with endoanal ultra sonography.
- Around 60–80% will have a good result and be asymptomatic at 12mths.
- For future deliveries they should be advised that the result may not be so good from a 2nd repair: if symptomatic they should be given the option of delivery by CS.

Further reading

RCOG. (2007). *Green-top guideline 29: Third- and fourth-degree tears—management.* ॐ http://www.rcog.org.uk/womens-health/clinical-guidance/management-third-and-fourth-degree-perineal-tears-green-top-29

Caesarean section: overview

Background
- CS involves delivery of the fetus through a direct incision in the abdominal wall and the uterus.
- The rates vary in different countries and populations:
  - the overall CS rate for nulliparous women in the UK has increased to about 24%
  - for multiparous women who have not previously had a CS the rate is <5%
  - for women who have had at least one previous CS the rate is increased to about 67%; most are elective.

Caesarean section

Associated with a higher incidence of:
- Abdominal pain.
- Venous thromboembolism.
- Bladder or ureteric injury.
- Hysterectomy.
- Very rarely maternal death.

Associated with a lower incidence of:
- Perineal pain.
- Urinary incontinence.
- Uterovaginal prolapse.
- Long-term effect of the last two are debated.

Some interventions to decrease morbidity from CS
- Preoperative haemoglobin check and correction of anaemia.
- Intraoperative prophylactic antibiotics given just before skin incision.
- Risk assessment and appropriate thrombo-prophylaxis (graduated stockings, hydration, early mobilization, and low molecular weight heparin).
- In-dwelling bladder catheterization during the procedure.
- Antacids and H_2 receptor analogues before surgery.
- Antiemetics as appropriate.
- Regional rather than general anaesthesia.
- The risk of hypotension can be reduced using:
  - intravenous ephedrine or phenylephrine infusion
  - volume preloading with crystalloid or colloid
  - lateral tilt of 15°.
- General anaesthesia for emergency CS should include preoxygenation and rapid sequence induction to reduce the risk of aspiration.

Vaginal birth after CS

- Uterine rupture is very rare but is increased with VBAC:
  - 50:10 000 with VBAC and spontaneous onset of labour
  - 1:10 000 with repeat CS.
- Intrapartum infant death is rare: 1:1000—the same as for primiparous women
- EFM is recommended during labour as FHR changes may be the earliest signs of scar rupture.
- Women should deliver in a unit where there is immediate access to CS and on-site blood transfusion.
- With induction of labour, there is increased risk of uterine rupture:
  - 8:1000 if oxytocin infusion is used
  - 24:1000 if prostaglandins are used.
- Women with both previous CS and a previous vaginal birth are more likely to give birth vaginally.

Caesarean section: indications

The main indications for CS are:
- Repeat CS.
- Fetal compromise.
- 'Failure to progress' in labour.
- Breech presentation.

✦ Maternal request accounts for 7% of CS, but is not, on its own, an indication for CS.

> ## Categories to determine the timing of CS
> - Immediate threat to the life of the woman or fetus (immediate, 'crash CS').
> - Maternal or fetal compromise, which is not immediately life-threatening (urgent).
> - No maternal or fetal compromise but needs early delivery (scheduled).
> - Delivery timed to suit woman and staff (elective).

⚠ In cases of suspected or confirmed acute fetal compromise, delivery should be as soon as possible. The accepted standard for category 1 (immediate) CS is within 30min.

Indications for category 1 CS
- Placental abruption with abnormal FHR or uterine irritability.
- Cord prolapse.
- Scar rupture.
- Prolonged bradycardia.
- Scalp pH <7.20.

Indications for category 2 CS
- Failure to progress with pathological CTG.

Indications for category 3 (scheduled) CS
- Severe pre-eclampsia.
- IUGR with poor fetal function tests.
- Failed induction of labour.

Indications for category 4 (elective) CS
- Term singleton breech (if ECV is contraindicated or has failed).
- Twin pregnancy with non-cephalic 1st twin.
- Maternal HIV.
- Primary genital herpes in the 3rd trimester.
- Placenta praevia.
- Previous hysterotomy or classical CS.

▶ Elective CS is usually carried out after 39wks unless indicated, as the risk of respiratory morbidity (transient tachypnoea of the newborn) is increased at lower gestational ages.

Caesarean section: types

Lower uterine segment incision

The two main types of skin incision are:
- *Pfannenstiel incision:* a straight horizontal incision 2cm above the symphysis pubis—superior cosmetic result.
- *Joel–Cohen incision:* also a straight horizontal incision, but higher, about 3cm below the level of the anterior superior iliac spines (ASIS)—allows quicker entry to the abdomen.

A transverse incision in the uterine lower segment is used in >90% of CS as it is associated with:
- Reduced adhesion formation.
- Decreased blood loss.
- Lower incidence of scar dehiscence in subsequent pregnancies.

However, if the lower segment is poorly developed, a low transverse incision carries a risk of lateral extension into the uterine vessels and haemorrhage.
Following delivery of the fetus and completion of the 3rd stage, the lower uterine segment is closed in one or two layers.

◆ Double-layer closure is usually practiced, but research comparing single- with double-layer has no long-term results to compare scar integrity, although short-term morbidity showed no difference.

Classical CS

This involves a vertical incision into the upper uterine segment. It is rarely performed, but indications may include:
- Structural abnormality of the uterus.
- Difficult access to the lower uterine segment due to fibroids or severe adhesions over the lower segment.
- Postmortem CS delivery (if the fetus is viable).
- Anterior placenta praevia with abnormally vascular lower uterine segment.
- Contraction ring.
- Very preterm fetus (especially breech presentation) where the lower segment is poorly formed.
- Elective Caesarean hysterectomy.
- Transverse lie of the fetus with ruptured membranes.

This incision allows rapid delivery and has a lower risk of bladder injury. However, the closure is more complicated and time-consuming and there is a higher incidence of infection and adhesion formation.

⚠ There is a greater risk of uterine rupture in subsequent pregnancies with a greater risk of the fetus being expelled into the peritoneal cavity. For these reasons, a classical incision is an absolute contraindication to a trial of a vaginal delivery (VBAC).

Caesarean section: complications

Intraoperative complications

Major complications are most common with an emergency CS and 82% of anaesthesia-related maternal deaths occurred in women undergoing CS, most frequently with general anaesthesia.

▶ Intraoperative complications occur in 12–15% of women and include:
- Uterine or uterocervical lacerations (5–10%).
- Blood loss >1L (7–9%).
- Bladder laceration (0.5–0.8%).
- Blood transfusion (2–3%).
- Hysterectomy (0.2%).
- Bowel lacerations (0.05%).
- Ureteral injury (0.03–0.09%.).

Risk factors predisposing to uterocervical lacerations include:
- Low station of the presenting part and full dilatation.
- Birth weight >4000g.
- ↑ Maternal age.
- Category 1 CS.

Risk factors predisposing to intraoperative haemorrhage include:
- Placenta praevia or abruption.
- Extremes of fetal birth weight.
- BMI >25.

Postoperative complications

▶ Postoperative complications occur in up to 1/3 of women and include:
- Endometritis (5%).
- Wound infections (3–27%).
- Pulmonary atelectasis.
- Venous thromboembolism.
- Urinary tract infections.

Risk factors independently associated with infection are:
- Preoperative remote infection.
- Chorioamnionitis.
- Maternal severe systemic disease.
- Pre-eclampsia.
- High BMI.
- Nulliparity.
- ↑ Surgical blood loss.

Long-term effects of CS

In subsequent pregnancies there is a higher risk of:
- Uterine rupture (1:200 with spontaneous labour).
- Placenta praevia (47% ↑ of background risk).
- Placenta accreta.
- Antepartum stillbirth: risk doubles with a previous CS.

Women undergoing multiple CS (≥3) are at higher risk of:
- Excessive blood loss (8%).
- Difficult delivery of the neonate (5%).
- Dense adhesions (46%).
- The risk of any major complication is higher (9%).
- Complications are ↑ with ↑ number of CS:
  - 4% for 2nd
  - 8% for 3rd
  - 13% for 4th.

Prelabour rupture of membranes at term

> ## Definition
> Prelabour rupture of membranes (PROM) at term is defined as leakage of amniotic fluid in the absence of uterine activity after 37 completed weeks of gestation.

Incidence
8% of term pregnancies (2–3% before 37wks).

Aetiology
- Unknown.
- Clinical or subclinical infection.
- Polyhydramnios.
- Multiple pregnancy.
- Malpresentations.

Clinical assessment
It is important to establish a correct diagnosis to plan further management. If unnecessary interventions are undertaken there is a risk of increased maternal and fetal morbidity.

History
Women give a history of a sudden gush of fluid leaking from the vagina, recurrent dampness, or constant leaking.

Examination
- There is no need to carry out a speculum examination with certain history of ruptured membranes at term with liquor seen on the pad or undergarments.
- If the history is uncertain, a speculum examination should be offered (liquor should be seen pooling in the upper vagina or trickling through the cervical os):
  - coughing or straining (Valsalva manoeuvre) may help to demonstrate leaking fluid
  - note the colour of the liquor (?blood or meconium stained).
- Temperature, pulse, and BP.
- Obstetric examination of abdomen (including lie and presentation).
- CTG.

▶ If conservative management is planned, avoid digital examination as it increases the incidence of chorioamnionitis, post-partum endometritis, and neonatal infection.

⚠ Any concern regarding fetal well-being is an indication to deliver.

⚠ Signs of chorioamnionitis should prompt treatment with antibiotics and rapid delivery.

Clinical features of chorioamnionitis
- Fetal tachycardia.
- Maternal tachycardia.
- Maternal pyrexia.
- Rising leucocyte count.
- Rising CRP.
- Irritable or ↑ tender uterus.

Prelabour rupture of membranes: management

If there are no contraindications to waiting, women should be offered the choice between immediate induction and expectant management.

Expectant management vs. immediate induction

- 60% of women will labour spontaneously within 24h.
- No evidence of a difference in the mode of delivery for either.
- 1% risk of serious neonatal infection (compared with 0.5% for women with intact membranes).

With expectant management

- Women are more likely to develop chorioamnionitis and endometritis with expectant management of >24h.
- Baby is more likely to be admitted to SCBU: no evidence of a difference in eventual neonatal outcome (morbidity/mortality) with expectant management of <24h.

▶ The NICE guidelines recommend induction after 24h.

Conservative management advice

If the woman opts for this she should be advised to:

- Record her temperature every 4h (during waking hours).
- Urgently report any change in colour or offensive smell.
- Avoid sexual intercourse (showering and bathing is okay).
- Report any ↓ in fetal movements.
- Deliver in a unit with neonatal services and remain in hospital for >12h after delivery to allow close observation of the baby.
- Consider induction if not in labour by 24h.
- Seek medical advice if any concerns regarding the baby's well-being in the 1st 5 days of life (especially in the first 12h).

⚬ Use of antibiotics is controversial. NICE does not recommend prophylactic antibiotics for either mother or baby in absence of symptoms, even if her membranes have been ruptured for >24h.

▶ In labour, regular maternal observations are essential to pick up signs of infection early. Fetal heart rate monitoring should be carried out as it may be tachycardic in the presence of infection.

⚠ If there is clinical evidence of infection a full course of broad spectrum IV antibiotic therapy should be started after blood cultures have been sent.

Known group B streptococcus carriers

See ▢ Group B streptococcus, p. 172.

- Immediate induction should be encouraged (↓ neonatal infection).
- Mothers should be offered benzylpenicillin in labour.
- Neonates should be screened soon after birth.

Further reading

NICE. (2007). *Intrapartum care*, guideline September 2007. ℘ http://www.nice.org.uk/Search.do?x= 17&y=18&searchText=Intrapartum+care&newsearch=true#/search/?reload

Abnormal lie: transverse and oblique

Transverse and oblique lie occur in 1:300 pregnancies and result in a shoulder, limb, or cord presentation. If this persists, vaginal delivery is not feasible (Fig. 2.4).

Diagnosis

- The maternal abdomen is unusually wide and the fundus is lower than expected for the gestation.
- Neither fetal pole is palpable entering the pelvis.
- Fetal head is identifiable at one side.
- On vaginal examination the pelvis is empty.
- A limb or cord may prolapse through the cervix.

Management

When this presents in labour, fetal well-being should be established and a USS performed to try to identify the cause.

⚠ Exclude placenta praevia before attempting vaginal examination.

- CS is indicated in almost all cases.
- An unstable lie at term due to multiparity alone may warrant a gentle attempt at ECV if the following criteria are met:
  - the membranes must be intact
  - labour not advanced
  - the fetus must have no signs of compromise.
- If ECV is successful cord presentation or prolapse should be excluded before labour is allowed to establish.
- CS for transverse lie, especially with placenta praevia or fibroids, requires an experienced obstetrician and cross-matched blood.
- Vertical uterine incision on the uterus or acute tocolysis with a transverse incision may be necessary for safe delivery of fetus.

Malpresentations in labour: overview

- >95% of fetuses at term present with vertex (area subtended by two parietal eminences, anterior, and posterior fontanelle).
- Malpresentation describes any presentation other than vertex lying in close proximity to internal os of the cervix and includes:
  - breech (most common malpresentation with an incidence of 3–4% at term; see 📖 Breech presentation: delivery, p. 86)
  - brow
  - face
  - shoulder
  - arm
  - cord.

Some causes of malpresentation

Maternal
- Multiparity.
- Pelvic tumours.
- Congenital uterine anomalies.
- Contracted pelvis.

Fetal
- Prematurity.
- Multiple pregnancy.
- Intrauterine death.
- Macrosomia.
- Fetal abnormality including:
  - hydrocephalus
  - anencephaly
  - cystic hygroma.

Placental
- Placenta praevia.
- Polyhydramnios.
- Amniotic bands.

Malpresentations: brow and face

Brow presentation

Incidence ranges between 1:1000 and 1:3500 deliveries. The head occupies a position midway between full flexion (vertex) and full extension (face). It can revert to a face or vertex presentation, but if it persists vaginal delivery is not usually possible (see Fig. 6.11a).

Diagnosis
- Often diagnosed in advanced labour (may be suspected on abdominal palpation when both occiput and chin are palpable).
- The head does not descend below the ischial spines.
- Vaginal examination is diagnostic as the frontal sutures, anterior fontanelle, orbital ridges, eyes, and the root of nose are palpable.

Management
- Watch and wait: may become a vertex or face presentation.
- If progress is slow or if the brow persists then CS is indicated.

Face presentation

Incidence of face presentation is between 1:600 and 1:1500 deliveries. It is due to hyperextension of the fetal neck (see Fig. 6.11b).

Diagnosis
- Face presentation is diagnosed in labour on vaginal examination.
- The orbital ridges, nose, malar eminences, mentum, gums, and mouth can be distinguished.

▶ It may be mistaken for a breech, but presence of gum margins will help to differentiate between a mouth and an anus.

Management
- 90% are mentoanterior (MA) and head can flex to allow vaginal delivery.
- Expectant management should be considered with mentoposterior (MP) as about 20–30% will rotate on reaching the pelvic floor.
- Persistent MP face presentations cannot deliver vaginally as it would require the head to overextend.
- If there is poor progress or failure to rotate, CS is indicated.
- Fetal monitoring should be external and fetal blood sampling is contraindicated.
- The use of ventouse is absolutely contraindicated but forceps delivery is possible with an MA position well below spines.

⚠ Attempts to convert face presentations manually into vertex or use of forceps to rotate persistent MP positions can lead to complications of cord prolapse and fetal cervical cord injury.

📖 See Figs 1.6 and 1.7.

Cord presentation

This occurs when one or more loops of cord lie below the presenting part and the membranes are still intact. It is associated with malpresentation, abnormal lie, and a high head. The risk is of cord prolapse when the membranes rupture. This is an obstetric emergency (see 📖 Cord prolapse, p. 401).

Diagnosis

- The diagnosis of cord presentation is often made on USS, but may be found on VE in labour.
- It can be suspected clinically when persistent variable fetal heart decelerations occur early in labour.
- ARM is contraindicated as it will cause cord prolapse.

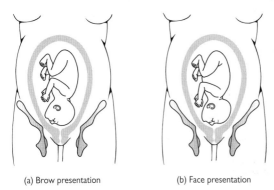

(a) Brow presentation   (b) Face presentation

Fig. 6.11 Malpresentations: (a) brow presentation; (b) face presentation.

Retained placenta and placenta accreta

Retained placenta should be suspected if it is not delivered within 30min of the baby in an actively managed 3rd stage and 1h in a physiological 3rd stage.

⚠ Care must be taken as blood can gather behind placenta leading to significant occult blood loss—beware of high uterus full of blood!

Management of retained placenta
- IV access, FBC, and cross-match.
- If it was physiological management, revert to active management:
  - give Syntometrine® or oxytocin
  - try controlled cord traction.
- If the oxytocin is not effective within 30min, transfer to theatre for regional block and manual removal of the placenta.
- Intraoperative prophylactic antibiotics should be given.

✎ The use of a 40IU IV oxytocin infusion to help deliver the placenta is controversial. The NICE guidelines do not recommend using it before the placenta is delivered.

Placenta accreta, increta, and percreta

Abnormal placentation occurs in about 1:7000 pregnancies, but is much more common if there have been prior Caesarean deliveries. The placenta is normally separated from the myometrium by the decidua basalis. However, if the decidua is abnormal the villi may invade further through the uterine wall. There are three types, but they are all often referred to as just accreta:
- *Placenta accreta:* placental villi are attached to the myometrium.
- *Placenta increta:* villi invaded into >50% of the myometrium.
- *Placenta percreta:* villi pass through the whole myometrium up to the serosa, potentially involving other viscera (bladder or bowel).

Risk factors for placenta accreta may include:
- Uterine surgery such as CS or myomectomy.
- Repeated surgical termination of pregnancy.

Management of placenta accreta post delivery
- With heavy bleeding:
  - blood replacement
  - tamponade with balloon (e.g. Rusch)
  - hysterectomy.
- With minimal bleeding, leaving the placenta *in situ* is an option, with close monitoring.

How to perform manual removal of placenta (MROP)

- One hand is placed on abdomen to steady uterus (reduces the risk of perforation).
- Other hand is gently inserted through cervix into uterus.
- Fingers are used to identify plane between placenta and uterine wall, and gently separate it.
- Placenta should be removed in one piece and inspected to ensure it is complete.
- Uterine cavity is then explored again to make sure it is completely empty.
- Oxytocin infusion is continued for 4h prophylactically.
- IV antibiotics are given.
- Mother observed for bleeding or infection by observing vaginal bleeding, fundal height, change in pulse, BP, temperature, urinary output, and Hb%.

Post-partum haemorrhage

- *Primary PPH* is defined as blood loss of 500mL or more from the genital tract occurring within 24h of delivery.
- *Secondary PPH* is defined as 'excessive' loss occurring between 24h and 6wks after delivery.

- Major cause of maternal morbidity and mortality: globally >125 000 women die of PPH each year.
- Major cause of maternal deaths in the UK (often after CS).
- Incidence is 2–11% in the UK.
- With a low BMI or low Hb, <500mL loss may cause haemodynamic disturbance requiring prompt and appropriate management.

Causes of primary PPH
- Uterine atony.
- Genital tract trauma.
- Coagulation disorders.
- Large placenta.
- Abnormal placental site.
- Retained placenta.
- Uterine inversion.
- Uterine rupture.

Uterine atony (90%)
Caused by failure of uterus to contract effectively after delivery. May be due to many factors—overdistended uterus with twins or polyhydramnios, prolonged labour, infection, retained tissue, failure to actively manage 3rd stage of labour, or, rarely, due to placental abruption (diffuse bleeding into uterine muscle preventing contraction).

Genital tract trauma (7%)
Tears, episiotomy, lacerations of the cervix, and rupture of uterus.

Coagulation disorders
Severe PET, placental abruption, and sepsis may contribute to PPH. Autoimmune diseases, liver disease, and inherited or acquired coagulation disorders are rare causes. Sometimes patients may be on heparin, which can lead to excessive bleeding.

Abnormal placental site
Placenta praevia, accreta, and percreta are associated with PPH. Appropriate preplanning is needed to avoid morbidity and mortality.
  Uterine inversion and rupture are rare causes of excessive bleeding.

For management see \square Massive obstetric haemorrhage: medical management, p. 386.

Antenatal risk factors for PPH

- Previous PPH.
- Previously retained placenta.
- Maternal Hb ≤8.5g/dL at onset of labour.
- ↑ BMI.
- Para 4 or more.
- Antepartum haemorrhage.
- Overdistention of uterus (multiple pregnancy or polyhydramnios).
- Uterine abnormalities.
- Low-lying placenta.
- Maternal age >35yrs.

⚠ The presence of any risk factors for PPH should lead to the woman being advised to deliver in an obstetric unit (facilities for blood transfusion and surgical management of PPH).

Intrapartum risk factors for PPH

- Induction of labour.
- Prolonged 1st, 2nd, or 3rd stage.
- Use of oxytocin.
- Precipitate labour.
- Vaginal operative delivery.
- CS.

Home birth: overview

Home birth can be safe for women screened as low risk, and emotionally satisfying for the mother and her family. For women identified as having risk factors, hospital delivery is safer. Debates about the safety of home births focus on risk of preventable perinatal morbidity and mortality, and on broader issues of appropriate screening and referral.

The numbers

- Proportion of births at home fell from 80% in 1930 to 1% in 1990.
- As a result of Government committee recommendation (HMSO 1993), stating that a full choice including home births should be offered, further enhanced by 'Maternity matters', a Government white paper (2007), the UK home birth rate is increasing and is now about 2–3%.
- Some studies suggest that 10–14% of women would choose home birth if given the opportunity.
- In some regions where there is difficulty in geographical accessibility to a hospital the home birth rate could be about 10%.
- In women booked for home births:
  - change to hospital care is nearly 29%
  - transfer in labour is up to 15% in multiparae and 30% in nulliparae.
  - most of these transfers are for failure to progress or pain relief.
- The risk of intrapartum fetal death in appropriately selected low-risk women is 1:1000.
- It is difficult to compare directly the perinatal mortality rates for home and hospital, as more complex deliveries occur in hospital.
- Recent prospective study suggests a slight increase in perinatal mortality with home births.

Discussion points when considering home birth

- In the presence of obvious risk factors (hypertension, diabetes, placenta praevia) the advice must be to deliver in hospital.
- If mother is low-risk and wishes to have home birth, she should be counselled appropriately with full information about the very slight increase in perinatal mortality and possibility of transfer in labour.
- If a risk arises before birth, the booking should be changed.
- If risk is minimal, the lead professional in charge should offer the woman and her partner the opportunity to review their choice and respect their decision.

Reasons for women to choose home birth

- Wish for a familiar setting where they feel relaxed and in control.
- Fear of hospital setting.
- To have a continuing relationship with a known midwife.
- To be with more family members who provide support.
- Previous home birth.
- To avoid intervention.

Further reading

Maternity Matters: choice, access and continuity & care in a safe service. ℘ http://www.dh.gov.uk/en/publicationsandstatistics/publications/publicationspolicyandguidance/DH_073312

Home birth: risks and GP involvement

The potential risks of home birth are rare, but should be discussed with the woman as part of her decision. These include:

- Should a complication occur, transfer to hospital may be required.
- Should there be a delay in transfer, response to acute complications, such as intrapartum fetal hypoxia or post-partum haemorrhage, may be delayed, potentially leading to a worse outcome although such complications are rare.
- The facilities for neonatal resuscitation will be limited but the midwife should be well trained in basic neonatal resuscitation.
- Inadequate lighting and analgesia may make diagnosis of the extent of perineal tears difficult, necessitating transfer to hospital.

Discussion of the risks and other factors, including type of pain relief available, will help the woman to make an informed choice. Clear documentation of these discussions in the antenatal period is essential for the mother not to regret her choice and for medico-legal reasons.

The role of the GP

- The GP should be fully informed about the local options for place of birth, and will then be in a position to provide the options to the woman in a clear, understandable, and balanced manner.
- GPs who do not wish to provide care for home births should refer women to the community midwife, supervisor of community midwives at the district maternity unit, or a GP who provides this care.
- In case of any unfortunate event occurring with intrapartum care of a woman being looked after by her GP and if the case proceeds to a litigation, the GP would not be judged by the standards of a consultant obstetrician, but by those of a GP with similar skills and standing (the Bolam test).
- The GP does not have to attend a home birth even when the woman has been accepted by the GP for full maternity care, unless asked to do so by the midwife.
- The GP should provide support to the woman and midwife, help identify any deviations from normal course of labour, and arrange for hospital care.
- Where the midwife feels that the GP is supportive, the likelihood of transfer to hospital is reduced.
- In current practice very few GPs offer care in labour and delivery services.

Further reading

The GP's guide to home birth. ℘ http://www.medicine.ox.ac.uk/bandolier/band32/b32-8.html

Home birth: the evidence

Meta-analysis of several methodologically sound observational studies comparing the outcomes of planned home births (irrespective of the eventual place of birth) with planned hospital births for women with similar characteristics showed that there was no increase in maternal mortality. The rate is unlikely to be different as the maternal mortality is generally low, and good midwifery and ambulance services help to avoid such deaths, although occasional cases have been described.

Recent home birth study in the UK showed:
- Slightly increased perinatal mortality, but when all studies in literature are considered there is little statistically significant difference. This is partly due to the complexity of such studies, some being retrospective or prospective descriptive.
- In the home births group there were significantly fewer medical interventions (including in women transferred to hospital).
- Fewer babies had low Apgar scores, neonatal respiratory problems, and instances of birth trauma with home births.

Further randomized controlled trials are needed to resolve this controversy over relative safety of home and hospital births. Because maternal and perinatal mortality and morbidity are so low in low-risk pregnancies, to observe differences in these primary outcome measures large numbers need to be studied.

Home birth: general points

GPs and midwives have the responsibility for creating the right circumstances for safe and satisfying home births.

This means:
- Selecting women without risk factors.
- Establishing an infrastructure for safe obstetric care including:
  - hygiene during delivery
  - keeping the baby warm
  - care of the eyes.
- Providing support and care during labour, delivery, and in immediate postnatal period.
- Arrangements for transfer to hospital in the event of any unforeseen complication.
- Care should be provided based on prearranged protocol that provides guidance as to conduct of labour and what action needs to be taken should the woman need help.

Obstetric anaesthesia

Pain relief in labour

Uterine contractions in labour are associated with pain. Professionals can help to reduce women's fears by giving precise, accurate, and relevant information antenatally including the types of analgesia available in their unit.

Ideal pain relief in labour

Should
- Provide good analgesia.
- Be safe for the mother and baby.
- Be predictable and constant in its effects.
- Be reversible if necessary.
- Be easy to administer.
- Be under the control of the mother.

Should not
- Interfere with uterine contractions.
- Interfere with mobility.

Non-pharmacological methods

- Education regarding what to expect may help reduce fear and the sense of loss of control.
- A trusted companion present throughout labour and birth reduces the need for pain relief.
- Warm bath, acupuncture, hypnosis, and homeopathy are also helpful.

Transcutaneous electrical nerve stimulation (TENS) is a safe form of analgesia. It may help with short labour and postpone the need for stronger analgesia, but may not be adequate as labour advances.

Pharmacological methods

Nitrous oxide (Entonox®)

Entonox® is premixed nitrous oxide and oxygen as a 50:50 mixture. It is self-administered and has quick onset of action and a short half-life. Side effects can include feeling faint, nausea, and vomiting.

Narcotic agents

- *Pethidine:* administered at a dose of 50–150mg; onset of action is 15–20min. It lasts about 3–4h and can be repeated. It is usually given with an antiemetic. If given within 2h of delivery, it can cause neonatal respiratory depression and naloxone may be needed.
- *Diamorphine:* is also used in some units at a dose of 2.5–5mg. There is controversy about the extent and timing of neonatal respiratory depression, but it may be up to 3–4h after the last dose.
- *Meptazinol:* is an opioid that may cause less respiratory depression. The onset of action starts in 15min and lasts for about 2–7h.

Pudendal nerve block and local perineal infiltration

- Pudendal nerve block is used for operative vaginal delivery and is performed by the obstetrician: lidocaine (lignocaine) is injected 1–2cm medially, and below the right and left ischial spines; this is done transvaginally with a specially designed pudendal needle.
- Local anaesthetic such as lidocaine (lignocaine) is infiltrated in the perineum before performing an episiotomy at the time of delivery, or before suturing tears and episiotomies.

Epidural analgesia: overview

Safe and effective analgesia for labour is still something that is not available for the vast majority of women in the world today. Although the provision of epidural analgesia during labour has been one of the greatest advances in the care of women during this difficult and distressing time, it still carries a small, but definite complication rate.

Consent for analgesia in labour

Women in labour present a particular group of patients in whom obtaining fully informed consent may be difficult because of a variety of factors such as pain, fatigue, or the effects of narcotic analgesia administered previously. Ideally anaesthetists should try to explain the risks and benefits of epidural analgesia to women in the antenatal period.

Anatomy

The epidural space lies between the spinal dura and the vertebral canal (Fig. 7.1). The superior margin is the foramen magnum, inferiorly the sacrococcygeal membrane. Posteriorly lies the ligamentum flavum and the anterior surfaces of the laminae, anteriorly the posterior longitudinal ligament. Within the epidural space lie the spinal nerve roots as well as the spinal arteries and extradural veins. The usual distance between skin and the epidural space in the lumbar region in adults is about 4–5cm. It is important to realize that the epidural space is continuous the whole way down the back. The lumbar region is chosen for the provision of labour analgesia as this is where the nerve roots involved in the production of pain during labour are found.

The pain of the first stage of labour is caused by uterine contractions and is referred by afferent Aδ and C fibres mainly to dermatones T10–L1, and by distension of the perineum during the second stage of labour to S2–4.

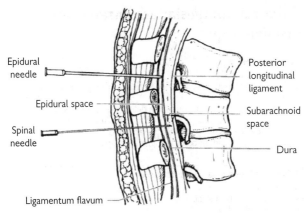

Fig. 7.1 Subarachnoid and epidural spaces. Reproduced from Allman KG, McIndoe A, Wilson I. (2011). *Oxford Handbook of Anaesthesia*, 3 edn. With permission from Oxford University Press.

Epidural analgesia: advantages and disadvantages

Advantages
- Effective analgesia in labour.
- Reduced maternal catecholamine secretion (thought to benefit fetus).
- Can be topped up for an operative delivery or any other complications, e.g. retained placenta or difficult perineal repair.
- Can provide effective postoperative analgesia.
- Can be used to aid BP control in pre-eclampsia.

Disadvantages and complications
- Failure to site, or a patchy, or incomplete block.
- Hypotension from sympathetic blockade.
- Decreased mobility.
- Tenderness over the insertion site.

▶ There is no association between epidural analgesia and long-term backache.
- *Inadvertent dural puncture:*
  - incidence <1:100
  - may develop a post-dural puncture headache, characterized by ↑ on sitting up or standing
  - may need treatment with an epidural blood patch.
- *Respiratory depression:*
  - from the catheter migrating into the subarachnoid space followed by bolus of local anaesthetic (total spinal)
  - from accumulation of epidurally administered opiates.
- *Extremely rare complications resulting in neurological deficits:*
  - epidural abscess formation
  - epidural haematoma
  - damage to individual nerves or the spinal cord itself.
- Increased risk of operative delivery.

An alternative to epidural: remifentanil patient-controlled analgesia

There are a few women in whom epidural analgesia is contraindicated and who are not able to obtain adequate analgesia from more conventional methods such as nitrous oxide. Remifentanil, a powerful opiate which is rapidly metabolized and unable to cross the placenta, may be used via a patient-controlled IV system (patient-controlled analgesia (PCA)).

Contraindications to epidural analgesia

- Septicaemia.
- Infection at site of insertion.
- Coagulopathy/thrombocytopaenia (platelet count < 75 × 10^9).

⚠ Beware of a falling count over the past few days—always check the platelet count if this has occurred.

If the platelet count is between 75 and 100 × 10^9, clotting studies should be performed before proceeding with the epidural.

- Raised intracranial pressure.
- Haemorrhage and cardiovascular instability/hypovolaemia.

▶ There may be limited circumstances where an epidural is appropriate in these cases.

- Known allergy to amide (lidocaine-type) local anaesthetic solutions or opioids.
- Fixed cardiac output states, e.g. severe aortic stenosis, hypertrophic obstructive cardiomyopathy (HOCM).

Technique for siting an epidural

- The procedure should be explained and consent sought.
- There should be no clotting abnormalities.
- Establish wide-bore IV access.
- Position the woman either on her side or sitting, with the back curved to open intervertebral spaces.
- Full aseptic technique must be followed.
- A suitable interspace, usually L3/4, is identified and lidocaine (lignocaine) 1% injected.
- The epidural space is identified by a loss of resistance technique, usually to saline 0.9%.
- Once the space is identified, a catheter is threaded in and the needle withdrawn and the catheter firmly fixed to the skin.
- A test dose of local anaesthetic, usually bupivacaine, can be given to check that the epidural catheter has not inadvertently entered the subarachnoid space.
- Various regimens exist for the delivery of local anaesthetic to the epidural space either involving bolus administration or infusions.
- Careful monitoring is mandatory following epidural top-up doses including BP reading every 5min for 20min following the administration of a top-up dose.
- Block height and degree of motor block should be recorded.
- Continuous electronic fetal monitoring is required if an epidural has been sited.

Further reading

♫ http://www.youtube.com/watch?v=1evFwMXnGil

Anaesthetic techniques for Caesarean section: spinal

Regional anaesthetic techniques are undoubtedly safer for the woman and most anaesthetists would counsel women having a CS to opt for one of them. However, the choice of anaesthetic technique may be influenced by the urgency of the CS. Facilities for conversion to GA, such as drugs and endotracheal tubes must always be available, as conversion to GA may be required if the block wears off during surgery, or is too high, or if the woman requests it due to pain or discomfort.

Spinal anaesthesia
- Accounts for the majority of CS performed in the UK.
- Fasting and antacid precautions are ideal, as GA may be required if the block is unsatisfactory.
- Good IV access is essential to provide fluids rapidly to counteract hypotension that may occur. Vasopressor drugs, such as phenylephrine or ephedrine, should also be available.
- Hyperbaric bupivacaine 0.5% in a dose of 12.5–15mg is usually used, together with an opiate such as fentanyl (20 micrograms) or damorphine (around 250 micrograms).

Advantages and disadvantages

Advantages
- Technically relatively easier than epidurals to perform.
- Enable mother to bond immediately with baby.
- The most reliable option for establishing a dense, bilateral block.

Disadvantages
- May cause severe hypotension.
- May wear off if surgery is unexpectedly prolonged.

⚠ Hypotension is common due to sympathetic blockade and inadequate tilt leading to aortocaval pressure, and must be prevented by the use of fluids, adequate left lateral tilt, and vasopressors if appropriate.

▶ Patients must be warned of the risk of intra-operative pain and the small chance of conversion to GA.

▶ The full extent of the block must be tested and recorded by the anaesthetist, prior to the commencement of surgery.

Anaesthetic techniques for Caesarean section: epidural

Conversion of a functioning epidural from analgesia to anaesthesia is the choice if a woman requires an operative or instrumental delivery, provided there is sufficient time (it takes about 20min or longer).

Advantages and disadvantages

Advantages
- Can be topped, should the surgery be extended.
- Can be used for good postoperative analgesia.

Disadvantages
- More likely than spinal anaesthesia to produce patchy or unilateral blockade.
- Takes longer to establish an adequate block.
- Can be technically difficult, with a higher incidence of headache in the event of inadvertent dural puncture.
- The catheter can migrate into the subarachnoid or subdural space, resulting in unpredictable and possibly fatal complications if large doses of local anaesthetic are administered.
- Larger doses of local anaesthetic agents are required, leading to the possibility of toxicity if the catheter has migrated intravenously.

Anaesthetic techniques for Caesarean section: combined spinal epidural

These are usually performed by inserting a spinal needle through an epidural needle, although two separate injections may be performed.

▶ Combined spinal epidural (CSE) anaesthesia combines the advantages of spinal anaesthesia, i.e. speed of onset and dense block, with the ability to prolong the period of anaesthesia and analgesia via the epidural route.

Advantages and disadvantages

Advantages
- The epidural component can be used to top-up the block.
- A smaller volume of local anaesthetic can be used intrathecally and the block extended gradually with the epidural component (this may cause less cardiovascular instability and be useful in women with cardiac disease).
- The epidural component can provide postoperative analgesia.

Disadvantages
- There is a higher risk of failure of the intrathecal component.
- Possible higher risk of meningitis than with either spinal or epidural alone.
- The epidural component of the technique is untested and any local anaesthetic agents must be given in small boluses, in case the catheter is in the subarachnoid space.

Anaesthetic techniques for Caesarean section: general anaesthesia

There has been a general trend throughout the developed world away from using GA for CS. However, it is still necessary in the presence of contraindications to regional anaesthesia or in an emergency.

Problems with GA

- *Potential airway difficulties:* incidence of failed intubation in pregnant women is approximately 1:300 compared with 1:3000 in the general surgical population.
- Pulmonary aspiration of gastric contents.
- *Awareness:* rare with modern anaesthetic techniques, but may occur if inadequate levels of inhalational agents are used.

Technique for GA in pregnancy

- Adequate assessment of the airway is essential, as well as questioning about relevant medical, obstetric, and drug treatment, and allergies.
- Antacid prophylaxis must be administered.
- Left lateral tilt maintained at all times to prevent aortocaval compression.
- Adequate preoxygenation must precede induction of GA, regardless of the obstetric indications for the CS.
- ECG, pulse oximetry, and capnographic monitoring must be available.
- For full discussion of GA for CS, readers are advised to consult a specialist anaesthetic text.

⚠ Emergency GA is associated with increased maternal morbidity and mortality.

▶ There are few absolute indications for GA for CS.

Neonatal resuscitation

Overview

Most babies establish normal respiration and circulation without help after delivery. However, all babies should be assessed at delivery. Newborn infants who are born at term, have clear liquor, and are breathing and crying with good tone will only require drying and keeping warm. Less than 1% of babies need resuscitation. Anticipation of problems before delivery is the key to success.

It is prudent, where possible, to call for specialist skilled personnel to attend deliveries where need for additional support may be anticipated. These situations include:

- Preterm deliveries.
- Emergency Caesarean deliveries.
- Vaginal breech birth.
- Thick meconium-stained liquor.
- Major fetal abnormality.
- Other concerns (multiples, signs of significant fetal compromise).

All trained personnel attending a delivery have a responsibility for initiating resuscitation at birth and should possess the appropriate knowledge and skills to approach the management of the newborn infant during the first 10–20min in a competent manner. The environment should be warm, draught free, and well lit, with a flat surface available for resuscitation. Equipment should be checked on a daily basis and before each delivery.

Some of the important items are:

- A warmed flat surface (Resuscitaire with radiant warmer) (see Fig. 8.1).
- Source of air and oxygen with pressure-limited gas delivery.
- Appropriate size face masks, oropharyngeal airways, endotracheal tubes.
- Suction device with different size suction catheters.
- Stethoscope.
- Laryngoscope with straight laryngeal blades.
- Instruments for clamping and cutting the umbilical cord.
- Emergency resuscitation box for advanced resuscitation.
- Clock or stopwatch.

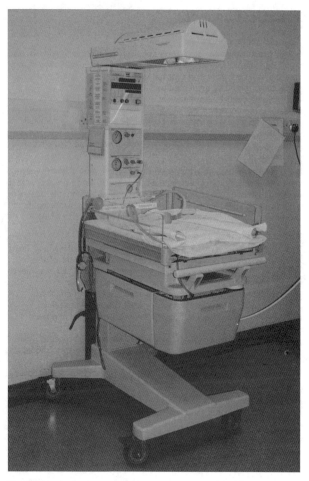

Fig. 8.1 Neonatal radiant warmer (Resuscitaire). Reproduced with permission of Dräeger Medical UK, 2008.

Practical aspects

Temperature control

Hypothermia can lower oxygen tension, increase metabolic acidosis, lead to hypoglycaemia, and inhibit the production of surfactant. Low temperature is associated with poor neonatal outcome.

Heat loss should be prevented by:
- Protecting the baby from draught.
- Keeping the delivery room warm.
- Drying the term baby immediately after delivery, covering the head and body with warm towel to prevent further heat loss.
- Placing baby on warm surface under radiant warmer, if resuscitation is needed.

▶ For a preterm baby born before 28wks of gestation (<~1kg birth weight), the most effective way of keeping the baby warm is not to dry and wrap it in warm towels, but to cover the head and body (apart from the face) with a plastic bag before placing under a radiant heater. Plastic wrapping should therefore be available at all deliveries of extremely preterm infants.

Initial assessment at delivery

The immediate assessment includes colour, tone, breathing, and heart rate. Apgar scoring is often used for the initial assessment of the baby. However, it is a retrospective, highly subjective tool and was never intended to identify babies needing immediate resuscitation.

- *Colour:* baby may be centrally pink, cyanosed, or pale (peripheral cyanosis is common and does not by itself indicate hypoxaemia).
- *Tone:* a very floppy baby is likely to be unconscious, and may need respiratory support.
- *Breathing:* the rate, depth, and symmetry of respiration together with any abnormal breathing pattern such as grunting and gasping should be noted.
- *Heart rate:* best evaluated by auscultating with a stethoscope (palpating the umbilical cord is often effective, but can be misleading).

After the initial assessment, infants can be generally classified into one of four groups and further management guided by this (Table 8.1).

Further reading

How to perform an Apgar score. ℘ http://www.youtube.com/watch?v=hdNVhDuD4wU

Table 8.1 Classification of babies at birth with appropriate action

	Assessment	Clinical condition	Action
Group 1	Healthy	Vigorous baby Crying Becoming pink Good tone Heart rate >100	Dry and warm Hand to mother for skin to skin contact
Group 2	Primary apnoea	Apnoeic or inadequate breathing Remaining blue Reduced tone Heart rate >100	Dry and warm Tactile stimulation Facial oxygen Consider mask ventilation if not improving
Group 3	Terminal apnoea	Apnoeic Blue or pale Floppy Heart rate <100	Dry and warm Mask ventilation If no improvement may need intubation, ventilation, and chest compressions if heart rate not improving
Group 4	Fresh stillbirth	Apnoeic Pale floppy No heart rate	Full cardiopulmonary resuscitation

Airway, breathing, and circulation (ABC)

⚠ Call for skilled help as soon as a problem is identified.

Airway

The head should be placed in neutral position. This is different from the head position for adult resuscitation because of the relatively large occiput of babies. Overextension of the neck can occlude the airway. A jaw thrust may be helpful, but care must be taken not to compress the airway under the chin. Use of an appropriately sized Guedel airway can be considered, particularly in infants with micrognathia. Suction of the airway is only required if there is blood or particulate material in the oropharynx. Aggressive pharyngeal suction should be avoided and suction should always be done under direct vision with a laryngoscope.

⚠ Blind suction is not helpful; even in the presence of meconium-stained liquor. It may lead to trauma and induce bradycardia or laryngospasm.

Breathing

Mask ventilation may be necessary if the infant is apnoeic, has irregular breathing, or is bradycardic. The aim is to achieve adequate lung inflation and to deliver oxygen. In most cases mask ventilation is as effective as intubation in the initial resuscitation scenario.

It is essential to use the correct-sized mask. The mask should cover the nose and mouth, but should not extend beyond the chin or over the orbits. Mask ventilation can be performed using a bag and mask, or via a constant flow T-piece system (Fig. 8.2).

The lungs of newborn infants are fluid-filled immediately after birth and the first 5 breaths given should sustain an inflation pressure of approximately 30cm of water (for a term infant) for 2–3s (inflation breaths). These long breaths aim to displace the lung fluid and expand the lungs. If effective, chest wall movement and improvement of heart rate should be seen. If the heart rate rises, but baby is still not breathing, continue to ventilate at 30–40 breaths/min (maintain the inflation for ~1s for each breath).

⚠ If there is no improvement, the airway should be checked again. Help should be sought and early additional assistance will be beneficial if there is no improvement.

Circulation

⚠ Chest compressions are effective only if the lungs have been successfully inflated.

Chest compressions aim to deliver oxygenated blood to the heart allowing the circulation to recover. Chest compressions should be commenced if the infant remains bradycardic despite adequate ventilation.

How to perform chest compressions in the neonate
- Both thumbs should be placed over the lower 1/3 of the sternum, encircling the chest with both hands; other fingers lie behind the baby supporting the back.
- For effective chest compressions, the chest is compressed to a depth of 1/3 the anteroposterior diameter allowing the chest wall to return to its relaxed position between compressions.
- 3:1 ratio of compression and ventilation is used, i.e. 90 compressions and 30 breaths/min, each breath lasting for 1s.
- The quality of compressions and ventilation are more important than the rate.
- Recheck the heart rate after 30s and every 30s after that.

Video teaching basic neonatal resuscitation to midwifery students. ℛ http://www.youtube.com/watch?v=TWaZBcjmxu8

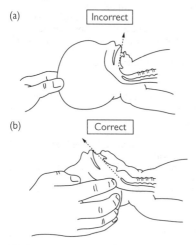

(a) | Incorrect

(b) | Correct

Fig 8.2 Neonatal resuscitation. (a) Incorrect head position. Neonates have a prominent occiput and in the prone position will naturally adopt flexed head posture, compromising the airway. (b) Correct 'neutral' head position. Neutral position is neither extended nor flexed, but opens the airway to allow effective inflation breaths.

Drugs

Drugs are rarely indicated in neonatal resuscitation. They should be considered only if adequate ventilation and effective chest compression have failed to increase the heart rate above 60 beats/min. In the resuscitation situation, drugs should be given via an umbilical venous catheter.

Drugs used in neonatal resuscitation
- *Adrenaline:* 1:10 000, dose 0.1–0.3mL/kg equivalent to 10–30 micrograms/kg; route through umbilical venous catheter or IV.

▶ Adrenaline should not be given down the endotracheal tube (ETT).
- *Sodium bicarbonate:* dose 1–2mmol/kg (2–4mL/kg of 4.2% $NaHCO_3$); route through IV or UVC. Reversing the intracardiac acidosis may help bump-start the heart.

▶ Repeated doses of $NaHCO_3$ should be avoided without proper evidence of metabolic acidosis from blood gas analysis.
- *Glucose 10%:* dose 2mL/kg/dose (200mg/kg/dose), route through IV or UVC. Glucose should be given if there is hypoglycaemia.
- *Volume replacement:* crystalloid (0.9% saline, 10mL/kg/dose) is the preferred fluid if the infant appears to be in shock. Blood should be given if there is evidence of hypovolaemia and evidence of acute blood loss.
- *Naloxone:* is no longer kept in the resuscitation trolley.

Actions in the event of a poor response to resuscitation

Check for a technical problem
- Is the gas flow connected?
- Is there a leak in the circuit? Check the tubing.
- Is the ETT in the trachea? If in doubt remove ETT, give breaths by mask, and replace ETT if necessary.
- Is the ETT blocked? If in doubt remove ETT, give breaths by mask, and replace ETT if necessary.
- Check the blow-off valve pressure (30cm of water for term infant).

Does the baby have other pathology?
- Pneumothorax.
- Congenital lung problem, e.g. diaphragmatic hernia.
- Lung hypoplasia.
- Hydrops fetalis.
- Perinatal asphyxia.

Recent advances

Delayed cord clamping

For uncompromised babies, a delay in cord clamping of at least 1min from complete delivery of the infant is now recommended.

Infants with meconium-stained liquor

There is now evidence that suctioning of the meconium from the infant's airway after delivery of the head but before delivery of the shoulder is not beneficial and so it is no longer recommended.

▶ No suctioning should be performed if the infant is active, vigorous, and crying.

If an infant is born through thick meconium and is floppy and depressed after birth, it is reasonable for a skilled person to inspect the larynx directly with a laryngoscope and suction the oropharynx and trachea. There is no role for bronchial lavage.

Preterm infants

It is easier to maintain the preterm infant's temperature by placing it into a food-grade plastic wrap or bag (while wet, leaving the face uncovered) and then under a radiant heater. This is more effective than drying and wrapping for infants <28wks gestation. For these infants the delivery room temperature should be at least 26°C.

Also, preterm infants usually require less pressure to inflate their lungs and therefore the blow-off valve on the Resuscitaire should be initially set at 20–25cm of water (rather than 30cm of water for term infants). In addition, exogenous surfactant is important in the initial stabilization of extremely preterm infants.

Use of air vs. oxygen in resuscitation

☛ There is evidence that using air for the resuscitation of near-term and term babies is as effective as using oxygen, although there is still active debate. It is therefore reasonable to resuscitate infants in air, with supplemental oxygen available if needed and its use guided by pulse oximetry.

Confirmation of tracheal tube placement

Detection of exhaled carbon dioxide in addition to clinical assessment is recommended as the most reliable method to confirm placement of a tracheal tube in neonates with spontaneous circulation.

Therapeutic hypothermia

Newly born infants born at term or near term with evolving moderate to severe hypoxic-ischaemic encephalopathy should, where possible, be offered therapeutic hypothermia. This does not affect immediate resuscitation, but is important for post-resuscitation care.

Communication with parents

Resuscitation decisions

If resuscitation is required, parents should be fully informed of the procedure undertaken and the purpose.

The decision to resuscitate an extremely preterm infant should be a combined decision of parents, and paediatric and obstetric staff. This is a difficult conversation, but one that is best had early. The obstetricians caring for any woman who has a strong probability of delivering very prematurely must raise the issue early and actively involve their paediatric colleagues. The decision taken about resuscitation should also influence the level of fetal monitoring in labour.

The decision to discontinue resuscitation should involve senior paediatric staff. Proper birth plans should be in place in cases of severe congenital malformations. All communication with parents should be documented in the mother's notes and later in the baby's notes after delivery.

Stopping resuscitation

If there are no signs of life after 10min of continuous and effective resuscitation, it is appropriate to consider stopping ongoing attempts as the outcome is universally poor. The decision should be made by the resuscitation team and the most senior staff available. Local and national guidelines are very helpful in making such decisions.

Further reading

Biarent D, Binghma R, Richmond S, et al. (2005). European Resuscitation Council Guidelines for resuscitation. *Resuscitation* **67**(S1): S97–S133.

Resuscitation Council (UK). (2011). Resuscitation at birth. Newborn life support course provider manual, 3rd edn. London: Resuscitation Council (UK).

Richmond S, Wyllie J. (2010). European Resuscitation Council Guidelines for Resuscitation (2010). Section 7: Resuscitation of babies at birth. *Resuscitation* **81**: 1389–9.

Postnatal care

Normal changes in the puerperium

The puerperium begins after delivery of placenta and lasts until reproductive organs have returned to their pre-pregnant state—usually about 6wks.

Hormones
- *Human placental lactogen and beta hCG (BhCG):* levels fall rapidly; by 10 days neither should be detectable.
- Oestrogen and progesterone: non-pregnant levels are achieved by 7 days post-partum.

Genital tract
- *Uterus:* undergoes rapid involution. Weight of the uterus falls from 1000g post-delivery to about 500g at the end of a week. By 2wks, it returns to pelvis and is no longer palpable abdominally.
- *Vagina:* initially vaginal wall is swollen, but rapidly regains tone, although remaining fragile for 1–2wks. Gradually, vascularity and oedema decrease, and by 4wks rugae reappear, but are less prominent than in a nullipara.
- *Cervix:* cervical os gradually closes after delivery. It admits 2–3 fingers for the first 4–6 days and by the end of 10–14 days is dilated to barely more than 1cm.

Perineum
Perineal oedema persists for some days. It may take longer if there was a prolonged second stage, especially with a long period of pushing, operative vaginal delivery, or perineal tears that needed repair.

Lochia
Lochia consists of sloughed-off necrotic decidual layer mixed with blood. It is initially red (lochia rubra), becomes paler as bleeding reduced (lochia serosa), and finally becomes a yellowish white (lochia alba). The flow of lochia may last for 3–6wks.

Breasts
Between 2nd and 4th days, breasts become engorged, vascularity increases, and areolar pigmentation increases. Enlargement of lobules results from an increase in number and size of the alveoli.

Cardiovascular system
After the 3rd stage of labour, cardiac output initially increases due to return of blood from the contracted uterus. Plasma volume, which expanded by 40% during pregnancy, rapidly decreases as a result of diuresis and returns to normal by 2–3wks post-partum. Heart rate decreases and returns to pre pregnancy rate, and is partly responsible for reduced cardiac output. Blood loss at delivery, excretion of extracellular fluid, and reduction of plasma volume due to changes in hormonal status are responsible for alterations in the blood volume.

Major postnatal problems

The three major causes of morbidity in the postnatal period are:
- 2° PPH (Box 9.1; 📖 Post-partum haemorrhage, p. 322; 📖 Massive obstetric haemorrhage: causes, p. 380).
- VTE (Box 9.2; 📖 Venous thromboembolism: overview, p. 390).
- Puerpural pyrexia.

Puerperal pyrexia is defined as the presence of fever in a mother ≥38°C in the first 14 days after giving birth.

Box 9.1 Secondary PPH
- Any 'abnormal' bleeding occurring 24h to 6wks postnatally.
- In developed countries, 2% of postnatal women are admitted to hospital with this: 50% undergo surgical evacuation.
- In developing countries it is a major cause of maternal death.
- Caused by retained products, endometritis, or a tear.
- Management depends on the cause (📖 Post-partum haemorrhage, p. 322; 📖 Massive obstetric haemorrhage: causes, p. 380).

Box 9.2 VTE
⚠ Second major cause of direct maternal death in the UK (see 📖 Venous thromboembolism: overview, p. 390). May be asymptomatic until it presents with a PE, but signs and symptoms may include:

Deep vein thrombosis
- Leg pain or discomfort (especially in the left leg).
- Swelling.
- Tenderness.
- Erythema, increased skin temperature and oedema.
- Lower abdominal pain (high DVT).
- Elevated white cell count.

Pulmonary thromboembolism
- Dyspnoea.
- Collapse.
- Chest pain.
- Haemoptysis.
- Faintness.
- Raised jugular venous pressure (JVP).
- Focal signs in chest.
- Symptoms and signs associated with DVT.

⚠ In the postnatal period there should be a high level of suspicion for women presenting with any of the above symptoms, and urgent investigation is warranted starting with pulse oximetry, ECG, and chest X-ray (CXR).

Puerperal pyrexia: overview

- Puerperal sepsis was the most common cause of maternal mortality before the mid-1930s, accounting for >40% of all maternal deaths.
- Control and cure of puerperal infection began in 1935 with introduction of the first sulphonamides.
- Resurgence of puerperal infection as major cause of direct maternal deaths was reported in the last UK confidential enquiries (2006–2008).

Puerperal sepsis CEMAC recommendations

- Management of pregnant or post-partum women with acute severe illness needs a team approach, e.g. sepsis with circulatory failure, severe pre-eclampsia, eclampsia, and massive PPH.
- Trainees should seek help early from senior medical staff, including anaesthetic and critical care colleagues.
- In acute emergencies, telephoning a senior colleague to discuss the case would be valuable.
- Follow RCOG guidelines on the responsibilities of the consultant.
- Recently delivered women with unexplained pain who require opiate analgesia require urgent senior review.
- High-dose IV broad-spectrum antibiotics should be commenced as early as possible, i.e. within 1h—the longer the delay, the greater the morbidity and mortality.
- Recently delivered women should be given verbal and written information on personal hygiene, risks, signs and symptoms of infection.
- Hand washing after toilet use, cleaning the perineum, and change of pad should be emphasized especially when the mother or her close relatives at home have upper respiratory tract infection.
- Staff should adhere to infection control protocols and the mother should be urgently referred for hospital care when there is suspicion of sepsis.

Puerperal pyrexia: genital causes

Uterine infection (endometritis)

Predisposing factors
- Caesarean section—more with failure to use prophylactic antibiotics.
- Prelabour rupture of membranes—incidence increases with the latency to onset of labour.
- Intrapartum chorioamnionitis.
- Prolonged labour.
- Multiple pelvic examinations.
- Internal fetal monitoring—use of scalp electrodes/ intrauterine pressure catheters.
- Other risk factors, e.g. anaemia, low socio-economic status.

Signs and symptoms
- Fever usually in proportion to the extent of infection.
- Foul smelling, profuse, and bloody discharge.
- Subinvolution of uterus.
- Tender bulky uterus on abdominal examination.

Perineal wound infection
- Includes infection of episiotomy wounds and repaired lacerations.
- Perineum becomes painful and erythematous.
- May cause breakdown of wound.

> **Complications of pelvic infection**
> - Wound dehiscence.
> - Adnexal infections.
> - Pelvic abscess.
> - Septic thrombophlebitis.
> - Septicaemia.
> - Subsequent subfertility.

> **Factors predisposing to puerperal pyrexia**
> ### Antepartum
> - Anaemia.
> - Duration of membrane rupture.
>
> ### Intrapartum
> - Duration of labour.
> - Bacterial contamination during vaginal examination.
> - Instrumentation.
> - Trauma, e.g. episiotomy, vaginal tears, CS.
> - Haematoma.

Puerperal pyrexia: non-genital causes

Breast causes (mastitis, breast abscess)
- About 15% of women develop fever from breast engorgement.
- Fever may be as high as 39°C.
- Associated with painful and hard breast.
- Antibiotics may be needed in presence of infection.
- Breast-feeding should be continued.
- Abscess may need surgical drainage.

Urinary tract infection
- About 2–4% of women develop UTI post-partum.
- Hypotonic bladder may result in stasis and reflux of urine.
- Catheterization, birth trauma, pelvic examinations during labour.
- *Presenting symptoms*: increased frequency of micturition, dysuria, or urgency. High fever, rigors, loin pain, and tenderness may be present in pyelonephritis.
- Most common organisms involved: *E. coli*, *Proteus*, and *Klebsiella*.

Thrombophlebitis
- Superficial or deep venous thrombosis of legs may cause pyrexia.
- Caused by venous stasis.
- Diagnosis made by the observation of a painful, swollen leg, usually accompanied by calf tenderness.

⚠ High risk of post-partum DVT and PE—be vigilant and carry out appropriate investigations urgently.

Respiratory complications
- Usually seen within the first 24h after delivery.
- Almost invariably in women delivered by CS.
- Complications due to atelectasis, aspiration, and/or bacterial pneumonia.

Abdominal wound infection
- Incidence following CS is about 6%.
- With prophylactic antibiotics, the rate of infection could be <2%.
- Recent guidelines recommend antibiotics prior to skin incision (e.g. cefuroxime 1.5g IV; if sensitive then clindamycin 900mg IV. Co-amoxiclav best avoided for fear of necrotizing enterocolitis in the neonate).
- Risk factors include:
  - obesity
  - diabetes
  - corticosteroid therapy
  - poor haemostasis at surgery with subsequent haematoma.

⚠ VTE can also cause low-grade pyrexia and must always be considered in the differential diagnosis.

Puerperal pyrexia: management

Investigations

Investigations should be aimed at identifying the most likely source of infection, causative organism, and antibiotic sensitivity, and may include:

- FBC.
- Blood cultures.
- MSU.
- Swabs from cervix and lochia for *Chlamydia* and bacterial culture.
- Wound swabs.
- Throat swabs.
- Sputum culture and chest radiograph.

Management

Supportive

- Analgesics and anti-inflammatory drugs (NSAIDs).
- Wound care in cases of wound infection.
- Ice packs for pain from perineum or mastitis.

Antibiotics

- A regimen with activity against the *Bacteroides fragilis* group and other penicillin-resistant anaerobic bacteria is better than one without.
- There is no evidence that any one regimen is associated with fewer side effects, except that cephalosporins are associated with less diarrhoea.
- No specific recommendations can be made for the treatment of women who develop endometritis after receiving antibiotic prophylaxis for CS.
- Combination of clindamycin and an aminoglycoside (such as gentamicin) is appropriate for the treatment of endometritis.
- Tetracyclines should be avoided in breast-feeding women.
- Involvement of microbiologists is indicated in women who fail to respond to antibiotics.

Surgical

- Incision and drainage of breast abscess.
- Secondary repair of wound dehiscence.
- Drainage of pelvic haematomas and abscesses.

Prevention
- Women with suspected UTI during the antenatal period should be investigated and any infection treated vigorously.
- Advice should be offered with regard to breast-feeding and care of breasts during the antenatal period.
- Prevention and treatment of pre-existing anaemia (especially important in women from developing countries).
- Rigid antiseptic measures taken during labour and delivery also help to eliminate infection, including:
  - hand washing and use of alcohol hand gel by midwives and doctor before examining the patient
  - examining in a sterile environment and using sterile instruments
  - use of antiseptic creams and lotions
  - catheterizing only when it is indicated and using all sterile precautions while introducing the catheter.
- Prophylactic antibiotic administration at CS.
- Treatment with broad-spectrum antibiotics while waiting for the culture results.

Further reading

French LM, Smaill FM. (2004). Antibiotic regimens for endometritis after delivery. *Cochrane Database of Systematic Reviews* **18**(4): CD001067.

Other postnatal problems

Pain

- 'After-pains' due to uterine contractions cause lower central abdominal pain mainly during the first 3–4 days.
- Perineal pain could be severe, especially after instrumental delivery, episiotomy, or vaginal tears:
  - increasing pain may be a sign of infection
  - if infected, antibiotics are prescribed depending on the local policy.

▶ Randomized controlled trials of oral analgesia for perineal pain show that paracetamol and NSAIDs are as effective as oral narcotic medications. Some may find topical application of local anaesthetic (e.g. 1% lidocaine gel) helpful.

Bladder problems

- *Urinary retention:* occurs commonly with an epidural as bladder sensation and the desire to void is masked. Instrumental delivery or extensive tears (especially peri-urethral), perineal pain, and oedema can cause voiding difficulties and retention. Reassurance along with analgesics is helpful in most situations.
- Occasionally, catheterization is required to protect from over-distention. It may be best to leave indwelling for 24–48h.
- *UTI:* has low threshold for suspicion; confirm with MSU and treat with appropriate antibiotics and plenty of oral fluids.

⚠ An in dwelling catheter should be used after a spinal, until full sensation returns to protect the bladder from damage by over distension.

Bowel problems

- Lack of fluid and food, and dehydration during labour lead to constipation, which may continue into the puerperium.
- Pain and fear of wound disruption following perineal tears could further exacerbate the problem, as can opiate analgesia.
- Advice should be offered to increase the intake of fibre and fluids.
- Osmotic laxatives such as lactulose may be helpful.
- Women with 3rd or 4th degree tears should be prescribed stool softeners and laxatives (see 📖 Third- and fourth-degree tears, p. 304).

Symphysis pubis discomfort

- Symptoms include severe pubic and groin pain exacerbated by weight bearing.
- Most cases resolve by 6–8wks.
- Conservative approach includes rest, a belt that wraps around the femoral trochanters to discourage separation, weight-bearing assistance, and analgesics.
- Rarely surgical assistance may be needed.

Maternal obstetric paralysis

- This is very rare but manifests as intrapartum foot drop due to lumbosacral trunk compression by the fetal head at the pelvic brim.
- Placing the legs on lithotomy wihout protection at the region of the head of the fibula can compress the peroneal nerve and cause palsy.
- The primary pathology is predominantly demyelination, and recovery is usually complete in up to 5mths.
- Referral for neurological assessment and input is recommended.

Identifying mental health problems

- Lack of social and psychological support during puerperium is a common problem and may occur in 7–30% of women in developed countries.
- Psychological well-being of women should be carefully and continually assessed in the postnatal period.
- Enquiry should be made of every mother about past mental health.
- Close liaison between midwives, general practitioners, and obstetricians is essential to provide appropriate care.

⚠ Mental illness is one of the leading causes of maternal death in the UK.
- The majority of these deaths are the result of suicide, which is itself most strongly associated with perinatal depression.
- Over half of suicides occur between 6wks prenatally and 12wks postnatally and are sudden and of a violent nature and hence the need to provide appropriate treatment to avoid such occurrences (see Postnatal depression, p. 454).

Other postnatal care issues

Lifestyle

Both care and information provided should be culturally appropriate. The cultural practices of women from ethnic minority groups should be incorporated into their postnatal care. Advice should be given regarding diet, exercise, breast-feeding, weight and shape, rest, and support for coping with changes.

Post-partum contraception

- Discussion of contraception should be a routine part of post-partum care.
- Contraception is not needed in the first 3wks.
- Breast-feeding (lactational amenorrhoea) may be used as contraception (see 🕮 Breast-feeding, p. 362).
- Breast-feeding women can start POP without the need for additional contraceptive protection.
- The COCP should be avoided in lactating women as it can affect milk composition and increase the incidence of breast-feeding failure.
- Bottle-feeding women can start COCP 21 days post-partum.

▶ There may be an increased risk of VTE with earlier commencement of COCP.

Maternal immunization

Rubella

Women found to be seronegative on antenatal screening for rubella should receive rubella vaccination after delivery, before discharge from the maternity unit. Breast-feeding is not a contraindication for rubella immunization, but women should be warned to avoid conceiving in the following 3mths, although the risk is only theoretical.

Anti-D

The RCOG recommends the administration of anti-D 500IU to every non-sensitized RhD –ve woman within 72h after the delivery of an RhD +ve infant (see 🕮 Rhesus isoimmunization (immune hydrops), p. 135).

Hepatitis B

There are no specific recommendations for post-partum vaccination against HBV. However, it could be offered to individuals who are at increased risk because of their lifestyle or occupation. Neither pregnancy nor lactation should be considered a contraindication for hepatitis B vaccination of susceptible women. Neonatal vaccination is recommended for the babies of women at risk or who already have the virus.

Breast-feeding: overview

Breast-feeding confers several advantages to the newborn and is supported by healthcare institutions. WHO and UNICEF launched the Baby-Friendly Hospital Initiative (BFHI) in 1992, to strengthen maternity practices to support breast-feeding. The foundation for the BFHI are the 10 steps to successful breast-feeding described in *Protecting, Promoting and Supporting Breast-feeding*: a Joint WHO/UNICEF Statement. Breastmilk provides enormous medical and physical benefits to the infant.

During the years 2005–2010, initiation of breast-feeding rates in England was 78–83%, in Wales 67–71%, and in Scotland 70–74%. The latest figures are available at ℘ www.unicef.org.uk/babyfriendly

Colostrum

- Thick yellow fluid produced from around 20wks gestation.
- It has a high concentration of secretory IgA.
- It is rich in proteins that play an important part in gut maturation and immunity for the infant.
- It is produced in small quantities following the birth of the baby.

Human milk

- The amount of milk produced rapidly ↑ to ~500mL at 5 days post-partum.
- It has 57–65kcal/dL (2.4–2.7mJ/L) and is more energy efficient than formula milk.

Initiation and frequency

Initiation

- Skin-to-skin contact should start as soon as possible after delivery and is provided as 'Kangaroo care' from birth.
- Early contact ↑ breast-feeding within the first 2h after birth and ↑ duration of breast-feeding when compared with delay of 4h or more.

Frequency

- Varies widely.
- Demand feeding should be encouraged because of its benefits of less weight loss in the immediate post-partum period and ↑ duration of breast-feeding subsequently.
- Frequent feeding is associated with less hyperbilirubinaemia during the early neonatal period.
- For mothers, demand feeding helps to prevent engorgement, and breast-feeding is established more easily.

Demand feeding: facts and figures

- Exclusively breast-fed term infants feed a median of 8 times/day—
  6 times during the day, and twice in the night.
- Feeds tend to be infrequent in the first 24–48h and could be as
  few as 3 feeds in the first 24h (this should not cause concern in an
  otherwise well baby).
- The frequency increases gradually and reaches a peak around the 5th
  day of life.
- WHO recommends exclusive breast-feeding for 4–6mths, with
  introduction of appropriate complementary foods after this period.

Further reading

WHO. (1998). *Evidence for the ten steps to successful breast feeding.* ℘ http://.www.who.int/
    maternal_child_adolescent/documents/9241591544/en

WHO/UNICEF. (1989). *Protecting, promoting and supporting breast-feeding.* WHO, Geneva.

Breast-feeding: benefits

Human breastmilk contains numerous protective factors against infectious disease and may influence immune system development. Includes effect of colostrum on immunity, fewer diarrhoeal diseases, benefits of omega-3 fatty acids on visual developments in small infants, improved bonding, and reduced risk of breast disease for mother.

For the infant

Gastrointestinal illness Infants who are exclusively breast-fed for 6mths experience less morbidity from gastrointestinal infection than those who are mixed breast-fed at 3–4mths.

UTIs Breast milk is a part of the natural defence against UTIs.

Respiratory infection Exclusive breast-feeding protects against chest infections.

Atopic illness Breast-fed babies are less likely to have atopic illnesses, such as eczema and asthma.

Leukaemias Breast-feeding associated with a reduced risk of childhood acute leukaemia, acute lymphoblastic leukaemia, Hodgkin's disease, and neuroblastoma in childhood.

Giardiasis Children born to non-immune mothers are at significantly higher risk of acquiring *Giardia* infection and developing giardiasis with more severe symptoms compared with children of immune mothers.

Intelligence It remains unclear whether the child's intelligence is affected by breast-feeding, although it remains an unequalled way of providing ideal nutrition.

For the mother

Uterine involution Breast-feeding helps in uterine involution and reduces risk of post-partum haemorrhage.

Amenorrhoea and contraception
- Lactational amenorrhoea, and full or nearly full breast-feeding for up to 6mths is nearly 99% effective as contraception.
- At 12mths the effectiveness during amenorrhoea dropped to 97%.
- Amenorrhoea can be helpful for anaemia in developing countries.

Other benefits
Breast-feeding protects the mother against premenopausal breast cancer, ovarian cancer, and osteoporosis.

Breast-feeding: potential problems

Inadequate milk supply
- <1% of women are physiologically incapable of producing an adequate milk supply.
- Treatment for insufficient milk includes: adequate fluids, nutrition, secure and private environment, dopamine antagonists, thyrotropin-releasing hormone, and oxytocin.

Problems with milk flow
Breast engorgement, mastitis, and breast abscess
- Limitations on feeding frequency and duration.
- Problems with positioning the baby at the breast.
- Allowing the baby unrestricted access to the breast is the most effective method of treating.

See Box 9.3.

Sore or cracked nipples
- It could be because of incorrect attachment of the baby to the breast.
- It may be necessary to rest the breast and express the breastmilk manually until the crack has healed.

Lactation after breast cancer
- There will be little or no enlargement of the treated breast during pregnancy.
- The ability to lactate and breast-feed from an untreated breast remains normal.
- Tamoxifen inhibits milk production.

Drugs that may reduce milk production
- Progestins.
- Oestrogens.
- Ethanol.
- Bromocriptine.
- Ergotamine.
- Cabergoline.
- Pseudoephedrine.

Box 9.3 Breast problems

Mastitis (non-infective)
- Results from obstruction of milk drainage from one section of the breast, which may be due to:
  - restriction of feeding
  - a badly positioned baby
  - blocked ducts
  - compression from fingers holding the breast or from wearing too small a bra.
- Characterized by swollen, red, and painful area on breast, tachycardia, pyrexia, and an aching, flu-like feeling, often accompanied by shivering and rigors.
- Resolves with relieving the obstruction by continuing to breast-feed with correct positioning of the baby.

Mastitis (infective)
- If non-infective mastitis is not managed appropriately, it may become infected.
- *Staphylococcus aureus* is the most common organism involved.
- The antibiotics that should be used include penicillinase-resistant penicillins (e.g. cloxacillin, flucloxacillin, co-amoxiclav) or cephalosporins (cefalexin, cefadrine, cefaclor).
- Breast-feeding should be continued.

Breast abscess
- Possible complication of inappropriately managed infective mastitis.
- It may need surgical drainage under anaesthetic.
- In severe cases breast-feeding may have to cease on the affected side.

Drugs and breast-feeding

Almost all drugs, to some extent, pass in breastmilk. The effect of the drug depends on degree of passage into milk, amount of milk ingested by the infant, absorption of the drug, and whether the drug affects the infant. There are limited human studies to advise on which drugs are contraindicated in pregnancy.

▶ Prescribe medication only when absolutely indicated. Choose ones with shorter half-lives, less toxicity, those commonly used in infants, and those with reduced bioavailability. Only a few medications are unsafe.

Medications with poor bioavailability and low risk
- Heparin.
- Insulin.
- Aminoglycoside antibiotics.
- Third generation cephalosporins.
- Omeprazole and lansoprazole.
- Inhaled steroids and beta agonists.

Drugs generally contraindicated in breast-feeding mothers
- Amiodarone.
- Antineoplastic.
- Chloramphenicol.
- Ergotamine.
- Cabergoline.
- Ergot alkaloids.
- Iodides.
- Methotrexate.
- Lithium.
- Tetracycline.
- Pseudoephedrine.

Viruses and breast-feeding

Human immunodeficiency virus (HIV)
HIV can be transmitted through breastmilk. Risk factors are:
• Maternal viral load.
• Duration of breast-feeding.
• Oral lesions in infant and maternal breast lesions.

⚠ In developed countries, breast-feeding by HIV-infected mothers should be avoided.

Human lymphotropic virus (HTLV-1)
Breast-fed babies of HTLV-1-infected mothers are likely to become infected, especially with prolonged breast-feeding.

⚠ HTLV-1 seropositive women are advised not to breast-feed.

Hepatitis B virus (HBV)
Infants born to HBV +ve mothers, already exposed to maternal blood, amniotic fluid, and vaginal secretions during delivery, may be breast-fed. Babies of all mothers +ve for HBV surface antigen should be immunized at birth. Babies of mothers +ve for HBVe antigen are also given immunoglobulins as additional protection.

▶ Breast-feeding does not appear to increase the rate of infection among infants.

Herpes simplex virus
If there are no breast lesions, breast-feeding should be encouraged.

Chickenpox/varicella
If the mother contracts chickenpox while breast-feeding, she should continue to breast-feed, because the antibodies in her milk confer immunity against chickenpox to her baby. This passive immunization may even spare the baby from symptoms of chickenpox.

Cytomegalovirus
CMV is possibly the most commonly detectable virus in human milk. No serious illness or clinical symptoms in neonates 2° to breast-feeding has been reported.

Rubella
Can be passed on to infant if mother has active infection. However, infant does not become ill as transmission of maternal antibodies serves as natural vaccine. If mother is immunized to rubella post-partum, breast-feeding infant will not show symptoms of the illness.

Drugs to avoid in breast-feeding mothers
- Acebutolol.
- ACEIs (except captopril).
- Alcohol.
- Caffeine.
- Cocaine.
- Marijuana.
- Fluoxetine.
- Iodine.
- Sulphonamides.

Obstetric emergencies

Sudden maternal collapse

⚠ **Immediate maternal resuscitation is vital**
- **A** *Airway*: open airway with head tilt and chin lift; jaw thrust may be required (care must be taken if a cervical spine injury is suspected).
- **B** *Breathing*: assess for chest movements and breath sounds; feel for breathing. If no breathing, put out cardiac arrest call and give 2 rescue breaths.
- **C** *Circulation*: check carotid pulse; optimize circulation by aggressive IV fluids and blood transfusion if indicated.

▶ Cardiopulmonary resuscitation (CPR) should be initiated as necessary.

▶ If CPR required at >20wks, CS within 5min of arrest in a left lateral position is essential for maternal resuscitation.
- **D** *Drugs*: to maintain circulation, combat infection, antidotes if drug overdose, anticoagulants in cases of massive embolism.
- **E** *Environment*: avoid injury (eclampsia), ensure safety of patient and staff.
- **F** *Fetus*: if CPR is required at >20wks, unless there is immediate reversal, immediate CS (at the location of the arrest) must be performed. If CPR is not required, assess fetal well-being and plan delivery as appropriate once maternal condition is stable.

General investigations
- *History:* from the patient or her relatives.
- *Observations:* BP, pulse, respiration, oxygen saturation, temperature, and urine output every 15min.
- *Bloods:* FBC, coagulation profile, U&Es, LFTs, uric acid, group and save or cross-match, and blood glucose.

Specific investigations
- If a cardiorespiratory cause is suspected: ECG, CXR, ABG.
- If pulmonary embolism is suspected: Doppler ultrasound of calf veins, ventilation (Q) scan or ventilation/perfusion (V/Q) scan.
- If intracranial pathology is suspected: cerebral imaging (CT/MRI).

Treatment
Specific treatment depends on the cause. Important to ensure multidisciplinary input early to optimize outcome. Anaesthetic and ICU assistance urgently required. If focal neurological signs are present, early neurosurgical input may save lives.

Some causes of sudden maternal collapse

Obstetric

- Massive obstetric haemorrhage (⚠ may be concealed):
  - placenta praevia
  - placental abruption
  - PPH
  - uterine rupture
  - supralevator haematoma following genital tract trauma.
- Severe pre-eclampsia with intracranial bleeding.
- Eclampsia.
- Amniotic fluid embolism.
- Neurogenic shock due to uterine inversion.
- Surgical complications:
  - bleeding after CS
  - pelvic/broad ligament haematoma.
- Severe sepsis, e.g. chorioamnionitis.
- Cardiac failure, e.g. peripartum cardiomyopathy.

Medical/surgical

- Massive pulmonary embolism.
- Cardiac failure:
  - pre-existing cardiac disease
  - myocardial infarction.
- Shock:
  - anaphylactic
  - septic.
- Intra-abdominal bleeding:
  - hepatic
  - splenic
  - aortic rupture.
- Intracerebral haemorrhage.
- Overdosage or substance abuse.
- Metabolic/endocrine: diabetic coma.
- Cerebral infection:
  - encephalitis
  - cerebral malaria.

Shoulder dystocia: overview

Defined as any delivery that requires additional obstetric manoeuvres after gentle downward traction on the head has failed to deliver shoulders. Complicates about 1:200 deliveries, and has potential for serious fetal complications.

Complications of shoulder dystocia

Fetal
- Hypoxia and neurological injury (cerebral palsy).
- Brachial plexus palsy.
- Fracture of clavicle or humerus.
- Intracranial haemorrhage.
- Cervical spine injury.
- Rarely, fetal death.

Maternal
- PPH.
- Genital tract trauma including 3rd and 4th degree perineal tears.

Mechanism

- Usually the anterior shoulder is impacted against the symphysis pubis, often due to the failure of internal rotation of the shoulders.
- Rarely, the posterior shoulder may be impacted against the sacral promontory, resulting in bilateral impaction, causing problems at delivery.
- Fetal deterioration is rapid, often without cord acidosis, largely due to cord compression and trauma.

Risk factors

Prediction of shoulder dystocia by use of risk factors has poor predictive value. Estimated that only 50% of shoulder dystocia is associated with a birth weight of >4kg. However, it is important to be aware of antepartum and intrapartum risk factors, so that shoulder dystocia may be anticipated and to allow senior input to be available.

Shoulder dystocia can often be anticipated by limited or slow delivery of the head and McRoberts' manoeuvre is often used prophylactically. Attempts at delivery, however, should not occur before next contraction.

Risk factors for shoulder dystocia

Antenatal

- Previous history of shoulder dystocia.
- Fetal macrosomia.
- BMI >30 and excessive weight gain in pregnancy.
- Diabetes mellitus.
- Post-term pregnancy.

Intrapartum

- Lack of progress in late first or second stage of labour.
- Instrumental vaginal delivery (especially rotational deliveries).

Shoulder dystocia: management

- Prompt, skillful, and well-rehearsed manoeuvres may improve outcome.
- A mnemonic *'HELPERR'* (ALSO course) has been suggested to aid in remembering the sequence.
- Main objectives are to facilitate the entry of anterior (or posterior) shoulder into pelvis and to ensure rotation of shoulders to larger oblique or transverse diameter of the pelvis.

- **H** Call for help (including additional midwife, senior obstetrician, neonatologist, anaesthetist).
- **E** Episiotomy—remember shoulder dystocia is a bony problem, but an episiotomy may help with internal manoeuvres.
- **L** Legs into McRoberts' (hyperflexed at hips with thighs abducted and externally rotated).
- **P** Suprapubic pressure applied to posterior aspect of anterior shoulder (must know which side fetal back is on) to dislodge it from under symphysis pubis; if continuous pressure fails, a rocking movement may be tried.
- **E** Enter pelvis for internal manoeuvres, which include:
  - pressure exerted on the posterior aspect of anterior shoulder to adduct and rotate the shoulders to the larger oblique diameter (Rubin II)
  - if this fails combine it with pressure on the anterior aspect of the posterior shoulder (Woods' screw)
  - if this fails, reversing manoeuvre may be tried with pressure on the anterior aspect of anterior shoulder and posterior aspect of posterior shoulder in opposite direction (reverse Woods' screw).
- **R** Release of posterior arm by flexing elbow, getting hold of fetal hand, and sweeping fetal arm across chest and face to release posterior shoulder.
- **R** Roll over to 'all fours' may help aid delivery by the changes brought about in the pelvic dimensions (Gaskin manoeuvre).

▶ In practice, 80% of babies will deliver with suprapubic pressure and McRoberts' manoeuvre. If these fail, delivery of posterior arm is probably the best next manoeuvre.

Other manoeuvres

- *Zanvanelli:* replacement of head into the vagina by reversing the mechanism of labour (i.e. flexion and 'de-restitution') and performing a CS may be a last resort. Tocolysis may be required to facilitate this procedure.
- *Symphysiotomy:* may be performed to 'open up' pelvic girdle, but can result in severe maternal morbidity (urethral injury, incontinence, altered gait, and chronic pelvic pain). Urethral injury should be avoided by displacing urethra with a metal catheter at time of symphysiotomy.

Other considerations in the event of a shoulder dystocia

⚠ Essential not to exert traction on head without disimpaction of shoulders as this increases risk of brachial plexus injury.

- Time-keeping is essential and it is good practice to allocate a member of the team to document the timeline of events.
- Paediatric team must be called urgently as a need for neonatal resuscitation should be anticipated.
- PPH should also be anticipated and prophylactic measures considered, such as a 40IU oxytocin infusion.
- The genital tract should be carefully examined for trauma.
- Carefully document the timing and sequence of events, who was involved, and what each person did, as soon as possible afterwards.
- Important to explain delivery and discuss outcome with parents after the event.
- An incident report form should be filled for risk management.
- If an injury has occurred, it may become a medico-legal issue, making documentation even more important.

Further reading
Advanced Life Support in Obstetrics (ALSO) course. ⅀ www.also.org.uk

Massive obstetric haemorrhage: causes

This is an important cause of maternal morbidity and mortality. Identification of risk factors, institution of preventive measures, and prompt and appropriate management of blood loss are likely to improve outcome. It is also important to remember that all bleeding can be concealed.

▶ Massive obstetric haemorrhage refers to the loss of 30–40% (generally about 2L) of the patient's blood volume. This may be caused by an insult leading to hypovolaemia (then coagulopathy) or rarely from direct coagulation failure (leading to hypovolaemia).

Consequences of massive obstetric haemorrhage

- Acute hypovolaemia.
- Sudden and rapid cardiovascular decompensation.
- DIC.
- Iatrogenic complications associated with fluid replacement and multiple blood transfusions.
- Pulmonary oedema.
- Transfusion reactions.
- Adult respiratory distress syndrome (ARDS).
- Sheehan's syndrome (hypopituitarism).

Causes of massive obstetric haemorrhage

Antepartum
- Placental abruption.
- Placenta praevia.
- Severe chorioamnionitis or septicaemia.
- Severe pre-eclampsia (including hepatic rupture).
- Retained dead fetus.

Intrapartum
- Intrapartum abruption.
- Uterine rupture.
- Amniotic fluid embolism.
- Complications of CS; angular or broad ligament tears.
- Morbidly adherent placenta (accreta/percreta).

Post-partum
- Primary PPH is usually due to:
  - atonic uterus ('tone')
  - genital tract trauma ('trauma')
  - coagulopathy ('thrombin')
  - retained products of conception ('tissue').
- Secondary PPH is due to:
  - infection (often associated with retained products of conception)
  - rarely, gestational trophoblastic disease or uterine arteriovenous malformation including a pseudo-aneurysm.

Massive obstetric haemorrhage: pathophysiology

Pregnancy is associated with an increase in blood volume (see 📖 Physiology of pregnancy: haemodynamics, p. 26). The blood flow to the pregnant uterus at term is about 500–800mL/min with the placental circulation accounting for about 400mL/min. It is therefore quite easy for a large proportion of the circulating volume to be lost in a short time.

A loss of about 500–1000mL (10–15% of blood volume) is usually well tolerated by a fit, healthy young woman, as she is able to maintain her cardiovascular parameters by effective compensatory mechanisms until about 30–40% of the blood volume is lost (Table 10.1).

> **Blood loss >1000mL may result in:**
> - Acute hypovolaemia.
> - Shock with sudden reduction in perfusion to vital organs.
> - Loss of clotting factors ('washout phenomenon').
> - DIC.
> - Hypoxia leading to anaerobic metabolism, accumulation of lactic acid, and metabolic acidosis.
> - Multi-organ dysfunction/failure.

Pulse rate, rather than BP, is more useful in assessing the degree of blood loss, especially with occult loss such as concealed abruption or scar rupture. In these situations, the degree of haemodynamic instability may be out of proportion to the visually estimated blood loss. Table 10.1 shows cardiovascular responses to blood loss.

Disseminated intravascular coagulopathy

The main cause of DIC is massive blood loss, but it can occur with other conditions such as amniotic fluid embolism. It occurs due to the depletion of fibrinogen, platelets, and coagulation factors that are consumed or lost with the blood. Infusions of replacement fluids further dilute the remaining coagulation factors and combined with hypotension-mediated endothelial injury may trigger DIC.

The most useful tests to diagnose DIC are fibrin degradation products (FDPs), fibrinogen, partial thromboplastin time (PTT), and APTT. Early involvement of a senior haematologist is vital to advise on appropriate replacement of blood products.

- *Fresh frozen plasma (FFP):* contains all the clotting factors required. Ideally, 1U of FFP should be given with each unit of rapidly transfused blood.
- *Cryoprecipitate:* contains more fibrinogen but lacks antithrombin III which is often depleted in massive obstetric haemorrhages.
- *Platelet concentrate:* rarely indicated, but may be required if surgical intervention is planned.
- *Recombinant activated factor VII:* used successfully in severe coagulopathy but is expensive and not always readily available.
- Consider tranexamic acid 1g IV.

Table 10.1 Blood loss and cardiovascular parameters

Blood loss	Heart rate	Systolic BP	Tissue perfusion
10–15%	Increased	Normal	Postural hypotension
15–30%	Increased +	Normal	Peripheral vasoconstriction
30–40%	Increased ++	70–80mmHg	Pallor, oliguria, confusion, restlessness
40%+	Increased+++	<60mmHg	Collapse, anuria, dyspnoea

Massive obstetric haemorrhage: resuscitation

Massive obstetric haemorrhage is a life-threatening emergency requiring swift and appropriate treatment. Most units will have a local guideline for its management, with a detailed protocol and hospital alert system once blood loss has reached 2000mL. This should include such details as who to contact, agreed timescales for laboratory results, and designated responsibilities of key staff.

Management should consist of immediate resuscitation with restoration of the circulating volume and rapid treatment of the underlying cause in order to stop ongoing blood loss.

Initial measures for resuscitation
- Call for help; include alerting the senior obstetrician, anaesthetists, haematologist, hospital porter, blood bank, and theatres.
- Left lateral tilt if antepartum, to relieve venocaval compression and improve venous return.
- High-flow facial oxygen (regardless of oxygen saturation).
- Assess airway and respiratory effort—intubation may be indicated to protect airway if there is decreased level of consciousness due to hypotension.
- Two large-bore IV cannulae (14 gauge):
  - take blood whilst cannulating for FBC, cross-match, U&Es, LFTs, coagulopathy screen
  - start IV crystalloids to correct hypovolaemia.
- Catheterize and measure hourly urine output.
- *Blood transfusion:* O rhesus –ve blood can be used immediately until cross-matched blood is available.
- *Replace clotting factors:*
  - FFP (1U for every 1U of blood once 2U of blood given)
  - consider cryoprecipitate and platelets.
- As soon as appropriate in the resuscitation process, transfer the woman to a place where there is adequate space, lighting, and equipment to continue treatment (usually theatre).
- Assess need for a CVP line.

⚠ One member of the team should be assigned to record the vital signs, urinary output, type and quantity of fluid replacement, drugs given, and timeline of events.

▶ Once the bleeding has been stopped and the woman stabilized, she should be managed in HDU or ICU.

Massive obstetric haemorrhage: medical management

The exact management plan will depend on the cause of the bleeding. The most common cause is uterine atony, often secondary to retained tissue, but genital tract trauma and underlying coagulation disorders must also be considered.

⚠ Call for senior obstetric and anaesthetic help and inform haematologists.

Principles for stopping the bleeding
- Empty uterus (fetus or tissue).
- Treat uterine atony (physically, medically, surgically).
- Repair genital tract trauma.

Medical management of uterine atony
⚠ Should be accompanied by physical attempts to contract uterus, such as rubbing up contractions and bimanual compression.
- 500 micrograms of ergometrine is given IV (may be given IM if difficulties with IV access).
- Start oxytocin infusion (40IU).
- If the bleeding does not stop, 10U of oxytocin may be given IV.
- If the bleeding still persists (or ergometrine is contraindicated) then 800 micrograms of misoprostol (tablets) is given rectally.
- If the atony continues, carboprost 250 micrograms IM is given in the thigh or directly into the myometrium and repeated at 15min intervals up to a total of 4 doses.

▶ If all these measures fail, examination under anaesthesia with possible further surgical management is indicated without delay.

General interventions in the management of massive obstetric haemorrhage

- Empty uterus:
  - deliver fetus
  - remove placenta or retained tissue.
- Massage uterus (to 'rub up' a contraction).
- Give drugs to ↑ uterine contraction:
  - oxytocin 40IU infusion
  - ergometrine 500 micrograms IV or IM
  - misoprostol 800–1000 micrograms
  - carboprost 250 micrograms.
- Apply bimanual compression.
- Repair any genital tract injuries (including cervical tears).
- Uterine tamponade with a Rusch balloon.
- Laparotomy:
  - if bleeding from placental bed, may need oversewing and insertion of a Rusch balloon
  - if uterus is atonic, not responding to drug treatment but the bleeding is ↓ with compression, a B-Lynch or vertical compression suture should be placed
  - internal iliac or uterine artery ligation (proceeds to hysterectomy in 50% of cases)
  - uterine artery embolization may be helpful but is not always an option in emergency situations
  - total or subtotal hysterectomy.

▶ Compression of the aorta may be used to gain temporary control while a definitive treatment gets under way.

Massive obstetric haemorrhage: surgical management

Interventions after laparotomy

> **Tamponade test**
> A Rusch ballon catheter, Sengstaken–Blakemore tube, or Cooke's bal-
> loon is inserted into the uterine cavity and filled with 100–500mL of
> warm saline (warm saline accelerates the clotting process). If the bleed-
> ing is controlled then the balloon is left *in situ* for 12–24h and removed.
> This test is therapeutic as it stops bleeding in 80% of cases, and prog-
> nostic in revealing within 15min whether further surgical intervention
> is needed.

- ⚠ Ensure that the uterine cavity is definitely empty as even very small
  pieces of retained tissue can cause atony.
- If the bleeding is from large placental sinuses following CS then
  undersewing the placental bed ± insertion of a Rusch balloon may
  control the bleeding.
- If the bleeding is from uterine atony unresponsive to drug treatment,
  but which ↓ with manual compression, a B-Lynch or vertical
  compression suture should be attempted (this provides continuous
  compression and reduces the blood flow into the uterus).
- Systematic pelvic devascularization by ligation of uterine, tubal branch
  of the ovarian, or anterior division of internal iliac arteries:
  - ligation of uterine artery and utero-ovarian artery anastomosis will
    not control the bleeding from the vaginal branch of the internal iliac
    artery which supplies the lower segment of the uterus
  - internal iliac artery ligation will help in controlling both the uterine
    artery and the vaginal branch bleeding (bilateral ligation results in
    85% reduction in the pulse pressure and 50% reduction in blood
    flow, and bleeding is reduced by 50%).
- Hysterectomy is the last option:
  - sub-total hysterectomy is safer and quicker to perform
  - if the bleeding is from the lower segment (placenta praevia, accreta,
    or tears) then total hysterectomy is carried out.

⚠ The decision to carry out hysterectomy should not be unduly delayed
as this can result in the death of the mother.

Arterial embolization for massive obstetric haemorrhage

Advantages
- Less invasive than laparotomy.
- Helps to preserve fertility.
- Can target individual bleeding vessels.

Disadvantages
- Only available in a few centres.
- It may not be possible to get the required equipment to the obstetric theatres or to transfer a woman to the radiology department.
- Appropriately trained interventional radiologists must be available.

Method
- A catheter is inserted through the femoral artery and advanced above the bifurcation of the aorta and a contrast dye is injected to identify the bleeding vessels.
- The catheter is then directed to the bleeding vessel and embolized with gelatin sponge, which is usually reabsorbed in about 10 days.

▶ If excessive bleeding is anticipated (e.g. major placenta praevia with accreta), prophylactic interventional radiology can be a planned procedure where balloons are placed in the internal iliac or uterine vessels in advance if embolization is required.

Venous thromboembolism: overview

Background

VTE is a leading cause of maternal morbidity and mortality in developed countries. In the UK, VTE accounted for 18 maternal deaths in 2006–2008. Thromboembolic events include venous thrombosis (DVT) of the leg, calf, or pelvis, and PE.

- Incidence of pregnancy-associated VTE is 1–2:1000 pregnancies.
- Incidence of DVT is 3 times higher than that of PE.
- Emergency CS is associated with a higher incidence of DVT than elective CS or vaginal delivery.
- Thromboembolic disease can occur at any point in pregnancy:
  - antenatal DVT is more common than post-partum DVT
  - the event rate of VTE is higher in the puerperium.
- DVT leads to PE in approximately 16% of untreated patients.

Women with past history of VTE

The risk of VTE in pregnancy is ↑ in women with past history of VTE.

- For a single previous thrombosis with no known thrombophilia, the risk of VTE in pregnancy is increased from about 0.1 to 3%.
- The risk is higher if the woman has thrombophilia or if the previous VTE was in an unusual site or unprovoked.
- Women with previous VTE should be screened for thrombophilia before pregnancy.

Inherent pregnancy-associated risk factors for VTE

Pregnancy itself is a risk factor for VTE, due to:

- Venous stasis in the lower limbs.
- Possible trauma to the pelvic veins at the time of delivery.
- Changes in the coagulation system including:
  - ↑ in procoagulant factors (factors X, VIII, and fibrinogen)
  - ↓ in endogenous anticoagulant activity
  - suppression of fibrinolysis
  - significant ↓ in protein S activity.

▶ All pregnant women are at risk of thrombosis from early in the first trimester until at least 6wks post-partum. Some women are at even higher risk during pregnancy because they have one or more additional risk factors.

Other risk factors for VTE

Pre-existing risk factors

- Previous VTE.
- Congenital thrombophilia:
  - antithrombin deficiency
  - protein C deficiency
  - protein S deficiency
  - factor V Leiden
  - prothrombin gene variant.
- Acquired thrombophilia (antiphospholipid syndrome):
  - lupus anticoagulant
  - anticardiolipin antibodies.
- Age >35yrs.
- Obesity (BMI >30) either before pregnancy or in early pregnancy.
- Parity >4.
- Gross varicose veins.
- Paraplegia.
- Sickle cell disease.
- Inflammatory disorders, e.g. inflammatory bowel disease.
- Medical disorders, e.g. nephrotic syndrome, cardiac diseases.
- Myeloproliferative disorders, e.g. essential thrombocythaemia, polycythaemia vera.

New onset or transient risk factors

- Ovarian hyperstimulation syndrome.
- Hyperemesis.
- Dehydration.
- Long-haul travel.
- Severe infection, e.g. pyelonephritis.
- Immobility (>4 days bed rest).
- Pre-eclampsia.
- Prolonged labour.
- Mid-cavity instrumental delivery.
- Excessive blood loss.
- Surgical procedure in pregnancy or puerperium, e.g. evacuation of retained products of conception, post-partum sterilization.
- Immobility after delivery.

Further reading

Cantwell R, Clutton-Brock T, Cooper G, et al. (2011). Saving mothers' lives. Reviewing maternal deaths to make motherhood safer: The 8th report of the confidential enquiries into maternal deaths in the UK. Br J Obstet Gynaec **118**(suppl. 1): 1–203.

RCOG. (2007). Thrombosis and embolism during pregnancy and the puerperium. Reducing the risk. Green-top guideline 37b. ♒ http://www.rcog.org.uk/files/rcog-corp/GTG37aReducingRiskThrombosis.pdf

Venous thromboembolism: prevention

- LMWHs are the agents of choice for antenatal thromboprophylaxis.
- They are as effective as unfractionated heparin (UFH) in pregnancy, and safer.
- Monitoring anti-Xa levels is not usually required when using LMWH for thromboprophylaxis.
- In antithrombin deficiency, anti-Xa monitoring is critical, as higher doses of LMWH may be necessary.

Indications and minimum duration of thromboprophylaxis

- *Previous provoked/non-oestrogen-related VTE:* LMWH for 6wks post-partum.
- *Previous unprovoked or oestrogen-related VTE, or recurrent VTE or previous VTE and family history (1st-degree) of VTE:* LMWH antenatally and for ≥ 6wks post-partum.
- *Previous VTE and thrombophilia:* LMWH antenatally and for ≥6wks post-partum.
- *Asymptomatic inherited or acquired thrombophilia:* thromboprophylaxis depends on specific thrombophilia and presence of other risk factors.
- *Antithrombin III deficiency:* merits higher doses of LMWH as it is associated with a 30% risk of VTE in pregnancy.
- *Three or more persisting 'moderate' risk factors:* LMWH for 5 days post-partum.

▶ Women should be reassessed before, during, and after labour for risk factors for VTE using mandatory, often electronic, 'scoresheets'. An individual's score will guide management (Fig. 10.1).

Thromboprophylaxis: other considerations

- All women should undergo an assessment of risk factors for VTE in early pregnancy.
- Repeat if they develop any other problems and after delivery.
- Women with previous VTE should be screened for inherited and acquired thrombophilia, ideally before pregnancy.
- Immobilization and dehydration should be avoided.
- Antenatal thromboprophylaxis should begin as early as practical.
- Post-partum prophylaxis should begin as soon as possible after delivery (with precautions after use of regional anaesthesia).
- Excess blood loss and blood transfusion are risk factors for VTE, so thromboprophylaxis should be commenced or reinstituted as soon as the immediate risk of haemorrhage is reduced.

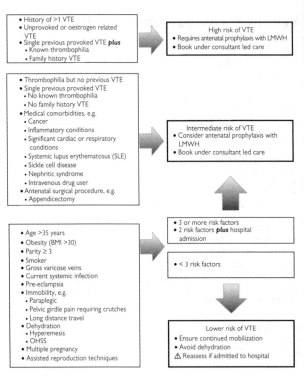

• History of >1 VTE
• Unprovoked or oestrogen related VTE
• Single previous provoked VTE **plus**
  • Known thrombophilia
  • Family history VTE

High risk of VTE
• Requires antenatal prophylaxis with LMWH
• Book under consultant led care

• Thrombophilia but no previous VTE
• Single previous provoked VTE
  • No known thrombophilia
  • No family history VTE
• Medical comorbidities, e.g.
  • Cancer
  • Inflammatory conditions
  • Significant cardiac or respiratory conditions
  • Systemic lupus erythematosus (SLE)
  • Sickle cell disease
  • Nephritic syndrome
  • Intravenous drug user
• Antenatal surgical procedure, e.g.
  • Appendicectomy

Intermediate risk of VTE
• Consider antenatal prophylaxis with LMWH
• Book under consultant led care

• Age >35 years
• Obesity (BMI >30)
• Parity ≥ 3
• Smoker
• Gross varicose veins
• Current systemic infection
• Pre-eclampsia
• Immobility, e.g.
  • Paraplegic
  • Pelvic girdle pain requiring crutches
  • Long distance travel
• Dehydration
  • Hyperemesis
  • OHSS
• Multiple pregnancy
• Assisted reproduction techniques

• 3 or more risk factors
• 2 risk factors **plus** hospital admission

• < 3 risk factors

Lower risk of VTE
• Ensure continued mobilization
• Avoid dehydration
⚠ Reassess if admitted to hospital

Fig. 10.1 Example of antenatal thromboprophylaxis risk assessment tool.

Further reading

RCG. Thrombosis and embolism during pregnancy and the puerperium, Reducing the risk, Green-top 37a. Available at: ℘ http://www.rcog.org.uk/files/rcog-corp/GTG37aReducingRiskThrombosis.pdf

Venous thromboembolism: diagnosis

Symptoms and signs of VTE

Deep vein thrombosis
- Leg pain or discomfort (especially in the left leg).
- Swelling.
- Tenderness.
- Pyrexia.
- Erythema, increased skin temperature, and oedema.
- Lower abdominal pain (high DVT).
- Elevated WBC.

Pulmonary embolism
- Dyspnoea.
- Collapse.
- Chest pain.
- Haemoptysis.
- Faintness.
- Raised JVP.
- Focal signs in chest.
- Symptoms and signs associated with DVT.

⚠ In pregnancy there should be a high level of suspicion for women presenting with any of the above symptoms and urgent investigation undertaken. If VTE is suspected, treatment should be commenced while diagnostic tests are awaited.

Investigations
- Thrombophilia screen.
- FBC, U&E, LFTs.
- Coagulation screen.

Diagnostic imaging
- Ultrasound (compression or duplex).
- Contrast venography with shielding of the uterus.
- MRI.

If PE suspected:
- ECG.
- CXR.
- ABG.
- Ventilation/perfusion lung scanning (V/Q or Q scan).
- Spiral CT/MRI scan.
- Bilateral duplex ultrasound leg examinations.

If diagnostic imaging reports a low risk of VTE, yet there is high clinical suspicion, anticoagulant treatment should be continued, with repeat testing in 1wk. Among women with clinically suspected VTE, <50% have the diagnosis confirmed as some of the symptoms and signs are commonly found in normal pregnancy.

D-dimers and pregnancy

- D-dimer is now used as a screening test for VTE in the non-pregnant woman, where it has a high –ve predictive value.
- D-dimer can be elevated due to the physiological changes in the coagulation system and particularly if there is a concomitant problem such as pre-eclampsia.
- Thus, a '+ve' D-dimer test in pregnancy is not necessarily consistent with VTE.
- However, low level of D-dimer is likely to suggest there is no VTE.

Venous thromboembolism: treatment

Anticoagulation

Unfractionated heparin

Has been the standard treatment in the initial management of VTE including massive PE. The regimen is:

- Loading dose of 5000IU, followed by continuous IV infusion of 1000–2000IU/h with an initial infusion concentration of 1000IU/mL.
- Measure APTT level 6h after the loading dose, then at least daily.
- The therapeutic target APTT ratio is usually 1.5–2.5× the average laboratory control value.
- Prolonged UFH use during pregnancy may result in osteoporosis, fractures, and allergic skin reactions.

Low molecular weight heparins

- More effective than UFH, with lower mortality and fewer haemorrhagic complications in non-pregnant subjects.
- LMWHs are as effective as UFH for treatment of PE.
- A bd dosage regimen for LMWHs is recommended in the treatment of VTE in pregnancy (enoxaparin 1mg/kg bd; dalteparin 100U/kg bd up to a maximum of 18 000U/24h).
- Long-term users of LMWHs have a lower risk of osteoporosis and bone fractures than UFH users.
- The peak anti-Xa activity (3h post-injection) should be measured to ensure the woman is appropriately anticoagulated.
- The target range for the anti-Xa level is 0.35–0.70IU/mL.

VTE: other considerations

- Therapeutic anticoagulation should be continued for at least 6mths.
- After delivery, treatment should continue for at least 6wks.
- Warfarin can be used postnatally and is safe for breast-feeding.
- The leg should be elevated and a graduated elastic compression stocking applied to reduce oedema; mobilization is recommended.
- Inferior vena caval filter may be considered for recurrent PEs, despite adequate anticoagulation or if anticoagulation is contraindicated.
- In life-threatening massive PE thrombolytic therapy, percutaneous catheter thrombus fragmentation or surgical embolectomy may be required.
- Where DVT threatens leg viability, surgical embolectomy or thrombolytic therapy may be considered.

Anticoagulation during labour and delivery

- The woman should be advised that once she thinks that she is in labour, she should not inject any further heparin.
- To avoid the risk of epidural haematoma:
  - regional anaesthesia should be avoided until at least 12h after the last dose of LMWH (24h if she is on a therapeutic dose)
  - LMWH should not be given for at least 4h after the epidural catheter has been removed
  - the epidural catheter should not be removed within 10–12h of a LMWH injection.
- Increased risk of wound haematoma following CS of ~2%.
- Wound drains should be considered.
- Skin incision should be closed with staples or interrupted sutures.
- Women on anticoagulant therapy at high risk of haemorrhage should be managed with UFH, as it has a shorter half-life and is more completely reversed with protamine sulphate.

Amniotic fluid embolism: overview

Amniotic fluid embolism (AFE) is a rare and often fatal maternal complication. It is not predictable or preventable, and is usually rapidly progressive. It accounts for 8% of the direct maternal deaths in the UK and 10% of all maternal deaths in the USA.

- Incidence 1:8000–30 000 births.
- Reported mortality ranges from 13% to 80%.
- Time from onset of symptoms to death varies from minutes to 32h.
- Causes permanent neurological sequelae in up to 85% of survivors.
- Tends to occur:
  - with spontaneous or artificial rupture of membranes (70%)
  - at CS (19%)
  - during delivery or within 48h (11%)
  - rarely during or after termination of pregnancy, manual removal of placenta, or amniocentesis.

Causes Presumed causal roles have been attributed to strong uterine contractions, excess amniotic fluid, and disruption of uterine vasculature.

AFE characteristics
Characterized by the acute onset of:
- Hypoxia and respiratory arrest (27–51%).
- Hypotension (13–27%).
- Fetal distress (17%).
- Convulsions (10–30%).
- Shock.
- Altered mental status.
- Cardiac arrest.

⚠ Although only 12% will present with DIC, virtually all cases will go on to develop it within 4h.

Risk factors for AFE
- Multiple pregnancy.
- Older maternal age.
- Caesarean or instrumental vaginal delivery.
- Eclampsia.
- Polyhydramnios.
- Placenta praevia.
- Placental abruption.
- Cervical laceration.
- Uterine rupture.
- Medical induction of labour.

Amniotic fluid embolism: diagnosis and management

Diagnosis

Diagnosis is clinical and essentially a diagnosis of exclusion. Differential diagnosis should include:

- Pulmonary embolism.
- Anaphylaxis.
- Sepsis.
- Eclampsia.
- Myocardial infarction.

⚠ In some patients, severe haemorrhage with DIC may be the first sign. Clinical diagnosis is supported by retrieval of fetal elements in pulmonary artery aspirate and maternal sputum. However, diagnosis is only definitively confirmed by the presence of fetal squamous cells and debris in the pulmonary vasculature at a post-mortem examination.

Investigations

- ABG.
- Electrolytes including calcium and magnesium levels.
- FBC (↑ WBC).
- Coagulation profile.
- CXR (pulmonary oedema).
- ECG (ischaemia and infarction).

Management of AFE

- Rapid maternal CPR and admission to ICU under multidisciplinary senior with input from obstetrics, anaesthetics, and haematology.
- Pulmonary artery wedge pressure monitoring will assist in the haemodynamic management. Blood aspirated via the catheter can be examined to aid with the diagnosis.
- Oxygen to maintain saturation close to 100% (helps to prevent neurological impairment from hypoxia).
- Fluid resuscitation is imperative to counteract hypotension and haemodynamic instability.
- For refractory hypotension, direct-acting vasopressors, such as phenylephrine, are required to optimize perfusion pressure.
- Inotropic support may be needed.
- DIC should be managed with the help of a haematologist (see 📖 Massive obstetric haemorrhage: medical management, p. 386).
- Plasma exchange techniques may be helpful in clearing fibrin degradation products from the circulation.
- If not yet delivered, continuous fetal monitoring is indicated: delivery by CS within 5min of cardiac arrest is recommended to facilitate CPR of mother.

Uterine inversion

Uterine inversion can cause serious maternal morbidity or death. The incidence is about 1:2000–3000 deliveries. Maternal mortality can be as high as 15%.

Risk factors for uterine inversion
- Strong traction on umbilical cord with excessive fundal pressure.
- Abnormal adherence of the placenta.
- Uterine anomalies.
- Fundal implantation of the placenta.
- Short cord.
- Previous uterine inversion.

Signs and symptoms
- Haemorrhage (present in 94% of cases).
- Severe lower abdominal pain in the 3rd stage.
- Shock out of proportion to the blood loss (neurogenic, due to increased vagal tone).
- Uterine fundus not palpable abdominally (or inversion may be just felt as a dimple at the fundus).
- Mass in the vagina on VE.

Management of uterine inversion
- Call for help (including a senior obstetrician and anaesthetist).
- Immediate replacement by pushing up the fundus through the cervix with the palm of the hand (the Johnson manoeuvre).
- IV access with 2 large bore cannulae.
- Bloods for FBC, coagulation studies, and cross-match 4–6U.
- Immediate fluid replacement.
- Continuous monitoring of vital signs.
- Transfer to theatre and arrange appropriate analgesia.
- If the placenta is still attached to the uterus it is left *in situ* to minimize the bleeding, and removal attempted only after replacement.
- Tocolytic drugs, such as terbutaline, or volatile anaesthetic agents may be tried to make replacement easier.
- If manual reduction fails then hydrostatic repositioning (O'Sullivan's technique) may be tried:
  - warm saline is rapidly infused into the vagina with one hand, sealing the labia (a silicone ventouse cup may be used to improve seal)
  - uterine rupture should be excluded first.
- Sometimes both manual and hydrostatic methods fail and a laporotomy is needed for correction (Haultain's or Huntingdon's procedure).

Cord prolapse

In cord prolapse the umbilical cord protrudes below the presenting part after rupture of membranes. This may cause compression of the umbilical vessels by the presenting part and vasospasm from exposure of the cord. These acutely compromise fetal circulation and if delivery is not immediate may lead to neurological sequelae or fetal death.

Predisposing factors for cord prolapse
- Abnormal lie or presentation (transverse lie, breech).
- Multiple pregnancy.
- Polyhydramnios.
- Prematurity.
- High head.
- Unusually long umbilical cord.

Prevention

When the presenting part is high or if there is polyhydramnios, a stabilizing induction (see 📖 Induction of labour: indications, p. 272) may be performed. During ARM, if cord presentation is detected (i.e. presence of cord below presenting part with intact membranes), the procedure should be abandoned and senior help summoned.

Management of cord prolapse
- ⚠ The fetus should be delivered as rapidly as possible; this may be by instrumental delivery or category 1 CS.
- Prevent further cord compression during transfer for CS by:
  - knee-to-chest position
  - fill the bladder with about 500mL of warm normal saline to displace the presenting part upwards (remember to unclamp the catheter before entering the peritoneal cavity at CS)
  - a hand in the vagina to push up the presenting part (may not always be practical).
- Prevent spasm by avoiding exposure of cord. Reduce cord into vagina to maintain body temperature and insert a warm saline swab to prevent cord coming back out.

⚠ It is important to avoid handling the cord as much as possible, as this provokes further spasms.
- Tocolytics (terbutaline 250 micrograms SC) may be administered to abolish uterine contractions and improve oxygenation to the fetus: may cause PPH at CS due to uterine atony; tackle with oxytocics but propranolol 1mg IV may be given if needed.
- Neonatal team must be present at delivery.

Fetal distress of second twin

See 📖 Multiple pregnancy: labour, p. 80.

Common causes of distress in the second twin
- Placental abruption (indicated by profuse bleeding).
- Cord prolapse.
- Excessive uterine contractions.

Fetal distress of the second twin can be iatrogenic (e.g. too much oxytocin, too hurried a delivery, too early amniotomy, or aortocaval compression).

Failure to adequately monitor a second twin is a common cause of problems. EFM is wise, if necessarily aided by ultrasound location of the best place to monitor, or a fetal scalp electrode.

▶ The second twin must be delivered by the fastest safe route.
- If it is *cephalic* and if the presenting part is at or below the ischial spines, an instrumental vaginal delivery may be attempted: with preterm babies (before 34wks), a ventouse delivery should be avoided.
- With a *breech* presentation, a 'breech extraction' may be attempted by an experienced clinician:
  - this involves grasping the feet of the fetus and gently pulling them through the vagina, aided by maternal effort
  - the arms will often become nuchal and Løvset's manoeuvre will then be required
  - in modern obstetric practice, a second twin with fetal distress is the only acceptable indication for this procedure.
- With a *transverse* lie, internal podalic version with breech extraction may be attempted.
- If vaginal delivery is not possible, immediate CS (category 1) should be performed.

Perinatal and maternal mortality

Perinatal mortality: overview

The role of modern maternity care is to ensure a safe maternal and fetal outcome at childbirth. A system whereby lessons can be learnt from adverse outcomes using analysis of databases and audits should improve outcome.

The first body established to do this in the UK was the Confidential Enquiry into Maternal Deaths (CEMD) in 1952 and subsequently the Confidential Enquiry into Stillbirths and Deaths in Infancy (CESDI) in 1992. The aim of these organizations was to undertake on-going national surveys of perinatal and infant deaths, identify risks, and make recommendations to improve clinical practice.

The Confidential Enquiry into Maternal and Child Health (CEMACH) was the successor to these, shortly followed by the setting up of the Centre for Maternal and Child Enquiries (CMACE). CMACE looks into the maternal, perinatal, and child health issues with extensive lay and voluntary sector involvement.

From 1954 to the mid-1990s, stillbirth and neonatal death rates in England and Wales fell steadily. In 1992 the gestation recognized for a stillbirth was decreased from 28 to 24wks.

Definitions

- *Late fetal loss:* a child delivering between 22+0 and 23+6wks of gestation who did not, at any time after being delivered, breathe or show any other signs of life.
- *Stillbirth:* a child delivered after the 24th week of pregnancy and who did not, at any time after being completely expelled from its mother, breathe or show any other signs of life.
- *Early neonatal death:* death of a live-born baby occurring less than 7 completed days from the time of birth.
- *Late neonatal death:* death of a live-born baby occurring from the 7th day of life and before 28 completed days from the time of birth.
- *Stillbirth rate:* number of stillbirths per 1000 live births and stillbirths.
- *Perinatal mortality rate (UK):* number of stillbirths and early neonatal deaths per 1000 live births and stillbirths.
- *Perinatal mortality rate (WHO):* number of late fetal losses, stillbirths, and early neonatal deaths per 1000 live births and stillbirths.
- *Neonatal mortality rate:* number of neonatal deaths per 1000 live births (this may be adjusted to take into account babies with congenital abnormalities, and then referred to as 'corrected neonatal mortality rate').

Classification of perinatal mortality
Primary cause of stillbirths and neonatal deaths in 2009, using the CMACE maternal and fetal classification (excluding termination of pregnancy)

Stillbirth (n=3373)
- No antecedent or associated obstetric factors 28%.
- Placental disorders conditions 12%.
- Ante- or intra-partum haemorrhage 11%.
- Major congenital anomaly 9%.
- Mechanical 8%.
- IUGR 7%.
- Hypertensive disorders of pregnancy 6%.
- Infection 5%.
- Maternal disorder 5%.
- Specific fetal conditions 4%.
- Associated obstetric factors (including preterm labour) 4%.
- Unclassified 2%.

Neonatal deaths (n=2115)
- Associated obstetric factors (including preterm labour) 27%.
- Major congenital anomaly 24%.
- No antecedent or associated obstetric factors 12%.
- Infection 10%.
- Ante- or intra-partum haemorrhage 9%.
- Specific fetal conditions 4%.
- Mechanical 3%.
- Hypertensive disorders of pregnancy 3%.
- Unclassified 3%.
- Maternal disorder 2%.
- IUGR 2%.
- Placental disorders conditions 1%.

Stillbirth rates since 1954
- 1954: 23/1000 total births.
- 1997: 5.3/1000 total births.
- 2001: 5.4/1000 live births.
- 2003: 5.7/1000 total births.
- 2005: 5.3/1000 total births
- 2007: 5.2/1000 total births.
- 2009: 5.2/1000 total births.

Neonatal mortality rates since 1954
- 1954: 18/1000 live births.
- 1997: 3.9/1000 live births.
- 2001: 3.7/1000 live births.
- 2003: 3.7/1000 live births.
- 2005: 3.4/1000 live births.
- 2007: 3.3/1000 live births.
- 2009: 3.2/1000 live births.

Perinatal mortality: key findings

- The stillbirth rate in the UK for 2009 was 5.2/1000 total births and has been showing a steady decline over the last 10yrs.
- 3/4 stillbirths deliver after 28wks gestation.
- Stillbirth and neonatal death rates are higher in socially deprived areas.
- 10% of mothers who had a stillbirth or neonatal death had a BMI >35. CMACE estimates that during 2009, the prevalence of this BMI in the pregnant population was 5%.

Risk factors for perinatal mortality
- Maternal age.
- Ethnicity.
- Social deprivation.
- Gestational age.
- Low birth weight.
- Multiple pregnancy.

Ethnicity as a risk factor
The stillbirth (SB) rates and neonatal mortality (NNM) rates were shown to be higher for babies of non-white mothers.
- *Black mothers:* SB 2.1 times and NNM 2.4 times higher than Caucasian mothers.
- *Asian mothers:* SB 1.6 times and NNM 1.6 times higher.

Low birth weight as a risk factor
42% of all stillbirths and 25% of all neonatal deaths were <10th birth weight centile.

Multiple births as a risk factor
Multiple births have a 3–4 times higher SB and 6–8 times higher NNM rate than singleton pregnancies.
    The cause of stillbirth is clearly different to singletons.
- *Specific fetal condition:* twins 21%, singletons 2%.
- *Major congenital abnormality:* twins 11%, singletons 9%.

Further reading
Centre for Maternal and Child Enquiries (2011). *Perinatal Mortality 2009*. London: CMACE.

Maternal mortality: definition

The 9th and 10th revisions of the International Classification of Diseases, Injuries, and Causes (ICD-9/10) define a maternal death as 'death of a woman while pregnant or within 42 days of the end of the pregnancy, from any cause related to or aggravated by the pregnancy or its management, but not from accidental or incidental causes'.

Maternal deaths

Direct maternal deaths

Result from obstetric complications of the pregnant state (pregnancy, labour, and puerperium), from interventions, omissions, incorrect treatment, or from a chain of events resulting from any of the above.

Indirect maternal deaths

Arise from pre-existing disease or disease that developed during pregnancy and which was not due to direct obstetric causes, but which was aggravated by the physiological effects of pregnancy and includes:
• Epilepsy.
• Cardiac disease.
• Diabetes.
• Hormone-dependent malignancies.

Maternal mortality ratio (MMtR)

This is defined as the number of direct and indirect maternal deaths per 100 000 live births.

ICD-10 new terms for maternal mortality

Pregnancy-related death

Death occurring in a woman while pregnant or within 42 days of termination of pregnancy, irrespective of the cause of the death (unlike maternal deaths, this includes accidental and incidental causes).

Late maternal death

Death occurring between 42 days and 1yr after termination of pregnancy, miscarriage, or delivery that is due to direct or indirect maternal causes.

Coincidental (fortuitous) maternal death

Includes accidental or incidental deaths, which would have happened even if the woman was not pregnant, and includes:
• Domestic violence.
• Road traffic accidents.

The Confidential Enquiry into Maternal Deaths

In 1949, the issue of reporting maternal deaths was raised at the 12th British Congress of Obstetrics and Gynaecology and this led to the establishment of a regional and national assessment by clinicians. A series of triennial reports were instituted to disseminate the findings and recommendations, with a view to reducing maternal deaths and to improve practice. In April 2003, the CEMACH for England and Wales came into existence. In 2009 this became an independent charity, the CMACE. It is commissioned mainly by the National Patient Safety Agency (NPSA) and the primary objective is to review mortality and improve maternal and child health. It assesses causes and trends in maternal deaths to identify avoidable and substandard factors that may have led to these deaths. Based on these findings it makes recommendations and suggestions concerning the improvement of clinical care.

Why is CEMACE important?
- Each year more than 20 million women experience ill health as a result of pregnancy, the lives of nearly 8 million are threatened, and over half a million women die as a result of pregnancy.
- It is estimated that 88–98% of maternal deaths in the world are avoidable with timely and effective care.
- The reporting of such deaths and their causes is important in order to identify avoidable causes and institute recommendations to improve practice.
- The recent world estimate of overall MMtR is around 400 per 100 000 live births: in the UK during 2006–08 the MMtR was 11.4:100 000.
- 261 maternal deaths were reported to the Enquiry:
  - 107 direct maternal deaths
  - 154 indirect deaths
  - 50 coincidental deaths
  - 33 late direct and indirect deaths.

Maternal death in the recent report is lower than in the previous triennium mainly due to the reduction in deaths due to thromboembolism and haemorrhage. However, there has been an increase in deaths due to sepsis and Sudden Adult/Arrhythmic Death Syndrome (SADS). Future reports should be able to ascertain whether this finding is a result of chance, improved case ascertainment or a real increase.

Digested data in this topic are reproduced from CEMACE. (2011). *Saving mothers' lives.* The 8th report on Confidential Enquiries into Maternal Deaths in the UK. With the permission of the Centre of Maternal and Child Enquires.

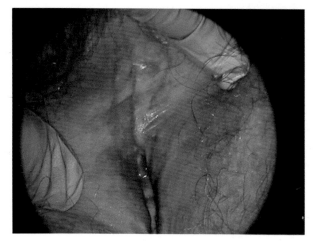

Plate 1 Lichen sclerosus (note the labial fusion and leukoplakia).

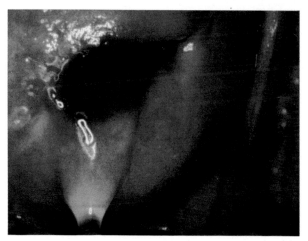

Plate 2 Colposcopy image 1: normal cervix.

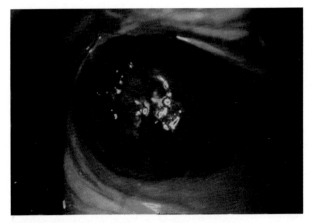

Plate 3 Colposcopy image 2: ectropion in a nulliparous woman.

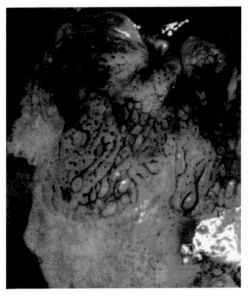

Plate 4 Colposcopy image 3: abnormal transformation zone (stained with acetic acid).

MACE: direct deaths I

tal tract sepsis

ulted in 26 direct deaths (and 3 late direct deaths).
e mortality rate from sepsis is 1.1:100 000 maternities.
gnant women with sepsis may present with a variety of symptoms
h as abdominal pain, diarrhoea, and vomiting.
e in deaths from sepsis is predominantly a result of community-
quired β-haemolytic streptococcus Lancefield Group A
eptococcus pyogenes).

Puerperal pyrexia: genital causes, p. 354.

sis: CEMACE recommendations

Be aware of sepsis—beware of sepsis.
aff must be aware of the signs and symptoms of critical illness.
nset may be insidious and carers need to be alert to changes that
ay indicate developing infection.
igh-dose broad-spectrum antibiotics should be started immediately
ithout waiting for microbiology results.
uidelines for detection, investigation, and management of suspected
epsis should be available to all healthcare professionals who deal
ith pregnant or post-partum women.

-eclampsia and eclampsia

re were 19 deaths recorded from hypertensive disease of pregnancy—14
cerebral causes, 3 from liver complications, 2 from multi-organ failure.

Pre-eclampsia: overview, p. 64.

e-eclampsia and eclampsia: CEMACH
commendations

Headache or epigastric pain is pre-eclampsia until proven otherwise.
Any discussions must explicitly mention the systolic BP.
Systolic BP ≥150mmHg requires effective antihypertensives.
Systolic BP of >180mmHg is a medical emergency.
Oxytocin not Syntometrine® should be used for 3rd stage.
Severe pre-eclampsia needs effective team communication.

nous thromboembolism

There were 18 deaths from VTE (and 4 late direct deaths): 16 from PE;
from cerebral vein thrombosis.
Risk factors were identified in 16 of the 18 women.

Venous thromboembolism: overview, p. 390)

ested data in this topic are reproduced from CEMACE. (2011). *Saving mothers' lives*. The 8th
rt on Confidential Enquiries into Maternal Deaths in the UK. With the permission of the
tre of Maternal and Child Enquires.

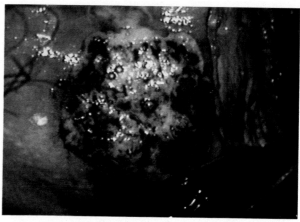

Plate 5 Colposcopy image 4: squamous cell carcinoma of the cervix.

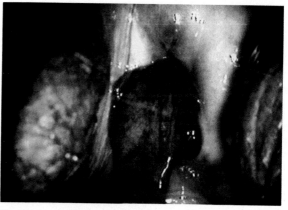

Plate 6 Colposcopy image 5: endocervical polyp.

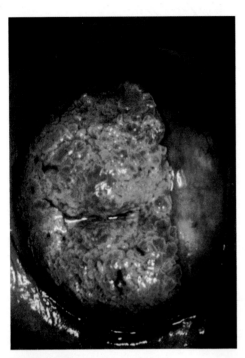

Plate 7 Colposcopy image 6: cervical wart.

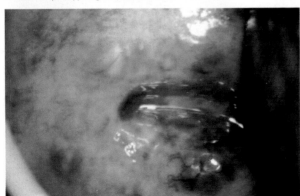

Plate 8 Colposcopy image 7: Nabothian follicles (note the regularly branching tree-like vessels often seen over the cysts).

'Top ten' CEMACE 2009 recommendations

- Preconception counselling should be provided for w pre-existing serious medical or mental health proble obesity.
- Professional interpretation services should be provid pregnant women who do not speak English.
- Referrals to specialist services in pregnancy should be urgent.
- Women with potentially serious medical conditions r immediate and appropriate multidisciplinary specialist
- Clinical staff must have improved training in identifica treatment of serious medical and mental health condi improved life support skills.
- Routine use of a national obstetric early warning chart pregnant or postpartum women.

⚠ Women who are pregnant or recently delivered wi pain severe enough to need opiate analgesia require review.

- All pregnant women with pre-eclampsia and a systolic 160mmHg or more require urgent and effective antihy treatment.
- All pregnant and recently delivered women need to be the risks and signs and symptoms of genital tract infecti to prevent its transmission.
- All maternal deaths must be subject to a high quality lo
- The standard of maternal autopsy must be improved.

CEMACE 2006–08: summary of direct causes of maternal death

- Genital tract sepsis (26).
- Hypertensive disease of pregnancy (19).
- VTE (18).
- Amniotic fluid embolism (13).
- Early pregnancy causes (11).
- Haemorrhage (9).
- Anaesthesia related (7).
- Acute fatty liver (3).
- Other (1).
- Late direct causes (9).

Further reading

Cantwell R, Clutton-Brock T, Cooper G, et al. (2011). Saving mothers' lives: rev deaths to make motherhood safer: 2006–2008. The 8th Report of the Confic into Maternal Deaths in the UK. *Br J Obstet Gynaecol* **118**(Suppl 1): 1–203.

VTE: CEMACE recommendations
- Obesity remains the most important risk for thromboembolism.
- Early risk assessment remains key in reducing mortality.
- Vulnerable women need help administering thromboprophylaxis.
- Chest symptoms appearing for the first time in at-risk women need careful assessment and low threshold for investigation.

CMACE 'back to basics'

Sepsis
- Red flag signs and symptoms requiring urgent hospital referral:
  - pyrexia >38°C
  - sustained tachycardia >100 beats/min
  - breathlessness—1 relative risk (RR) >20 is a serious symptom
  - abdominal or chest pain
  - diarrhoea and/or vomiting
  - reduced fetal movements or absent fetal heart
  - spontaneous rupture of membranes or significant vaginal discharge
  - uterine or renal angle pain and tenderness
  - if woman generally unwell or unduly anxious, distressed, panicky.
- A normal temperature does not exclude sepsis as pyrexia may be marked by paracetamol and other analgesics.
- Infection must be actively ruled out in a recently delivered woman with persistent bleeding and abdominal pain.
- Any concerns warrant referral back to a maternity unit.

Breathlessness
Red flag features requiring urgent hospital referral:
- Breathlessness of sudden onset.
- Breathlessness with chest pain.
- Orthopnoea or paroxysmal nocturnal dyspnea.

⚠ In normal women oxygen saturation does not fall below 95% on exercise.

⚠ Never assume that wheeze on auscultation represents asthma, it could be pulmonary oedema.

Headache
Red flag signs suggestive of sinister pathology associated with headache:
- Sudden onset.
- Neck stiffness.
- Any abnormal signs on neurological examination.

⚠ Headache that is 'the worst that the woman has ever experienced' is an indication for urgent brain imaging even in the absence of any other features because of concern about cerebral venous thrombosis.

CEMACE: direct deaths II

Amniotic fluid embolism

Amniotic fluid embolism: CEMACE recommendations

- Perform all maternal autopsies as soon as possible—if delayed, diagnosis becomes difficult if not impossible.
- The diagnosis must be confirmed using immunochemistry.
- If no squames can be found search for mucins.
- All cases suspected or confirmed should be reported to the National AFE register at ukoss@npeu.ox.ac.uk.
- 13 deaths were due to AFE (died since the last report).

See 📖 Amniotic fluid embolism: overview, p. 398.

Haemorrhage

There were 9 maternal deaths from haemorrhage reported (see 📖 Massive obstetric haemorrhage: medical management, p. 386).

Haemorrhage: CEMACE recommendations

- Regular training on identifying and managing haemorrhage.
- Early senior multidisciplinary team involvement.
- Clinicians must be aware of guidelines for management of women refusing blood products.
- MEOW charts should be used for 24h post-CS.
- Women with previous CS must have placental site determined with attempts to diagnose accreta or percreta (USS + MRI).
- Admit women with major placenta praevia who have bled from 34wks gestation.

▶ Anaemia magnifies effect of haemorrhage. Treat antenatally using parenteral iron therapy if unresponsive to oral iron.

Early pregnancy deaths

11 deaths resulted from early pregnancy causes: 6 due to ectopic pregnancy; 5 following haemorrhagic complications of spontaneous miscarriage.

Early pregnancy: CEMACE recommendations

- All women of reproductive age presenting to Emergency departments with gastrointestinal symptoms must have a pregnancy test.
- Clinical staff must be aware that gastrointestinal symptoms, particularly diarrhoea and dizziness, are important symptoms of ectopic pregnancy.
- Abandon term 'pregnancy of unknown location'. If no intrauterine sac seen on USS, active exclusion of ectopic pregnancy must begin.
- Abortion care must include strategy for minimizing risk of sepsis.

CEMACE: indirect causes of death

Cardiac disease is not only the most common cause of indirect maternal death, but also the commonest cause of death overall.

Cardiac disease in pregnancy (↑)
- 53 deaths were recorded that resulted from heart disease (↑ rate). A further 8 deaths are included in the late deaths.
- The leading causes of death are now:
  - SADS
  - myocardial infarction
  - dissection of the thoracic aorta
  - cardiomyopathy.
- Deaths from congenital heart disease continue to decrease (3).

See 🕮 Cardiac disease: management in pregnancy, p. 192.

> ### Cardiac disease: CEMACE recommendations
> - Women with cardiac disease must be cared for in a unit with a joint obstetric/cardiology clinic.
> - Low threshold for investigating women with symptoms of MI or aortic dissection especially if they are obese, smoke, or have hypertension.
> - ABGs showing hypoxaemia and a metabolic acidosis is a feature of reduced cardiac output secondary to cardiac disease.

Other indirect causes of death
88 other indirect deaths were recorded, including:
- Diseases of the central nervous system (34):
  - epilepsy (14)
  - subarachnoid haemorrhage (6)
  - intracerebral haemorrhage (5).
- Infectious diseases (7):
  - HIV infection (2).
- Diseases of the respiratory system (9):
  - asthma (5).
- Endocrine, metabolic, and immunity disorders (9):
  - diabetes (3).
- Diseases of the gastrointestinal system:
  - pancreatitis.
- Diseases of the blood (3).
- Diseases of the circulatory system (4).
- Indirect malignancies (3).
- Cause unknown (6).
- Other (2).

MI in pregnancy

- Ischaemic heart disease has become a common cause of death.
- All the women who died had identifiable risk factors, including:
  - obesity
  - age (>35) and higher parity (>3)
  - smoking
  - diabetes
  - pre-existing hypertension
  - family history of ischaemic heart disease.
- MI and acute coronary syndrome can have an atypical presentation in pregnancy (abdominal or epigastric pain and vomiting).
- A single normal ECG does not exclude ischaemia, especially if taken when the patient is pain free.
- There should be a low threshold for investigating symptoms especially in women with risk factors.
- There should also be a low threshold for emergency coronary intervention (such as angioplasty and stenting).

See 📖 Myocardial infarction and cardiomyopathy, p. 197.

Indirect deaths: some specific recommendations

- All women with serious medical conditions should receive prepregnancy counselling.
- All women with serious medical conditions should be referred to a specialist as early as possible.
- Lack of consultant involvement remains a problem; protocols should be developed specifying conditions that mandate consultant review.
- Anyone caring for unfamiliar conditions should consult experts.
- Medical conditions can cause symptoms that are more commonly obstetric related, e.g. epilepsy can cause fits as well as eclampsia.
- Multiple attendances are signs of serious undiagnosed disease or social problems.
- Undiagnosed pain requiring opiate analgesia demands immediate consultant input.
- Physicians not working directly with pregnant women need to know more about the interaction between their condition and pregnancy.
- Professional translation services must be made available to women who do not speak English.

Digested data in this topic are reproduced from CEMACE. (2011). *Saving mothers' lives*. The 8th report on Confidential Enquiries into Maternal Deaths in the UK. With the permission of the Centre of Maternal and Child Enquires.

CEMACE: psychiatric illness and domestic abuse

Deaths from psychiatric illnesses

- There were 29 deaths due to suicide during pregnancy and in the first 6mths post-partum.
- The majority died violently, e.g. hanging or jumping from a height.
- Over 50% of the maternal suicides were white, married, employed, living in comfortable circumstances, and aged 30yrs or older.

See ☐ Antenatal psychiatric disorders: overview, p. 446.

⚠ Care needs to be taken not to equate suicide risk with socio-economic deprivation.

Psychiatric causes: CEMACE recommendations

- All women should be asked about past history of psychiatric illness at booking, referred appropriately, and monitored for at least 3mths after delivery.
- Psychiatric services should have priority pathways for pregnant women.
- Risk assessment should be modified to take into account the distinctive picture of perinatal disorders and violent method of suicide.
- All mental health trusts should have specialized perinatal teams.
- Caution must be exercised when diagnosing a psychiatric cause for unexplained physical symptoms or distress and agitation.

▶ This is especially important when the woman does not speak English as a first language.

Domestic abuse

⚠ Domestic abuse is an important issue in obstetrics.
- 34 deaths from 'all causes' had features of domestic abuse:
  - many had self-reported domestic abuse
  - 38% were poor attenders or late bookers.
- 11 women were murdered, 7 by their partners.

Digested data in this topic are reproduced from CEMACE. (2011). *Saving mothers' lives.* The 8th report on Confidential Enquiries into Maternal Deaths in the UK. With the permission of the Centre of Maternal and Child Enquires.

Domestic abuse: CEMACE recommendations

- Enquiries about domestic violence should be routinely included at booking, with appropriate methods of recording in the notes that protects the woman from further harm, and further referral strategies.
- Women should be seen alone at least once in the antenatal period.
- Any member of the maternity team noticing an injury, e.g. a black eye, should ask sympathetically, but directly about domestic abuse.
- Information about local agencies and emergency helplines should be displayed in areas where women can have access to them.
- Women known to suffer from domestic violence are not 'low risk'.
- It must be remembered that healthcare professionals may themselves be victims: domestic abuse occurs across all social classes and within all ethnic groups.

Definition of domestic abuse

Any incident of threatening behaviour or abuse (psychological, physical, sexual, financial, or emotional) between adults who are or have been intimate partners or family members, regardless of gender or sexuality.

Some indicators of domestic abuse in maternity care

- Late booking and/or poor or non-attendance at antenatal clinic.
- Repeat attendance at antenatal clinic, GP surgery, or A&E for minor injuries, or trivial or non-existent complaints.
- Unexplained admissions.
- Non-compliance with treatment regimens or early self-discharge from hospital.
- Repeat presentation with depression, anxiety, self-harm, and psychosomatic symptoms.
- Injuries that are untended and of several different ages, especially to the neck, head, breasts, abdomen, and genitals.
- Minimalization of signs of abuse on the body.
- STIs and frequent vaginal or urinary tract infections and pelvic pain.
- Poor obstetric history:
  - repeated miscarriages or TOPs
  - stillbirth or preterm labour
  - preterm birth, IUGR, low birth weight
  - unwanted or unplanned pregnancy.
- The constant presence at examinations of the partner, who may be domineering, answer all the questions for her, and be unwilling to leave the room.
- The woman appears evasive or reluctant to speak or disagree in front of her partner.

Benign and malignant tumours in pregnancy

Fibroids in pregnancy

- Incidence in pregnancy varies from 0.1% to 3.9%.
- May be higher in women over 35, primigravida, and those of Afro-Caribbean origin.
- USS is usually used to make the diagnosis, but fibroids can be confused with solid ovarian or other tumours.
- Only 42% of fibroids in pregnancy are detected clinically.

Effects of pregnancy on fibroids

Whether fibroids increase, decrease, or stay the same after pregnancy remains controversial.

Effects of fibroids on pregnancy

Pain due to
- Red degeneration (necrobiosis).
- Torsion of a pedunculated fibroid.
- Fibroid impaction.
- △ Pain may be severe enough to require morphine via PCA.

1st and 2nd trimesters
- Risk of spontaneous miscarriage may be ↑: preconception myomectomy seems to improve likelihood of successful pregnancy with recurrent pregnancy loss, especially when no other cause found.
- May ↑ the risk of 2nd-trimester miscarriages.
- Invasive procedures, such as amniocentesis and CVS, may be technically difficult.

3rd trimester
- ↑ Risk of threatened preterm labour (reported rate up to 22%).
- Placentation over a fibroid is a strong risk factor for abruption.
- It is unclear whether fibroids are associated with IUGR.
- Large fibroids may exert pressure on the fetus, causing limb reduction defects, congenital torticollis, and head deformities (fetal compression syndrome).
- Very rare complications include disseminated intravascular coagulation, spontaneous haemoperitoneum, uterine inversion, uterine incarceration, acute renal failure, and urinary retention.

Delivery
- Incidence of CS is doubled, as malpresentations, dysfunctional labour, and obstructed labour are more common, especially when fibroids are in lower uterine segment.
- ↑ Risk of PPH.
- Higher incidence of retained placenta (may be due to lower-segment fibroids obstructing delivery of placenta).

Management of fibroids in pregnancy

- *Conservative management:*
  - symptomatic treatment of pain
  - monitoring of the fetus.
- Surgical procedures for fibroids during pregnancy carry risk of significant haemorrhage. Therefore myomectomy not performed in pregnancy.
- A myomectomy during CS is also avoided as it carries a high morbidity from haemorrhage: rarely, it may be necessary to remove a fibroid to gain access to the fetus or to facilitate uterine repair.

Ovarian cysts in pregnancy

- Incidence of 1–2%.
- The majority are small (3–4cm), persistent follicular cysts.
- Cysts ≥6cm occur in 0.5–2:1000 pregnancies.
- Most common ovarian cysts seen in pregnancy include:
  - functional ovarian cysts (follicular, corpus luteum, and theca-lutein)
  - benign cystic teratomas
  - serous cystadenomas
  - mucinous cystadenomas
  - endometriomas
  - malignant tumours (2–3%).

Effects of ovarian cysts on pregnancy

- Impaction of the cyst may lead to urinary retention.
- ↑ Risk of miscarriage or preterm delivery.
- May cause discomfort if very large.
- Large cysts may prevent engagement of the fetal head and predispose to malpresentation (rarely, may cause obstructed labour).

Complications are same as in non-pregnant state:

- Torsion most likely to occur at end of 1st trimester or in puerperium (risk of torsion is between 3 and 25%).
- Cyst haemorrhage may occur as a result of ↑ vascularity.
- Rupture (may follow impaction during labour).

Management of ovarian cysts in pregnancy

⚠ Acute complications should be treated by surgery at any gestation.

- Asymptomatic, non-enlarging cysts, cystadenomas, and dermoids should be managed conservatively.
- Cystectomy performed in patients with:
  - symptoms or acute complications (torted, haemorrhagic, ruptured)
  - suspicion of malignancy (if strong suspicion, unilateral oophectomy should be performed)
  - enlargement or large size (>8–10cm).
- Elective surgery should be performed at 16–20wks:
  - risk of miscarriage is lower
  - access to the pedicle is easy.
- The choice of laparotomy or laparoscopy is dependent on:
  - risk of malignancy
  - urgency of the procedure
  - skills of the surgeon.
- The risk of miscarriage after emergency surgery for ovarian torsion can be as high as 22.2%.
- If cyst causes obstruction of labour, delivery should be by CS and cyst dealt with at the same time.

Malignancy in pregnancy: overview

Cancer is rare under the age of 30. However, so are other causes of death, and therefore cancer is still the leading cause of death in England and Wales in this age group. Consequently, cancer in pregnancy is relatively rare. The last CEMD (2003–2005) reported 82 cancer-related deaths. However, upward shift in age of motherhood in the UK means that more women are now pregnant when incidence of cancer is starting to increase. During reproductive years, breast cancer is the most common cancer diagnosis being 10-fold more common than other cancers. This incidence increases dramatically in the over-40s. Principal cancers in younger women are melanoma and cervical cancer.

- Pregnancy-associated cancer is defined as a cancer diagnosis during pregnancy or within 12mths of a delivery.
- The incidence of cancer in pregnancy is about 1:6000 live births.
- This is about 50% lower than in non-pregnant women.
- Women diagnosed within the 12mth postnatal period are more likely to have advanced disease and a poorer prognosis is most likely due to a delay in diagnosis, either because the pregnancy masked signs and symptoms, especially true of breast cancer, or because of a reluctance to perform necessary investigations.
- There does not appear to be any difference in the stage-for-stage survival and mortality figures, and the prognosis.
- Some cancers, particularly hormone-dependent ones, can grow rapidly in pregnancy, but factors related to tumour growth in relation to the endocrine and physiological changes in pregnancy are still poorly understood.

Treating cancer in pregnancy

- Compromise between interest of fetus and mother.
- Some treatments cause fetal demise: pelvic radiotherapy (60Gy).
- Some are probably OK after 1st trimester, including chemotherapy.
  - carboplatin (avoid paclitaxel)
  - careful counselling regarding termination of the pregnancy should be undertaken.
- Each case has to be individualized, based on:
  - gestation
  - tumour histology
  - patient choice.

Cervical cancer in pregnancy: diagnosis

Most common cancer of the genital tract to present in pregnancy, with estimated incidence of 2.4/100 000 pregnancies. There has been a decline in invasive carcinoma of the cervix in developed countries, which may be attributed to cancer screening programmes (see 📖 Cancer screening in gynaecology: overview, p. 702).

Cervical screening and pre-invasive disease

- The UK National Cervical Screening Programme ensures the majority of women have routine screening with appropriate referral.
- Allows women to delay pregnancy if they have had abnormal cytology.
- May be more difficult to interpret cytology result in a pregnant woman and therefore routine screening deferred until >6wks post-partum, if previously adequately screened. Follow-up smears after treatment or abnormal smear should *not* be delayed.
- Where clinically indicated, referral for colposcopy should be made.
- At colposcopy, it is more difficult to interpret changes in colour following application of acetic acid and iodine in pregnancy.
- Biopsy of the cervix can lead to brisk bleeding and, where possible, should be avoided in pregnancy.
- Risk of miscarriage or preterm labour following biopsy is low.

Presentation and diagnosis

⚠ Cervical carcinoma can present as recurrent bleeding in pregnancy in a woman not up to date with her smear tests.

- Pregnancy does not accelerate progression of cervical intraepithelial neoplasia (CIN) to invasive.
- Prognosis may depend on duration from diagnosis to treatment.
- Delaying treatment to achieve fetal maturity is not known to worsen prognosis.
- Of those women with cervical cancer in pregnancy, nearly 7% are diagnosed at the time of their pregnancy confirmation.
- Most women are asymptomatic at presentation (up to 65%).
- Diagnosis may follow assessment of abnormal smear or colposcopy.
- Colposcopy and cervical punch biopsy are safe in pregnancy.

⚠ A large loop excision of the transformation zone (LLETZ) or knife cone biopsy carries a significant risk of haemorrhage and miscarriage.

Staging of the disease may be difficult when the uterus is enlarged:
- Avoid exposure of the fetus to ionizing radiation.
- MRI is safe in pregnancy.

Cervical cancer in pregnancy: management and prognosis

Management
Early invasive disease
- Risk of haemorrhage, infection, miscarriage, preterm labour, and prelabour rupture of membranes.
- 80% of pregnancies result in term deliveries and fetal survival is over 90%.

Stage 1a and b
- In the 1st and 2nd trimesters radical hysterectomy and lymphadenectomy may be performed with the fetus *in utero*.
- In late mid-trimester (>24wks) CS may be performed followed by radical hysterectomy and lymphadenectomy: a classical section reduces the risk of encroaching on the tumour.
- Little evidence to suggest any benefit, but if patient presents in labour, emergency CS may be performed to reduce dissemination of disease.

Advanced disease
- Treatment should not be delayed.
- If pregnancy is >24wks, management must be individualized according to mother's wishes; baby should be delivered at appropriate gestation, by classical CS, and radiotherapy instituted.

Prognosis
- There is no evidence to suggest that when early-stage disease is diagnosed in pregnancy, the prognosis is worse than for non-pregnant women.
- The 5yr survival in pregnant women with advanced disease is lower than for their non-pregnant counterparts: this difference could be due to radiation dosimetry during or soon after pregnancy.

See 📖 Cervical cancer: pathology and screening, p. 706.

Ovarian cancer in pregnancy

It is common to diagnose an ovarian mass in pregnancy, especially now that most women will have an early pregnancy ultrasound. Only 2–3% of the ovarian tumours that require surgery in pregnancy are malignant. Nearly 1/3 of these are dysgerminomas, teratomas, or germ-cell tumours (most likely due to the age of the patients).

- Most tumours are asymptomatic: <25% are >10cm.
- Some will present as abdominal pain due to cyst accident: torsion complicates 10–15% of tumours:
- Tumour markers not reliable in pregnancy.
- High incidence of germ cell tumours:
  - 30% germ cell tumours
  - 21% borderline tumours
  - 28% epithelial carcinomas
  - 3% krukenberg
  - 8% others.

Management of ovarian masses in pregnancy

- Ovarian cyst or mass identified in 1st trimester should be rescanned at 14wks (most corpus luteal cysts involute by then):
  - if it has not ↑ to >5cm, conservative management is appropriate
  - if >5cm, serial USS should be used to monitor any change in size or morphology (which may prompt surgery).
- Where there are signs of malignancy in the mass:
  - surgery can be limited to unilateral opherectomy, but a complete staging must be performed
  - if staging at laparotomy is suggestive of spread beyond the ovary, or if histology determines the need for chemotherapy, a multidisciplinary approach should be taken and treatment guided by patient wishes, after appropriate counselling.

Breast cancer in pregnancy

Breast cancer is the most common cancer associated with pregnancy in countries that have an effective cervical screening programme. The incidences from the literature are quoted as between 1 in 3000 and one in 10 000 pregnancies. There is evidence that diagnosis of breast cancer is delayed by pregnancy as associated symptoms are often attributed to pregnancy itself.

Prognosis
• Breast cancer in younger women has poorer prognosis.
• Pregnancy itself does not appear to worsen prognosis.

Diagnosis
Women presenting with breast lump during pregnancy should be referred to breast specialist team, and any imaging or further tests should be conducted in conjunction with multidisciplinary team.

Management
• Decision to continue pregnancy should be based on careful discussion of cancer prognosis, treatment, and future fertility with the woman and her partner, and multidisciplinary team.
• The multidisciplinary team review outcome should be forwarded to the obstetric team and family doctor.
• Surgical treatment should be same as non-pregnant woman:
  • wide local excision
  • modified radical mastectomy
  • reconstruction should be delayed until after delivery.
• Radiotherapy contraindicated until after delivery unless life-saving or to preserve organ function.
• Chemotherapy may be offered after 1st trimester.
  • there is no evidence for an ↑ rate of 2nd-trimester miscarriage or fetal growth restriction, organ dysfunction, or long-term adverse outcome with the use of chemotherapy
  • tamoxifen and trastuzumab are contraindicated in pregnancy.
• Birth of baby should be timed after discussion with woman and multidisciplinary team.
• Each case has to be individualized, based on gestation and patient choice.

Breast-feeding
• Reassure women that they can breast-feed from unaffected breast.
• Women should not breast-feed when taking trastuzumab or tamoxifen, as it is unknown whether these drugs are transmitted in breastmilk.

Further reading
RCOG. (2011). *Pregnancy and breast cancer*, Green top guideline 12. ✆ http://www.rcog.org.uk/files/rcog-corp/GTG12PregBreastCancer.pdf

Substance abuse and psychiatric disorders

Substance abuse in pregnancy

- The huge increase in drug and alcohol abuse in the UK since the 1980s has been disproportionately large in women of childbearing age.
- The prevalence of substance abuse is:
  - 4.7% for alcohol
  - 2.2% for drug dependence.
- It has a serious effect on the mother's health, as well as consequences for fetal well-being.
- There is under-identification because of:
  - inadequate history taking
  - reluctance to admit to substance abuse
  - late booking
  - poor antenatal attendance.
- Poor communication between GPs, social services, midwives, and obstetricians is a hindrance to adequate care.
- In the CEMACH report 2002–2005, there were 31 maternal deaths that were either directly or indirectly related to substance abuse:
  - social deprivation was a common factor
  - all but one pregnancy was unplanned.

Definitions relating to substance abuse

Problems associated with substance abuse are categorized in ICD-10 under the heading 'Mental and behavioural disorders due to psychoactive substance abuse'.

- *Harmful use:* a pattern of psychoactive substance use that is causing damage to physical or mental health.
- *Intoxication:* transient syndrome due to recent substance ingestion that produces clinically significant psychological/physical impairment.
- *Dependence syndrome:* cluster of physiological, behavioural, and cognitive phenomena in which the use of a substance or a class of substances takes on a much higher priority for a given individual than other behaviours that once had greater value.
- *Tolerance:* homeostatic adaptation to chronic administration of a drug; to ameliorate longer-term toxicity; and to allow the organism to continue functioning while chronically intoxicated.
- *Withdrawal:* characteristic pattern of signs and symptoms (psychological and physical) that occur when a drug is stopped after a period of chronic administration, or an antagonist to the drug is given.

Morbidity and mortality in substance abusers

Co-existing psychiatric disorders

There is a close association between substance misuse and other mental illnesses, such as personality disorder, depression, and anxiety.

Physical complications

- Substance misuse often accompanied by general neglect of health, with nutritional deficiency, poor hygiene, and generalized immunosuppression.
- As well as direct pharmacological consequences from the substance there are risks from route of administration.
- IV drug use may lead to:
  - HIV infection
  - hepatitis C (prevalence of between 50 and 80% in UK drug users) and hepatitis B (30–50%)
  - venous thrombosis
  - subcutaneous abscesses
  - bacterial endocarditis
  - septicaemia (may be fungal)
  - poor venous access in an emergency situation.

Withdrawal effects

Withdrawal symptoms can be distressing, but rarely life-threatening.

Social damage

- May lead to problems with employer and work-related accidents.
- Leads to financial strain with damaging effects on the family.
- Antisocial and criminal activities may arise from behavioural changes and need for money.
- May be child protection issues as a result of neglect or abuse.

Death

- Significant mortality (10–15% in opioid misusers over 10yrs).
- Mostly accidental due to overdose.
- Suicide is also a frequent cause of death.
- Deaths from HIV and hepatitis infection are becoming more common.
- Approximately 60% of deaths in drug addicts are related to drug use itself.

Perinatal morbidity and mortality with substance abuse

Risks of the following are increased:
- Preterm birth and prematurity.
- IUGR.
- Low birth weight.
- Symptoms of withdrawal from drugs.
- Increased stillbirth and neonatal mortality.
- Sudden infant death syndrome.
- Physical and neurological damage from drugs or violence.
- Fetal alcohol syndrome.

Substance misuse in pregnancy: management

Maternal issues

- To tailor proper ante- and postnatal care, a detailed history including use of illicit drugs, tobacco, and alcohol should be taken.
- Women using opiates should be prescribed substitution therapy (methadone).
- Women should not undergo opiate detoxification during pregnancy.
- Women on illicit drugs may be at risk of violence and abuse, and have other complex social, psychiatric, and psychological problems.
- Thus, they should be handled very sensitively, with dignity, in full confidence, and encouraged to attend for antenatal care.
- All patients should have multidisciplinary care with involvement of:
  - GP
  - social services
  - obstetric team (possibly including a specialist midwife)
  - local addiction services (possibly including a psychiatrist).
- Contraceptive advice should be offered where indicated.

Fetal issues

Most abusers will use more than one substance so there may be multiple risks to fetus. By definition, this is a high-risk pregnancy. General considerations should include:

- Detailed anomaly USS: consider the need for a later cardiac anomaly USS.
- Serial USS for growth and well-being: ↑ risk of IUGR.
- Increased awareness of the ↑ risk of obstetric complications such as:
  - preterm labour
  - placental abruption.

Alcohol abuse

Alcohol abuse is defined as drinking that causes mental, physical, or social harm to an individual.

- Alcohol consumption by women has increased over the last 15yrs.
- Excessive consumption of alcohol can lead to alimentary disorders, such as liver damage, gastritis, peptic ulcer, oesophageal varices, and acute and chronic pancreatitis.
- Damage to liver, including fatty infiltration, hepatitis, cirrhosis, and hepatoma, is particularly important.
- Neurological damage, such as peripheral neuropathy, epilepsy, and cerebellar degeneration, and cardiovascular complications, such as hypertension and stroke, are common.
- There may be child protection issues arising from potential neglect, as well as direct harm.

Fetal alcohol syndrome

There is evidence that this occurs in some children born to mothers who drink excessively (0.5–5:1000 live births). The exact relationship between alcohol and birth defects is a complex one, but there is no known safe lower limit for alcohol consumption; current recommendations limit consumption to 1U/day. Women drinking ≥18U/day have a 1 in 3 chance of fetal alcohol syndrome, characterized by pre- and postnatal retardation, developmental delay, and characteristic craniofacial dysmorphism, correlating with low IQ.

Features of fetal alcohol syndrome
- IUGR.
- Short stature.
- Developmental delay.
- Micro-ophthalmia.
- Short palpebral fissure.
- Short nasal bridge.
- Microcephaly with prominent forehead.
- Thin upper lip and small philtrum.
- Cleft palate.
- Maxillary hypoplasia.
- Gait abnormalities.
- Cardiac abnormalities.

Management of pregnancy in women abusing alcohol
- Attempt to reduce harm by:
  - counselling about risks and encouraging ↓ alcohol intake
  - encouraging antenatal attendance (ensure supportive, non-judgemental environment)
  - facilitating contact with support groups such as Alcoholics Anonymous (AA)
  - facilitating contact with social services (for help with benefits and improving housing)
  - screening for domestic abuse
  - offering help with smoking cessation if required.
- Detailed anomaly USS.
- Serial USS to assess growth and fetal well-being.
- Multidisciplinary team management with involvement of:
  - paediatric team
  - anaesthetic team
  - social services
  - local specialist alcohol support workers.
- May need child protection case conference.

Drugs of abuse: opiates

Routes of administration
Opiates (including morphine, heroin, methadone, buprenorphine) may be taken by snorting (intranasally), smoking, SC ('skin popping'), orally, or IV.

Maternal effects of opiates
- Act on the opioid receptors distributed throughout the CNS.
- They have many physical effects, including drowsiness, respiratory depression, nausea, hypotension, and papillary constriction.
- They act on pain receptors and may have significant mood-altering effects, producing a sensation of euphoria or intense pleasure.
- They are both physically and psychologically addictive.
- Withdrawal syndrome occurs within 4–12h after the last opiate dose, peaking at 48–72h, and subsiding by the end of 7–10 days.
- Characteristic symptoms of withdrawal include myalgia, arthralgia, dysphoria, insomnia, agitation, diarrhoea, and shivering.
- Withdrawal is not life-threatening.
- Annual mortality rate is about 1–2%, mostly due to overdose.

Effects of opiates on pregnancy
- Opiates not known to cause any specific congenital abnormalities.
- Babies of mothers abusing opiates are at ↑ risk of:
  - IUGR
  - stillbirth
  - sudden infant death syndrome.
- Withdrawal usually occurs within 24h of birth; symptoms include:
  - irritability and exaggerated startle response
  - jitteriness and tremors
  - poor feeding
  - hypotonicity.

Methadone maintenance treatment

- Methadone has a longer half-life than heroin, resulting in a more stable plasma concentration and allowing once-daily administration.
- Women already on replacement may need their methadone dose ↑ due to the physiological plasma dilution effect of pregnancy.
- Starting methadone may help with risk reduction by:
  - ↓ the physical risks of injecting
  - stabilizing lifestyle
  - ↓ the financial burden of purchasing street drugs
  - improving contact with healthcare professionals.
- Compliance with the treatment may:
  - ↓ neonatal mortality
  - ↑ birth weight.

⚠ Benefits can be lost if the mother also uses street drugs.

⚠ Withdrawal in pregnancy has a high risk to the fetus and should only be considered in highly motivated women with good social support.

Management of pregnancy in women abusing opiates

- Attempt to reduce harm by:
  - starting methadone
  - encouraging antenatal attendance (ensure supportive, non-judgemental environment)
  - facilitating contact with social services (for help with benefits and improve housing)
  - screening for domestic abuse
  - offering help with smoking cessation if required.
- Screening for STIs including HIV and hepatitis.
- Monitor injection sites for infection.
- Low threshold for antibiotics with symptoms of sepsis (may be atypical pathogens).
- High index of suspicion with any symptoms of VTE (may be unusual sites).
- Detailed anomaly USS.
- Serial USS to assess growth and fetal well-being.
- Multidisciplinary team management with involvement of:
  - paediatric team (baby will need admission to SCBU)
  - anaesthetic team (IV access may be difficult)
  - social services
  - local specialist drug support workers.
- Child protection case conference.

Drugs of abuse: cocaine

Routes of administration
- Intranasal is the major route.
- IV use either alone or with heroin has a high mortality rate.
- Smoking the freed alkaloid base as 'crack' is increasingly common in the UK.

Maternal effects of cocaine
- Inhibits the reuptake of neurotransmitters including dopamine.
- May result in euphoria, anorexia, verbosity, and sense of well-being.
- Also has stimulant effects from sympathetic overdrive.
- Deaths are mostly from accidents, cerebrovascular complications (intracranial bleed and emboli), and cardiac arrhythmias.

Effects of cocaine on pregnancy
- Teratogenicity
  - microcephaly
  - cardiac defects
  - possible genitourinary, limb, and gut defects.
- Vasoconstriction may cause abnormal placentation, resulting in:
  - ↑ risk of pre-eclampsia
  - ↑ risk of abruption
  - IUGR.
- Down-regulation of myometrial β-adrenoreceptors may cause:
  - miscarriage
  - uterine irritability
  - preterm labour.
- Neonates:
  - a limited withdrawal syndrome may occur
  - occasionally show hypotension and cardiac arrhythmias
  - are at ↑ risk of sudden infant death.

☛ Cocaine may have a detrimental effect on neurodevelopment, leading to developmental delay.

Management of pregnancy in women abusing cocaine

- Attempt to reduce harm by:
  - counselling about the risks and encouraging ↓ cocaine use
  - encouraging antenatal attendance (ensure supportive, non-judgemental environment)
  - facilitating contact with social services if needed
  - screening for domestic abuse
  - offering help with smoking cessation if required.
- Detailed anomaly USS.
- Fetal cardiac USS at 23–24wks.
- Serial USS to assess growth and fetal well-being.
- Multidisciplinary team management with involvement of:
  - paediatric team
  - anaesthetic team
  - social services
  - local specialist drug support workers.
- Child protection case conference.

Drugs of abuse: other stimulants

Amphetamine sulphate

Routes of administration
Illicit amphetamine can be taken orally, intranasally, or IV.

Maternal effects of amphetamine
- Enhances the dopaminergic neurotransmitter system.
- The stimulant properties are dose related and characterized by sympathetic overdrive (tachycardia, sweating, dry mouth, tremor).
- Effects on pregnancy.
- No proven syndrome of congenital abnormalities.
- Neonates occasionally show hyperactivity and poor feeding.

✒ May have similar risk of miscarriage, preterm labour, and IUGR as cocaine.

Ecstasy (MDMA)

Mode of action
- Like amphetamines, it increases the release of dopamine and also releases 5-hydroxytryptamine (5-HT), which may account for its hallucinogenic properties.
- It is selectively neurotoxic to fine serotonergic neurons.

Routes of administration
- Most commonly taken as a capsule in a dose of about 50–150mg.
- May also be injected or snorted.

Maternal effects
- Feelings of positive mood state, euphoria, sociability, and intimacy.
- Panic, paranoia, psychosis, and neuroses are also common and may extend to visual hallucinations, delusions, and suicidal feelings.

Effects on pregnancy
- Appears to have similar teratogenicity to cocaine, with reported ↑ in:
  - cardiac defects
  - limb and gut abnormalities.
- Neonates occasionally show hyperactivity and poor feeding.

✒ May have similar risk of miscarriage, preterm labour, and IUGR as cocaine.

Management of pregnancy in women abusing stimulants

- Attempt to reduce harm by;
  - counselling about the risks and encouraging ↓ drug use
  - encouraging antenatal attendance (ensure supportive, non-judgemental environment)
  - facilitating contact with social services if needed
  - screening for domestic abuse
  - offering help with smoking cessation if required.
- Detailed anomaly USS.
- If using ecstasy, consider fetal cardiac USS at 23–24wks.
- Serial USS to assess growth and fetal well-being.
- Multidisciplinary team management with involvement of:
  - paediatric team
  - anaesthetic team
  - social services
  - local specialist drug support workers.
- May need child protection case conference.

Drugs of abuse: sedatives and cannabis

Benzodiazepine and barbiturates

Since benzodiazepines first became available in the 1960s there have been many changes in the prescribing guidelines. Although the use of benzodiazepines as hypnotics has decreased, they are still prescribed as anxiolytics.

Mode of action They act on GABA-A receptors and enhance response to GABA.

Route of administration
- Given orally, bioavailability is almost complete, with peak plasma concentrations in 30–90min.
- Highly lipid soluble and diffuses rapidly through the blood–brain barrier and placenta; appears in breastmilk.
- IV or IM administration may lead to unpredictable absorption rate.

Maternal effects
- Tolerance develops after 2–3 days and is marked by 2–3wks.
- Tachyphylaxis has been reported.
- Onset of withdrawal is about 2–3 days after stopping (depending on the drug), peaking at 7–10 days and abating by 14 days.
- Symptoms of sensory disturbance, such as hyperacusis, photosensitivity, and abnormal body sensations are common.
- Anxiety symptoms and features of depression, psychosis, seizures, and delirium tremens are also seen.

Effects in pregnancy
- May cause increased congenital abnormalities, especially cleft lip and palate.
- Withdrawal symptoms in the baby include hypotonia, respiratory problems, and poor feeding (floppy baby syndrome).

Cannabis

Derived from the plant *Cannabis sativa*. It is consumed either as the dried plant in the form called marijuana or grass, or as the resin secreted by the flowers.

Mode of action Acts on the specific cannabinoid receptor (anandamide) in the CNS.

Route of administration Mostly smoked, often with tobacco, but may be ingested with food or in a herbal solution.

Maternal effects
- Like alcohol, it may cause either exhilaration or depression.
- It may also produce hallucinations and is an appetite stimulant.

Effects on pregnancy
- There is no definite evidence of teratogenicity.

Other drugs of abuse

Hallucinogens, lysergic acid diethylamide, and mescaline

- Usually consumed orally as small squares of blotting paper soaked in lysergic acid diethylamide (LSD), the drug causes hallucinations and visual illusions without lowering consciousness.
- Its action is mediated through the activation of the 5-HT$_2$ receptors.
- The physical actions of LSD are variable:
  - initially there is an increase in the heart rate and BP with adverse myocardial and cerebrovascular effects
  - however, overdosage does not have a significant physiological reaction.

👉 There may be a risk of miscarriage and congenital abnormalities among regular users.

Volatile substances ('glue sniffing')

- Volatile substance misuse is a widespread problem, mainly in the younger population.
- Substances used are generally solvents and adhesives (hence the term 'glue sniffing').
- Toluene, acetone, petrol, cleaning fluids, and aerosols are usually inhaled.
- Most often this is associated with other addictions, such as tobacco and alcohol.
- It can lead to sudden death from acute intoxication due to respiratory depression and cardiac arrhythmias.

👉 Little is known about the effects in pregnancy.

Tobacco

⚠ This is the most common substance of abuse and leads to complications including:
- ↑ Risk of miscarriage.
- ↑ Risk of placental abruption.
- Low birth weight.
- ↑ Risk of neonatal death and sudden infant death syndrome.

▶ Women should be advised to stop smoking, or at least cut down, in pregnancy.
- Help from specialist smoking cessation advisers should be available.
- Nicotine replacement therapy (patches or gum) may be used in pregnancy.

Antenatal psychiatric disorders: overview

Women of childbearing age carry a high burden of psychiatric disorders, particularly depression and anxiety. Although rates of psychiatric disorder during pregnancy appear similar to rates at other times in the life cycle (5–10%) the consequences are complicated by the additional risks to mother and fetus. Women with existing mental disorder require particularly careful management during pregnancy.

The importance of screening
⚠ Mental illness is one of the leading causes of maternal death in the UK.
- The majority of these deaths are the result of suicide, which is itself most strongly associated with perinatal depression.
- Over half of suicides occur between 6wks prenatally and 12wks postnatally, emphasizing the importance of early detection of antenatal psychiatric disorder and suicidal ideation.
- Most psychiatric disorders in pregnancy go unrecognized and unrecorded in the absence of systematic screening.
- Past history of mental illness is the best predictor of psychiatric disorder in pregnancy.
- Routine screening should include:
  - personal mental health history
  - other vulnerability factors, including substance misuse
  - family history of bipolar affective disorder (confers genetic vulnerability and a first episode is 7 times more likely to present in the immediate postnatal period).

Planning pregnancy with psychiatric disorders
Women suffering with recurrent and severe mental disorders who want to have children may benefit from pregnancy planning, as:
- Relapses are predicted by major life events.
- A medication holiday can be tried before conception, avoiding complications of relapse on pregnancy.
- Reproductive toxicology of essential medication can be minimized.
- Closer antenatal monitoring can be planned in advance.
- Contingency plans, including those for child protection, can be made with, and shared by, all the relevant agencies and caregivers.

Further reading
NICE. (2007). *Antenatal and postnatal mental health. Clinical management and service guidance*, NICE Clinical Guideline 45. London: National Institute for Health and Clinical Excellence. ♫ http://www.nice.org.uk/CG45

Antenatal psychiatric disorders: specific disorders

The classification and symptoms of psychiatric disorders appear in the ICD-10.

Anxiety disorders

- Panic disorder, generalized anxiety disorder, and obsessive–compulsive disorder are all relatively common in pregnancy.
- Symptoms include pervasive or episodic fearfulness, avoidance, and autonomic arousal.
- Excessive reassurance-seeking may be a presenting feature.
- Must identify any concurrent depression requiring treatment.
- Can be highly distressing and merit clinical attention, although evidence for an adverse effect on fetal outcome remains conflicting.
- High antenatal anxiety is a predictor for postnatal depression.
- Psychological management (including cognitive-behavioural therapy (CBT)) is preferable to anxiolytics, but access within the timescale of pregnancy may be limited.

⚠ Benzodiazepine use should be avoided.

Bipolar affective disorder

- Affects ~1% of women of childbearing age.
- Characterized by severe episodes of depression or mania (elevated mood, excitability, irritability, overactivity) often associated with psychotic symptoms. Can pose significant risk to mother and fetus.
- Associated with a 2-fold higher risk of admission postnatally than at other times.
- Decision to stop medication in existing patients when pregnancy is discovered should be made only after a careful risk/benefit review.

⚠ Associated with a high suicide rate.

Schizophrenia

- Affects ~1% of women of childbearing age.
- Clinical features vary, but include delusions, hallucinations, and abnormalities of affect, speech, and volition.
- Maintenance medication is usually required throughout pregnancy.
- Significant proportion of patients are unable to care for the child.
- The lifetime risk of schizophrenia for a child with one affected parent is in the order of 10%.

Eating disorders

- Bulimia nervosa affects 1% of women of childbearing age and anorexia nervosa 0.2%.
- Characterized by disturbances in eating behaviour and abnormalities in body image.
- Although anorexia nervosa is associated with reduced fertility and fecundity, patients with sub-threshold symptoms can become pregnant and require careful monitoring and management.
- Possible effects on fetal outcome include IUGR, low birth weight, prematurity, and a possible increase in congenital anomalies.

Depression

⚠ As common antenatally as it is postnatally.
- Characterized by:
  - low mood
  - lack of energy or increased fatigability
  - loss of enjoyment or interest in usual activities
  - low self-esteem
  - feelings of guilt, worthlessness, or hopelessness
  - poor concentration
  - change in appetite (leading to weight loss or gain)
  - suicidal ideation.
- Associated with an increased risk of suicide.
- Can be effectively treated with pharmacological and psychological therapy.

Further reading

WHO. (1992). *ICD-10 Classification of mental and behavioural disorders.* WHO, Geneva.

Psychiatric medications

Anticonvulsant mood stabilizers

Carbamazepine

Major malformation rate 2.2%:
- High rate of neural tube defects.
- Others include craniofacial abnormalities and distal digit hypoplasia.

▶ Breast-feeding is not recommended.

Lamotrigine

Major malformation rate 2.1%: high rate of cleft palate.

▶ Caution with breast-feeding (dermatological problems in infants).

Sodium valproate

Major malformation rate 6%:
- Very high rate of neural tube defects.
- Others include craniofacial abnormalities and distal digit hypoplasia.
- Significant neurobehavioural toxicity (22% of exposed infants develop low verbal IQ).

⚠ Should not be routinely prescribed to women with childbearing potential.

⚠ Should not be prescribed to women under 18 due to ↑ risk of developing polycystic ovary syndrome (PCOS) and ↑ risk of unplanned pregnancy.

Benzodiazepines

See 📖 Drugs of abuse: sedatives and cannabis, p. 444.

Lithium

- 50% of women with bipolar affective disorder stabilized on lithium relapse within 40wks of stopping it.
- *Early pregnancy:* risk of Ebstein's anomaly lower than previously estimated at 0.05–0.1% against a background risk of 0.0005%.
- *Late pregnancy:* levels need to be measured more frequently as plasma volume and GFR increase.
- *Labour:* reduced vascular volume and potential dehydration necessitates careful fluid balance and monitoring of serum lithium levels.
- *Neonate:* reported association with floppy baby syndrome, neonatal thyroid abnormalities, and nephrogenic diabetes insipidus.

⚠ Breast-feeding is not recommended.

▶ If women continue to take lithium, serum levels should be checked every 4wks until 36wks, then weekly.

▶ Women taking lithium should deliver in a consultant-led obstetric unit.

Antipsychotics
- Older antipsychotics (such as haloperidol) are preferred because more data are available with no strong evidence of ↑ malformations.
- May be an effective alternative to mood stabilizers in women with bipolar affective disorder.
- Clozapine is not routinely used in pregnancy and breast-feeding due to the theoretical risk of agranulocytosis in the fetus/neonate.

Antidepressants in pregnancy and lactation

When choosing an antidepressant, prescribers should bear in mind that the safety is not well understood, but take into account:
- Tricyclic antidepressants (amitriptyline, imipramine, and nortriptyline) have lower known risks than other newer antidepressants.
- Most tricyclics have a higher fat toxicity index than SSRIs.
- Fluoxetine is the SSRI with lowest known risk in pregnancy.
- No strong evidence of ↑ malformations with tricyclic drugs.
- Paroxetine may have association with cardiac malformations.
- SSRIs in late pregnancy have been associated with ↑ incidence of persistent pulmonary hypertension in infants.
- Venlafaxine may be associated with ↑ risk of high BP, ↑ toxicity in overdose, and ↑ difficulty in withdrawal.
- Serotonin and norepinephrine reuptake inhibitors (SNRIs) are relatively untested and so are not recommended as first-line drugs in pregnancy.

▶ Citalopram and fluoxetine are present in breastmilk at relatively high concentrations.

▶ Imipramine, nortriptyline, sertraline, and paroxetine have particularly low concentrations in breastmilk and are therefore recommended for breast-feeding mothers.

Considerations for managing psychiatric medications in pregnancy

- ⚠ Any decision to stop psychiatric medication for women with serious mental health problems should be made in consultation with a specialist, bearing in mind that the period of maximum vulnerability has often passed by the time pregnancy is identified. For example, an estimated 50% of women with bipolar affective disorder maintained on lithium will relapse during a 40wk pregnancy if it is stopped.
- Most psychiatric drugs are not associated with a significant increase in fetal anomalies.
- The risks of a relapse of psychiatric disorder during pregnancy tend to be underestimated.
- The risks of continuing medication need to be considered in terms of:
  - early fetal exposure
  - late fetal expose
  - delivery and neonatal withdrawal
  - breast-feeding
  - longer-term neurobehavioural toxicity.

Further reading

NICE. (2007). *Antenatal and postnatal mental health. Clinical management and service guidance*, NICE Clinical Guideline 45. National Institute for Health and Clinical Excellence, London. http://www.nice.org.uk/CG45

Postnatal depression

Over 10% of women are depressed in the postnatal period. Although the term 'postnatal depression' is both clinically useful and acceptable to women, there is no evidence that it is any different from depression at any other time in a woman's life. It should accordingly be taken seriously and not dismissed as a mild, self-resolving condition that does not require treatment. Emphasized by recent evidence of a link between postnatal depression and infant developmental problems when there are associated difficulties in the mother–infant relationship.

Diagnosis

Key features of depression are (see 📖 Antenatal psychiatric disorders: specific disorders p. 448):
• Tearfulness.
• Irritability.
• Anxiety.
• Poor sleep.

It can easily be missed if specific enquiries are not made, especially with milder cases. New mothers with depression are often embarrassed by their feelings and reluctant to admit to sadness at a time when they feel they are expected to be happy.

Screening for depression

NICE suggests the following questions are used to screen for depression both antenatally and at 4–6wks and 3–4mths postnatally:
• During the past month, have you often been bothered by feeling down, depressed, or hopeless?
• During the past month, have you often been bothered by having little interest or pleasure in doing things?
If the woman answers 'yes' to both of these:
• Is this something you feel you need or want help with?

Other screening questionnaires like the Edinburgh Postnatal Depression Scale (EPDS) are also helpful in identifying postnatal depression, and are routinely used by health visitors in many services.

Treatment and recovery

Mild to moderate depression may respond to self-help strategies and non-directive counselling ('listening visits' by a health visitor). Moderate to severe depression usually requires treatment with antidepressant medication and/or psychotherapy (CBT). Breast-feeding is not a contraindication for antidepressant treatment, but drugs with low excretion in breastmilk, such as sertraline, are preferred.

Women who have experienced postnatal depression have a high (>70%) lifetime risk of further depression and a 25% risk of depression following subsequent deliveries. For this reason, women who present in pregnancy with a history of postnatal depression are likely to benefit from closer postnatal follow-up.

Post-partum 'baby blues'

Over 50% of women experience a brief period of emotional instability starting around 3 days after delivery and resolving spontaneously within 10 days, characterized by:

- Tearfulness.
- Irritability.
- Anxiety.
- Poor sleep.

This usually responds to support and reassurance.

Puerperal psychosis

This is a commonly used term that describes a range of psychotic conditions presenting in the immediate postnatal period. Most cases are episodes of bipolar affective disorder, although severe unipolar depression, schizophrenia, and acute physical illness with associated organic brain syndrome can all present with psychotic symptoms.

Presentation

Puerperal psychosis presents rapidly (usually within 2wks of delivery), following approximately 1–2:1000 births. The associated suicide rate is in the order of 5% and the infanticide rate is up to 4%. Prediction and prevention are therefore key service priorities.

> **Risk factors**
> - Personal history of bipolar affective disorder.
> - Previous episode of puerperal psychosis.
> - 1st-degree relative with history of puerperal psychosis.
> - 1st-degree relative with bipolar affective disorder.

High-risk patients

⚠ A woman with bipolar affective disorder and a personal or family history of puerperal psychosis has a 60% risk of puerperal psychosis.

High-risk patients should be referred to specialist perinatal mental health services antenatally, so an appropriate care plan can be developed and the use of prophylactic medication, following delivery, may be considered.

Treatment and recovery

⚠ Women presenting with puerperal psychosis need urgent psychiatric assessment and treatment. They should be admitted, because of the risks to both mother and baby (neglect as well as direct harm): ideally this will be to a specialist mother and baby unit, where the maternal–infant relationship can be protected.

⚠ Any decision to admit a baby to a mother and baby unit must be child centred, and involve full consideration of the longer-term possibility of the baby remaining with the mother if the mental health problems have been long-standing.

Puerperal psychosis is treated according to diagnosis. This may involve:
- Antidepressant or antipsychotic medication.
- Mood stabilizers.
- Electroconvulsive therapy (ECT).

Most patients presenting with puerperal psychosis make a full recovery, but the 10yr recurrence rate (puerperal and non-puerperal) is up to 80% and the 10yr readmission rate is of the order of 60%.

Gynaecological anatomy and development

Gynaecological history: overview

▶ Always introduce yourself fully and explain what you are going to do; patients are often very apprehensive and nervous.

Personal information

- Name, date of birth, age.
- Relationship status.
- Occupation.
- Partner's details and occupation (relevant in subfertility patients).

Current problem

- Description of the problem.
- Severity, duration, relationship to menstrual cycle.
- Aggravating and relieving factors.
- Any previous investigations or treatment.

Menstrual history

- Date of *first day* of LMP.

⚠ Always *think*: is this patient pregnant or at risk of pregnancy?

Every woman you see (10–60yrs old) should be considered potentially pregnant until proved otherwise—then you will not miss it!

- Age at menarche/menopause.
- Menstrual pattern (number of days bleeding/length of cycle).
- Amount/character of bleeding (flooding, clots, double protection).

⚠ Always ask about intermenstrual (IMB) + postcoital bleeding (PCB).

⚠ Always ask about any postmenopausal bleeding (PMB).

- Any associated pain + pattern (dysmenorrhoea). Has this changed?
- Ask about pain at other times including dyspareunia.
- Current and recent contraception (or not!) and details.
- Current/future pregnancy plans—this may alter/limit therapeutic options, as many treatments are contraceptive.

Past obstetric history

All pregnancies must be recorded, including successful ones, miscarriages, ectopic pregnancies, TOPs, and molar pregnancies. Outcomes, gestation and mode of delivery, complications, birth weight, and current health of child(ren) should all be documented (see 📖 Obstetric history: current pregnancy, p. 2).

Past gynaecological history

- History of any other gynaecological problems especially endometriosis, fibroids, polycystic ovaries, and subfertility.
- All previous gynaecological surgery.
- Date of last cervical smear and result. Were they always normal?

Sexual history
- *Dyspareunia:* superficial on penetration or deep pain.
- Sexually transmitted infections or pelvic inflammatory disease (PID).
- Any abnormal vaginal discharge.

> **Key things to achieve in a gynaecological history**
> - A clear understanding of the presenting problem(s) including effect on quality of life. Most diagnoses are clear from a good history alone.
> - A good history will inform your examination and investigative rationale.
> - Exclude or confirm current pregnancy or risk of it. Offer contraceptive advice to the latter if they do not desire pregnancy!
> - Discover what current and near future pregnancy plans are.
> - Identify women at higher risk of malignancy or other serious pathology.
>
> ⚠ IMB, PCB, and PMB are all red flag symptoms warranting examination and investigation.
>
> Allow disclosure of a hidden agenda. Many women will disclose other issues regarding sex or abuse or fertility concerns if you establish a good rapport; if you sense there is another concern don't be afraid to ask ('You seem concerned about something. Is there anything else you would like to discuss?').

Gynaecological history: other relevant details

Micturition
General enquiry
If urinary symptoms disclosed then explore:
- Frequency (day and night).
- Pain or burning sensation (dysuria).
- Urgency.
- Urinary incontinence (stress or urge).
- Haematuria.
- Presence of 'something coming down' (prolapse related symptoms).

Bowel habit
General enquiry
If bowel symptoms are disclosed then explore:
- Regularity.
- Associated bloating, pain, or difficulty defecating.
- Use of laxatives.
- Any rectal bleeding.

Medical and surgical history
- All medical conditions, especially diabetes, hypertension, asthma, thrombo-embolism. Major effect if surgery is being considered.
- All previous abdominal surgery is important also.

Drugs and allergies
- Details of all medication (doses and duration of use).
- Allergies to medications and severity (anaphylaxis or rash?).
- Use of folic acid in early pregnancy.

▶ Consider the risks for all drugs in relation to pregnancy (see 📖 Drugs in pregnancy, p. 261).
- Possible teratogenesis.
- Altered pharmacodynamics and pharmacokinetics.
- Toxicity in breastmilk where appropriate.

Family history
- Especially diabetes, ↑ BP, and thrombo-embolism.
- Familial cancers should always be considered, as well as others with a genetic association including:
  - breast
  - ovarian
  - endometrial
  - bowel.

Social history
- Home conditions and relationships.
- Occupation.
- Smoking and alcohol intake.
- Lifestyle issues such as use of recreational drugs.

⚠ **Subtle symptoms of gynaecological malignancy**
- Change of urinary and/or bowel habit.
- Persistent bloating.
- Non-specific discomfort.
- Even upper GI dyspeptia-type.

These should always prompt further investigation, particularly in women >50yrs, when persistent.

Gynaecological examination

General examination
- Height and weight.
- BMI (=weight (kg)/[height (m)]²). ⚠ ↑ Risks with ↑ BMI.
- General, e.g. signs of anaemia, thyroid disease.

Abdominal examination
- *Inspection:* skin quality, abdominal distension, surgical scars (umbilical or Pfannensteil), any visible masses or distension.
- *Palpation:*
  - superficial palpation for guarding, tenderness, rigidity
  - deep palpation for any masses; if present determine if arising from the pelvis ('can I get below the mass?')
  - pelvic masses are compared to the equivalent sized pregnant uterus (e.g. 20/40 sized, firm, mobile fibroid uterus).
- *Percussion:* dull if the mass is solid, tympanic if distended bowel, shifting dullness and fluid thrill in cases of ascites.
- *Auscultation:* usually used postoperatively to detect bowel sounds.

Good practice for intimate examinations
- Full explanation of procedure and reasons for it should precede examination.
- Verbal consent should be obtained.
- A trained chaperone is mandatory.
- ⚠ Do NOT use partners, friends, or children as chaperones.
- The patient must be able to undress and dress in privacy and cover herself at all other times.
- Any students or extra personnel present should be introduced and consent obtained for their presence BEFORE procedure.

Further GMC guidance on intimate examinations can be found at: ℛ http://www.gmc-uk.org

---

Pelvic examination
- All equipment must be ready (speculum, KY jelly, swabs, cytobrush, pipelle, etc.) *before* the patient is exposed.
- *Position the woman:*
  - dorsal (most common in gynaecological outpatient setting)
  - lithotomy (used for vaginal surgery, the feet suspended from poles)
  - Sim's (examination of pelvic prolapse, type of the left lateral)
- *Inspection:* describe any swelling, inflammation, skin changes, lesions, or ulceration seen anywhere on the vulva. Do the same for the vagina and cervix once the speculum is passed.
- *Speculum examination:* see Box 14.1 for description of technique. Describe findings in vagina and on cervix.

▶ Don't forget to take any swabs required such as HVS for vaginal pathogens and flora or endocervical for Chlamydia +/or Gonorrhoea.
- *Bimanual (VE):* see Box 14.2 for description of technique.

Box 14.1 How to do a speculum examination

- Cusco's bivalve speculum is more frequently used, but Sim's speculum normally used in examination of pelvic organ prolapse.
- Use a warm and well-lubricated speculum.
- Part labia minora adequately with the left hand.
- Insert speculum upwards and backwards (direction of vagina).
- Advance into vagina fully (until it cannot advance any further).
- Directly visualize as you open blades exposing cervix: only open enough to see cervix fully.
- *If cervix not seen:* close blades, withdraw slightly, change direction (usually more anterior), and open again.
- *Speculum removal:* ensure the blades are open while sliding over cervix, avoiding trapping it—watch what you are doing!
- Blades should be closed at introitus, not trapping any vagina.

Common problems to avoid

- *Obvious non-familiarity with the speculum:* patients spot this a mile off and will automatically tense up.
- Inadequate labial parting leads to inversion and pain (start badly and all patient confidence quickly disappears).
- *The speculum is only partially inserted 'so as not to cause pain':* the cervix will usually not be seen, leading to repeated insertion.
- *Failure to find cervix first time:* likely to be more anterior and closer to the introitus—pull back and move anterior as above.
- Not watching for adequate opening of blades and continuing unnecessary wide opening.
- Not having control of closure and pulling out a still-open speculum.

Box 14.2 How to do a bimanual vaginal examination

- The lubricated index and middle fingers of the right hand are introduced into the vagina. The fingers of the left hand are on the abdomen above the symphysis pubis, and the uterus and adnexae are palpated between the two hands ('bimanual palpation').
- *Cervix:*
  - consistency (soft and smooth or irregular and hard)
  - tenderness
  - external os (?open during miscarriage).
- *Uterus:*
  - axis (anteverted, axial, or retroverted)
  - size (equivalent to gestational weeks of a gravid uterus)
  - consistency (soft in a gravid uterus, firm, or hard with fibroids)
  - mobility (may be fixed in endometriosis/adhesions).
- *Adnexae:*
  - normal ovaries are usually not palpable
  - any masses (cystic/solid) and describe approximate size.
- Direct digital pressure into the fornices assesses tenderness, and cervical excitation is elicited by moving the cervix laterally right and left.

▶ Uterine masses usually move with cervix, ovarian masses do not.
▶ Obese patients are usually difficult to palpate—consider ultrasound.

Anatomy: female reproductive organs

See 📖 The female pelvis, p. 10 for anatomy of the bony pelvis.

Vagina
- Fibromuscular tube, 7–10cm long.
- The cervix enters through the anterior wall.
- In the resting state the anterior and posterior walls are opposed.

Uterus
- Approximately 8 × 5 × 3cm in size (non-pregnant).
- Composed mainly of smooth muscle.
- Divided into the corpus and cervix uteri.
- Cylindrical and joins the uterine cavity at the internal os and the vagina at the external os.
- Anteverted in 80% of women (the remainder are retroverted or rarely axial).

Uterine (fallopian) tubes
- 10cm long; lie in the upper part of the broad ligament.
- *Divided anatomically into:*
  - isthmus (medial)—opens into the uterus at the ostia
  - infundibulum (lateral) with fimbrial end closely applied to the ovary
  - ampulla—in between (where fertilization takes place).

Ovaries
- Approximately 3 × 2cm during reproductive years.
- Attached to the posterior surface of the broad ligament by the mesovarium.
- Situated in the ovarian fossa at the division of the common iliac artery (the ureter runs immediately underneath).

See Fig. 14.1.

Supports of the uterus, vagina, and pelvic floor
- *Middle:*
  - transverse cervical ligaments (cardinal ligaments)
  - pubocervical ligament
  - uterosacral ligaments.
- *Lower:*
  - levator ani muscles and coccygeus
  - urogenital diaphragm
  - the superficial and deep perineal muscles with the perineal body.

▶ Defects and weaknesses of these supporting structures due to fascial tearing and denervation during parturition and surgery can cause organ prolapse and problems with urinary incontinence.

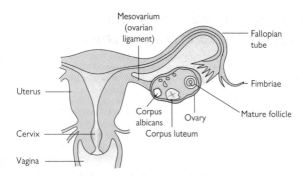

Fig. 14.1 Basic coronal view of the female pelvis. Adapted from Pocock G, Richards C. (2004). *Human physiology: the basics of medicine*, 2nd edn. Oxford: OUP. By permission of Oxford University Press.

Anatomy: blood supply and relationship to other structures

Blood supply

Uterus
- *The uterine artery:*
  - branches from the internal iliac
  - runs behind the peritoneum to enter the lateral border of the uterus, through two layers of the broad ligament
  - anastomoses with the ovarian and vaginal arteries.
- The venous drainage is to the internal iliac vein.

Ovaries
- *The ovarian arteries:* branches of the abdominal aorta from below the renal arteries.
- The right ovary drains directly into the inferior vena cava.
- The left ovary drains into the left renal vein.

Vagina
Supplied by
- Vaginal artery.
- Inferior vesical artery.
- Clitoral branch of the pudendal artery.

Urinary tract

Ureters
- Retroperitoneal throughout.
- Enter the pelvis in the base of the ovarian fossa.
- Run above the levator ani in the base of the broad ligament.
- Insert into the bladder posterolaterally.

> ⚠ The ureters are very close to the uterine artery near the lateral fornix and can be injured at hysterectomy.

Bladder
- Lies anterior to the uterus.
- *Three layers:* serous (peritoneal), muscular (detrusor smooth muscle), and mucosa (transitional epithelium).
- Supplied by superior and inferior vesical arteries (internal iliac artery).

Rectum
- Lies posterior to the uterus (separated from it by loops of small bowel lying in the pouch of Douglas).
- A thin rectovaginal septum separates the vagina and rectum.
- Supplied by superior, middle, and inferior rectal arteries (from the inferior mesenteric, internal iliac, and pudendal arteries respectively).

See Fig. 14.2.

Lymphatic drainage of the pelvic organs
- *Vulva and lower vagina* → inguinofemoral → external iliac nodes.
- *Cervix* → cardinal ligaments → hypogastric, obturator, internal iliac → common iliac, and para-aortic nodes.
- *Endometrium* → broad ligament → iliac and para-aortic nodes.
- *Ovaries* → infundibulopelvic ligament → para-aortic nodes.

⚠ Knowledge of lymphatic drainage is important when considering metastatic spread from genital tract cancer.

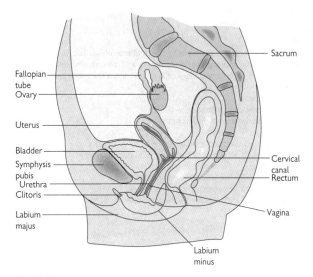

Fig. 14.2 Basic sagittal view of female pelvis demonstrating relationship to other pelvic organs. Adapted from Pocock G, Richards C. (2004). *Human physiology: the basics of medicine*, 2nd edn. Oxford: OUP. By permission of Oxford University Press.

Anatomy: external genitalia

Perineum
- The area inferior to the pelvic diaphragm can be divided into:
  - anterior urogenital triangle (pierced by the vagina and the urethra)
  - posterior anal triangle.
- The superficial and deep perineal fascias are continuous with the labia majora and are attached:
  - anteriorly to the pubic symphysis
  - laterally to the body of the pubis.
- The superficial perineal muscles are:
  - superficial transverse perineus
  - ischiocavernosus
  - bulbocavernosus.

Vulva
The external genital organs are known collectively as the vulva and are composed of the mons pubis, labia majora and minora, and clitoris.
- *Labia majora:* lateral boundary of the vulva from the mons pubis to the perineum.
- *Labia minora:*
  - anteriorly join to cover the clitoris
  - posteriorly form the fourchette.
- *Clitoris:*
  - composed of erectile tissue covered by a prepuce
  - supplied by a branch of the internal pudendal artery.
- *The vestibule:*
  - lies between the labia minora and the hymen
  - the urethra lies anterior in the vestibule
  - posteriorly and laterally lie the vestibular or Bartholin's glands.

See Fig. 14.3.

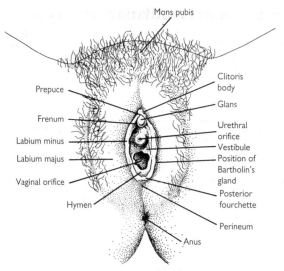

Fig. 14.3 External female genitalia. Reproduced from Collier J, Longmore M, Brinsden M. (2006). *Oxford handbook of clinical specialties*, 7th edn. Oxford: OUP. By permission of Oxford University Press.

Female genital mutilation: overview

Female genital mutilation (FGM) is defined by the World Health Organization (WHO) and the United Nations (UN) agencies as "the partial or total removal of the female external genitalia or other injury to the female genital organs for non-medical reasons" (See Table 14.1 for classification and Box 14.3 for complications).

Table 14.1 Classification of FGM (WHO)

Type I	'Sunna' or traditional circumcision with removal of prepuce with or without part or the entire clitoris.
Type II	Clitoridectomy with removal of prepuce and clitoris together with partial or total excision of labia minora.
Type III	Infibulation or 'clasp circumcision' with removal of part or all of external genitalia and stitching/narrowing of vaginal opening leaving a small aperture for passing urine and menstrual blood.
Type IV	Unclassified.

Box 14.3 Complications of FGM

Immediate complications
- Death.
- Shock and pain.*
- Haemorrhage.*
- Infection including septicaemia.*
- Adjacent organ damage.*
- Acute urinary retention.

Long-term complications affecting pelvic organs
- Failure of healing.
- Recurrent UTI and renal/bladder calculus formation.*
- Urethral obstruction and difficulty in passing urine.
- Pelvic infections and abscess formation.*
- Menstrual abnormalities and associated infertility.
- Sexual dysfunction.*
- Fistulae.

Long-term impact on reproductive health
- AIDS, HIV, and other blood borne diseases.
- Problems with pregnancy and childbirth.
- Psychological or psychiatric problems.

* Common complications.

Female genital mutilation: management

The management of girls and women affected by FGM is really determined by the complication that they present with, principally:

- *Problems with sexual intercourse and/or micturition*: de-infibulation under GA.
- *Problems during and/or following delivery*: obstructed labour and/or major tears or urethral injury—de-infibulation in the second stage of labour under local anaesthetic (LA)/regional block.
- *Individual problems*: such as infection, adjacent organ damage, and fistulae can be managed on an individual basis.

De-infibulation

- Obstructing skin divided in the middle.
- Anterior/upward episiotomy in labour.
- Edges of incised surfaces freshened and sutured.
- The urethra needs to be protected to avoid injury.
- Extensive reconstruction may be needed in severe cases.
- De-infibulation should be carried out by people experienced in dealing with this problem.

FGM overview

- Deeply rooted cultural tradition in 28 countries particularly northern, eastern, and western Africa.
- Highly complex social, religious, and political problem.
- WHO estimates 130–140 million women affected annually.
- Can occur at birth, infancy, childhood, teenage years, or in adulthood.
- May be carried out by a wide range of 'practitioners' mostly untrained with a variety of 'instruments'.
- Complications (as above) are common.
- Management is related to the individual complications/presenting symptoms: usually de-infibulation.
- Prevention of FGM is an ongoing major human rights issue.

⚠ An illegal practice in the UK and most parts of the world including areas where it is commonly practiced.

Malformations of the genital tract: overview

These congenital malformations range from asymptomatic minor defects to complete absence of the vagina and uterus. The prevalence is estimated to be as high as 3%.

Aetiology

They arise from failure of the paramesonephric (müllerian) ducts to form, fuse in the midline, or fuse with the urogenital sinus:

- *Complete failure to form:* Rokitansky syndrome.
- *Partial failure to form:* unicornuate uterus.
- *Failure of the ducts to fuse together properly:*
  - longitudinal vaginal septae
  - bicornuate uterus
  - uterus didelphys (complete double system).
- *Failure to fuse with the urogenital sinus:* transverse vaginal septae.
- *Remnants of the mesonephric (Wolffian) ducts may be present as lateral vaginal wall or broad ligament cysts:* usually trivial incidental findings and rarely of clinical significance.

⚠ Always look for renal and urinary tract anomalies (up to 40% co-existence).

Clinical features

Presentation often depends on whether it causes obstruction of menstrual flow.

- *Mayer–Rokitansky–Küster–Hauser (MRKH):* painless 1° amenorrhoea, normal 2° sexual characteristics, blind ending or absent vagina (dimple only).
- *Imperforate hymen:* cyclical pain, 1° amenorrhoea, bluish bulging membrane visible at introitus.
- *Transverse vaginal septum:* cyclical pain, 1° amenorrhoea, possible abdominal mass +/– urinary retention due to haematocolpos, endometriosis due to retrograde menstruation, not all obstructed, may present with dyspareunia.
- *Longitudinal vaginal septae and rudimentary uterine horns:* dyspareunia alone if no obstruction, but if one hemi-uterus or hemi-vagina is obstructed then increasing cyclical pain in the presence of normal menses +/– abdominal mass from haematocolpos, and endometriosis.
- *Uterine anomalies* (bicornuate uterus, arcuate uterus, uterine septae): often asymptomatic, incidental finding at CS, may present with 1° infertility, recurrent miscarriage, preterm labour, or abnormal lie in pregnancy (a causal relationship with these conditions is controversial).

Embryology of the female genital tract in a nutshell

- Genetic sex is determined at fertilization.
- Gender becomes apparent in the normal fetus by the 12th week of development.
- By the 6th week of life the following structures start to develop either side of the midline:
  - genital ridges (induced by primordial germ cells from the yolk sac)
  - mesonephric (Wolffian) ducts (lateral to the genital ridge)
  - paramesonephric (müllerian) ducts (lateral to the mesonephric ducts).
- In the female fetus the mesonephric ducts regress.
- The paramesonephric ducts go on to develop into:
  - the fallopian tubes (upper and middle parts)
  - the uterus, cervix, and upper 4/5 of the vagina (this results from the lower part of the ducts fusing together in the midline).
- The lower 1/5 of the vagina develops from the sinovaginal bulbs of the urogenital sinus, which fuses with the paramesonephric ducts.
- The muscles of the vagina and uterus develop from the surrounding mesoderm.

▶ Development of male genitalia is instigated by a single transcription factor encoded on the Y chromosome (*SRY* gene). This leads to the differentiation of the gonad to a testis, and production of testosterone and anti-müllerian hormone (AMH) with subsequent masculinization. In the absence of the *SRY* gene, fetus will develop female phenotype.

▶ The mesonephric ducts also sprout the ureteric buds (which go on to form the kidneys and ureters) and caudally develops into trigone of the bladder. Hence, close association between genital tract and urinary tract abnormalities.

Malformations of the genital tract: management

Investigations

- A thorough history and examination are required.
- Abdominal and TVS are invaluable, but not appropriate if not sexually active.
- MRI is the gold standard, especially if complex surgery is planned.
- Examination under anaesthesia +/– vaginoscopy, cystoscopy, and hysteroscopy may be required.
- Karyotyping to exclude 46XY female (androgen insensitivity syndrome) if uterus and upper vagina are absent.

⚠ Renal tract ultrasound +/– IV urography should always be undertaken because of high incidence of related renal tract abnormalities.

> **Aims for the management of genital tract malformations**
>
> - Minor anomalies usually need nothing more than reassurance, particularly if an incidental finding, as most are of no clinical significance.
> - Management should be a multidisciplinary approach including psychological help for the patient and her parents, as well as arranging correction of anomaly.
> - The aim of any treatment should be well defined.

Treatment

- *Imperforate hymen:* easily corrected by a cruciate incision in the obstructive membrane.
- *Vaginal septae:* should be removed surgically. Resection of longitudinal septae usually straightforward; transverse septae can be more complex, especially if high and thick, requiring surgical vaginoplasty.
- Obstructive uterine anomalies should also be surgically corrected or removed. This is usually performed laparoscopically. These procedures can be technically difficult and should only be performed in centres with expertise in this area.
- *Rokitansky:* vaginal dilation is first-line treatment for creating a functional vagina. If this fails, surgical vaginoplasty can be performed by several techniques. Timing should be related to when sexual activity is anticipated.
- Patients should be given information regarding their condition; support groups are often very helpful.

> **Aims for the treatment of genital tract malformations**
>
> - Creation of a vagina suitable for penetrative sexual intercourse.
> - Relief of menstrual obstruction and associated pain.
> - Prevention of long-term sequelae of endometriosis due to obstruction and retrograde menstruation.
> - Restoration or optimization of fertility wherever possible.

Disorders of sex development

Sex determination occurs in embryo, with female phenotype being default setting. Male genitalia require testosterone to develop; sex determining region (SRY) gene on Y chromosome principally responsible for development of testis, which in turn secretes AMH, causing regression of paramesonephric ducts. If any part of this process fails, resulting offspring may be genetically male, but phenotypically female.

> **Causes of disorders of sex development (DSD), classified according to karyotype**
>
> *46XX karyotype*
> • Virilizing forms of congenital adrenal hyperplasia (CAH).
> • Ovo-testicular DSD (previously termed true hermaphroditism).
> • Maternal virilizing condition or ingested drugs.
> • Placental aromatase deficiency.
>
> *46XY karyotype*
> • Androgen insensitivity syndrome (AIS).
> • Defects of testosterone biosynthesis (e.g. 5α-reductase deficiency, 17β-hydroxysteroid dehydrogenase deficiency).
> • Swyer syndrome (pure gonadal dysgenesis).
> • Partial gonadal dysgenesis 2° to single gene mutations.
> • Leydig cell hypoplasia.
>
> *Abnormal karyotype*
> • Turner syndrome (45XO): aneuploidy or mosaicism.
> • XO/XY mixed gonadal dysgenesis.

Later presentations of DSD
• DSD is not synonymous with ambiguous genitalia. Many conditions will present much later.
• Androgen insensitivity, Swyer syndrome, and Turner syndrome often present with 1° amenorrhoea.
• Although often associated with a degree of genital ambiguity, 5α-reductase deficiency and 17β-hydroxysteroid dehydrogenase deficiency may present with virilization at puberty.
• Ambiguous genitalia at birth.

Genitalia are said to be ambiguous when their appearance is neither that expected for a girl nor for a boy. Incidence approximately 1:4000 births. The extent ranges from mild clitoral enlargement to micropenis with hypospadias.

❶ Never guess the sex of a baby.

A full family history, drug history, and whether the mother has experienced any virilization during pregnancy should be ascertained.

Investigations

- Full assessment of the infant should occur looking for:
  - evidence of life-threatening salt-losing crisis (adrenal insufficiency), including hypovolaemia, hypoglycaemia, and hyperpigmentation

⚠ U&E are essential and must be sent urgently.
  - features of Turner syndrome or other congenital anomalies
  - full inspection of genitalia carefully recording the position of orifices.
- Urgent serum 17-hydroxyprogesterone (raised in CAH).
- 24h urine collection for steroid analysis.
- Karyotyping with urgent FISH for fragments of the Y chromosome.
- Ultrasound to locate gonads and presence of a uterus.
- Further investigations as deemed appropriate by multidisciplinary team.

Corrective surgery

🖝 Full disclosure is advocated and parents should be fully informed of the risks of surgery and anaesthesia. These include:
- Surgery as an infant may not be definitive.
- Each episode of surgery increases the risk of damage to sensitivity of the genitalia and dissatisfaction with sexual function in adult life.
- Such children may one day want to be the opposite sex to that assigned, because of hormonal influences on the fetal brain.

The need for gonadectomy should be discussed openly with regards to the risk of malignancy, especially for patients with gonadal dysgenesis (30% lifetime risk) or the presence of a Y fragment. In other conditions it may be advocated to prevent further virilization. In AIS, it is advised to delay gonadectomy until after puberty as the malignancy risk is much lower. In all cases parents should be given time to think.

Such children should be given age and developmentally appropriate information regarding their condition at an early stage, with psychological support as required leading up to full disclosure so they can be involved in decisions regarding their care.

Coping with a child with ambiguous genitalia

- Keeping parents informed and psychologically supported at a very difficult time is of prime importance.
- Referral to a dedicated multidisciplinary team is essential.
- Pressure to decide on sex of rearing should not be allowed to interfere with giving time to allow parents to come to terms with their child's condition or reach the correct diagnosis.
- Parents must be full partners in allocation of sex of rearing.
- Access to relevant support groups is invaluable.

Intersex Society of North America (ISNA). ℘ http://www.isna.org

Androgen Insensitivity Syndrome Support Group (AISSG). ℘ http://www.aissg.org

CAH Climb support group. ℘ www.livingwithcah.org

Surgery for ambiguous genitalia

✒ Timing of surgery is a difficult decision. Traditionally, surgery as an infant was advocated; however, emerging evidence from research and adult patients has led to surgery being deferred until adolescence.

- Aim of surgery is to improve cosmetic appearance of genital area and to provide potentially normal sexual function during adulthood.
- Feminizing genitoplasty is a very complex procedure that requires highly experienced surgeons in a specialized unit.
- As there is a risk of damaging clitoral sensation with surgery consideration must be given to deferring clitoral surgery, especially in mild or moderate clitoromegaly.
- Vaginoplasty can be achieved by a variety of techniques, including a 'pull-through' technique, skin flaps, skin grafts, or the use of bowel substitution. To avoid post-operative stenosis regular dilator use may be required. This is not recommended in children, so delaying surgery may be more appropriate.

Congenital adrenal hyperplasia

- An autosomal recessive condition of enzyme defects in the adrenal steroidogenesis pathways leading to:
  - cortisol deficiency
  - ↑ ACTH secretion with build-up of cortisol precursors
  - ↑ Androgen production.
- 90% is due to deficiency of 21-hydroxylase.
- If severe, aldosterone production is also affected leading to salt wasting.
- Incidence ~1:14 000 births (carrier rate of 1:80).
- The gene responsible is *Cyp21*, located on chromosome 6 (but up to 20% cases have no mutation detectable).

Clinical features of CAH (46XX)

CAH is the commonest cause of ambiguous genitalia at birth, responsible for up to 50% of cases (ranges from mild clitoral enlargement to a near normal male appearance). There is a wide spectrum of presentations including:
- Neonatal salt wasting crisis and hypoglycaemia.
- Childhood virilization and accelerated growth with early epiphyseal closure → restricted final height.
- Late-onset with hirsutism and oligomenorrhoea.

▶ Diagnosis is by detection of elevated plasma 17-hydroxyprogesterone levels and 24h urinary steroid analysis.

Fertility and CAH
- Menstrual irregularity occurs in:
  - ~30% of non-salt-losers
  - ~50% of salt-losers.
- Natural fertility:
  - ~60% women with non-salt-losing CAH
  - ~10% women with salt-losing CAH.
- Almost all have polycystic ovaries on ultrasound.
- Fertility treatment should be the same as for women without CAH.
- High levels of progesterone in poorly controlled CAH may be contraceptive by blocking implantation.

Management of CAH

- A multidisciplinary approach by paediatric urologists, endocrinologists, psychologists, and gynaecologists is required.
- Treatment requires replacement glucocorticoid to suppress ACTH and ↓ excess androgen production (whether dexamethasone, hydrocortisone, or prednisolone is used is a balance between risk of iatrogenic Cushing's syndrome and compliance, especially with teenagers).
- Salt-losing CAH requires fludrocortisone to replace aldosterone.
- Antiandrogens may be used to combat the effects of raised androgens with lower doses of glucocorticoids.
- In pregnancy, requirement is ↑ for both mineralocorticoid and glucocorticoid (placental aromatase converts testosterone to oestradiol protecting the fetus from virilization and destroys excess therapeutic hydrocortisone).
- Prenatal diagnosis is available if a previous child has CAH:
  - dexamethasone is started with a positive pregnancy test (it crosses the placenta and suppresses the fetal adrenal ↓ the severity of ambiguous genitalia)
  - if CVS then shows the fetus is male or negative for the gene mutation, it can be stopped.

Androgen insensitivity syndrome

- Caused by a mutation in the androgen receptor gene causing resistance to androgens in the target tissues:
  - in the embryo the testis develops normally, but the testosterone-dependent Wolffian structures do not
  - AMH is still secreted by the fetal testis, so regression of the müllerian structures also occurs.
- It has an X-linked recessive pattern in 2/3 of cases (up to 30% *de novo* mutations).
- If the mutation can be identified in a family then prenatal diagnosis can be offered with CVS.
- It can be complete (complete androgen insensitivity syndrome, CAIS) or partial (partial androgen insensitivity syndrome, PAIS).
- It is the commonest form of under-masculinization in an XY individual.
- Incidence of CAIS is thought to be about 1:20 000, that of PAIS is unclear.

Clinical features of AIS (46XY but appear female)

- CAIS individuals have:
  - female external genitalia
  - a short blind-ending vagina
  - absent uterus and fallopian tubes
  - normal breast development
  - sparse pubic and axillary hair.
- Presentation can be:
  - *Prenatally*—fetal karyotype (XY) does not match ultrasound findings
  - *after birth*—inguinal hernias or labial swellings, found to contain testes
  - *at puberty*: 1° amenorrhoea.
- PAIS includes a broad spectrum of under-masculinization ranging from ambiguous genitalia to simple hypospadias.
- The mildest form (mild androgen insensitivity syndrome (MAIS)) will not present until puberty with a high-pitched voice and gynaecomastia.

⚠ In CAIS physical appearance and core gender identity are both female.

▶ Individuals with PAIS raised as female have a higher than average dissatisfaction with gender identity (some studies show that >40% request gender reassignment).

▶ Diagnostic tests should include karyotype and pelvic ultrasound (to exclude müllerian structures and locate testes).

Management of AIS

⚠ The lifetime risk for malignancy within the testes is thought to be about 2% and therefore there is no need for immediate gonadectomy.
- If CAIS is diagnosed before puberty the testes may be left in to allow natural puberty without the need for hormone replacement therapy (HRT) in a child.
- *After puberty:*
  - gonadectomy should be offered because of the difficulty in monitoring intra-abdominal testes
  - HRT with oestrogens should be started following gonadectomy
  - some may require testosterone replacement to feel their best.
- Bone mineral density should be checked as, even with good compliance to HRT, a degree of osteopaenia is noted.
- Once sexual activity is anticipated then vaginal lengthening with the use of dilators should be offered.
- If dilators fail then consider surgical vaginoplasty.

Coping with the diagnosis of AIS

- The patient should be referred to a multidisciplinary team experienced in the management of DSD.
- Input from a psychologist should be offered with an open door policy (disclosure may need to be repeated on subsequent visits).
- The clinician should offer to explain the condition to the patient's relatives or boyfriend.
- Information should be given regarding her diagnosis and referral to patient support groups offered.

Androgen Insensitivity Syndrome Support Group (AISSG). ♫ http://www.aissg.org

Disorders of growth and puberty

Puberty is the development of 2° sexual characteristics in response to an ↑ in the pulsatile secretion of LH. In girls, breast budding with accelerated growth is usually the first sign, followed by development of pubic and axillary hair, with menarche occurring ~ 2yrs after breast budding. The average age for menarche is 12.7yrs.

Precocious puberty

This is the onset and progression of signs of puberty before the age of 8 or menarche before the age of 10yrs. Precocious puberty leads to early accelerated linear growth with premature epiphyseal closure resulting in restricted final height.

Causes of precocious puberty

- Central precocious puberty (gonadotrophin-dependent):
  - mostly idiopathic (74%)
  - congenital (e.g. cerebral palsy)
  - CNS space-occupying lesion.
- Peripheral precocious puberty (gonadotrophin-independent):
  - 1° hypothyroidism
  - hormone-secreting ovarian cysts
  - McCune–Albright syndrome
  - late-onset CAH (premature pubic hair).

Full history and examination

Should include documenting Tanner stage and enquiring about:
- Cerebral palsy.
- Previous diagnosis of intracranial space-occupying lesion.
- Exposure to sex steroids.

Investigations

Should include:
- Bone age (X-ray wrist).
- Cranial MRI.
- Pelvic USS.
- FSH/LH/oestradiol/17-hydroxyprogesterone.
- TFTs.
- Gonadotrophin-releasing hormone (GnRH) stimulation test.

Treatment

Should be for the underlying cause. If idiopathic chronic pelvic pain (CPP), injectable GnRH analogues are used as they:
- Have minimal side effects in children.
- Enable achievement of normal final height.
- Cause breast, uterine, and ovarian regression (so the child resembles its peers).
- Have no long-term effect on bone mineral density in this age group.
- Are safe to use for 4–5yrs.

Tanner stages

I   Prepubertal, basal growth rate, no breast or pubic hair development.
II Accelerated growth, breast budding, sparse straight pubic hair.
III Peak growth velocity, elevation of breast contour, coarse, curly pubic hair spreading on to mons pubis, axillary hair.
IV Growth slowing, areolae form 2° mound, adult pubic hair type, but no spread to inner thigh.
V   No further increase in height, adult breast contour, adult pubic hair type and distribution.

▶ Menarche usually occurs in stage III or IV.

Delayed puberty and primary amenorrhoea

Definition

The absence of menstruation and 2° sexual characteristics by age 14. 1° amenorrhoea also includes the absence of menstruation with normal 2° sexual characteristics by age 16 (see 📖 Menstrual disorders: amenorrhoea, p. 506).

Causes of delayed puberty

- Constitutional delay.
- Chronic systemic disease.
- Weight loss/excessive exercise.
- Hypothalamo-pituitary disorders (hypogonadotrophic hypogonadism, pituitary tumours).
- Ovarian failure (Turner syndrome, Swyer syndrome, iatrogenic).

History

Should include details of:
- Chronic illnesses.
- Anorexia.
- Excessive exercise.
- Family history of similar problems.

Examination

Should include assessment of:
- Height and weight.
- Pubertal (Tanner) stage.
- Visual fields (pituitary tumours).
- Hirsutism.
- Any stigmata of chronic disease.
- Signs of Turner syndrome.

Investigations

- LH/FSH, testosterone, TFTs, and prolactin.
- Karyotype.
- Pelvic ultrasound or MRI if müllerian anomaly suspected.
- Cranial MRI if prolactin >1500mU/L.

⚠ With *hCG* never forget pregnancy as a cause of amenorrhoea, even 1°.

▶ Puberty can be induced with low-dose oestrogen (oral or patches) and growth hormone. This is a specialist area for a paediatric endocrinologist.

Management
- Referral to an appropriate specialist is critical.
- Input may be required from endocrinologists, psychologists, and neurosurgeons.
- Treatment will depend on diagnosis.

Vaginal discharge: in childhood

Vaginal discharge is the commonest symptom in young girls and is often associated with itching or soreness. The history is usually from the carer, but the child should be engaged in the conversation and asked questions about her complaint, which should include:
- Duration, frequency, and quantity of the discharge.
- Colour and odour.
- Blood staining.
- Whether the child wipes 'front to back'.
- Use of bubble baths, soaps, washing powders.
- Previously tried creams or ointments.

Examination should be done carefully with the carer present. Frog-leg position or knee–chest position can be used and often seated in the mother's lap can be most reassuring for the child. A cotton-tipped swab may be used to collect a sample of discharge, for microbiological assessment, from the posterior vulva.

▶ If the discharge is bloodstained, particularly purulent or profuse, then examination under anaesthesia and vaginoscopy (with removal of any foreign body) are appropriate.

Differential diagnosis
- Vulvovaginitis.
- Foreign body (commonly small bits of toilet paper).
- Trauma (including sexual abuse).
- Rare tumours.
- Skin disease.

Vulvovaginitis
- Most common cause of vaginal discharge and soreness.
- Often occurs when girl starts to be responsible for going to toilet.
- Normally no specific organisms are isolated.
- Treatment based on simple measures:
  - wiping front to back
  - avoidance of perfumed soaps, bubble bath, and biological washing powder for underwear
  - loose cotton underwear (avoid tights, leggings, and pants at night)
  - a simple emollient such as nappy cream may be helpful.

⚠ Antifungal, antibiotic, or steroid creams are unhelpful and may cause further irritation.
- If these measures are unhelpful, a short course of oestrogen cream may be beneficial.
- The symptoms always improve at puberty.

Sexual abuse

⚠ Always needs to be considered, but it is an area fraught with difficulty. Seek senior advice if you have any concerns.

▶ Many chronically sexually abused girls show no signs on examination.

• Inspection of the hymen can be misleading for inexperienced doctor as irregularities, notches, and hymenal tags can all be normal findings.
• If STI is detected in a young girl it is normally an indicator of abuse, but not always.
• If abuse is suspected child should be referred to lead doctor responsible for child protection.
• Child should be examined by most experienced doctor available; if possible, refer to a local dedicated centre.

If abuse is suspected

⚠ It is your duty to disclose confidential information if there is an issue of child protection.

⚠ If swabs are to be useful medico-legally, set protocols for a chain of evidence needed to be followed. Seek senior advice urgently.

Vaginal discharge: in adolescence

Vaginal discharge in adolescents may be:
- Physiological leucorrhoea requiring explanation and reassurance only.
- A foreign body, such as a retained tampon.
- Due to any of the infections that affect adult women (see 📖 Sexually transmitted infections, p. 552).

The adolescent consultation

The adolescent consultation differs from that of an adult patient as obtaining a history may be more complicated.
- Usually the girl will be accompanied by a parent and unwilling to disclose information in front of them.
- It is important to give her an opportunity to talk to you away from her parent; this may be easily achieved by asking the parent to sit outside for the examination.
- Your manner should be frank and non-judgemental.
- She may need advice regarding contraception, as well as treatment for her presenting symptom.

▶ The girl may be very anxious about the examination and may be much more forthcoming with information once this is completed.

▶ Always explain what you are going to do, as this helps to allay anxiety.
The British Association for Sexual Health and HIV has specific guidelines for the treatment of infections and has a *pro forma* for consultations with the under 16s. See 🏵 http://www.bashh.org.

Sexually transmitted infections in adolescents

- The rates of STIs in teenagers are increasing rapidly.
- Teenagers are likely to have unprotected intercourse and are biologically more susceptible to infections than adults.

⚠ The risk of pelvic inflammatory disease in a sexually active 15yr-old may be up to 10 times that of a sexually active 25yr-old.

⚠ Always remember that a teenager having consensual sex may also be the victim of abuse.

Dermatological conditions in children and adolescents

Many dermatological conditions affect children and may well present on the vulva. Children will generally present with itching and soreness, with skin changes being noticed by a carer. Adolescents may be slow to present due to embarrassment and uncertainty of what are normal changes associated with puberty.

Labial adhesions

- The labia minora stick together due to the hypo-oestrogenic state.
- Usually asymptomatic:
  - noticed at nappy changing or bathing by the carer
  - occasionally may be associated with soreness (if an element of vulvovaginitis is present) or dysuria.
- Usually resolves spontaneously at puberty with no long-term problems.
- Treatment is not usually required. A short course of daily topical oestrogen cream can be useful if there is associated dysuria or pain. It may also be reassuring for the carer to see the adhesions disappear; however, they must understand that the adhesions are likely to reappear when treatment is stopped.
- Surgery is not indicated, unless the adhesions persist after puberty.
- USS to check for müllerian structures can be offered for reassurance if the adhesions are severe.

Lichen sclerosus

- Chronic inflammatory condition.
- Occurs in about 1:900 prepubertal girls.
- Usually presents with severe itching associated with dysuria and surface bleeding, but can be asymptomatic.
- Shiny, white crinkly plaques are classically distributed in a 'butterfly' pattern around the anogenital area. The vagina is spared.
- Diagnosis is usually by inspection alone in children.

See 📖 Vulval dermatoses: lichen sclerosus, p. 694.

⚠ Rubbing and scratching by the child leads to telangiectasia, purpura, fissures, and bleeding, with possible 2° bacterial infection. This can wrongly lead to suspicions of sexual abuse.

- Can be associated with other autoimmune diseases (careful examination is required for other signs of illness).
- Treatment is symptomatic relief with use of topical corticosteroids.
- Symptoms generally improve at puberty, although the condition will still be present.
- Long-term follow-up is required (association with squamous cell carcinoma in adulthood).

Other common dermatoses found in young people

Molluscum contagiosum
- Caused by *Molluscum contagiosum* virus, a member of the poxviruses.
- Common in nursery and primary school children.
- Lesions are typically 1–5mm, shiny pale pink, domed papules with a central depression, found on the trunk and limbs, but anogenital spread is common.
- Destruction of the papules is painful and can lead to scarring so is not recommended.
- Resolves spontaneously in 6–18mths (but may take up to 3yrs).

Irritant dermatitis
- Trigger factor is dependent on age group:
  - urine and faeces in infants.
  - bubble bath, soap, and sand in toddlers and young girls
  - shampoo and shower gels in adolescents.
- Check no secondary infection with *Candida*.
- Advise avoidance of triggers and use of a simple barrier cream.

Threadworms
- Common in schoolchildren with poor hand hygiene.
- Worms migrate from the anus and cause anogenital itching.
- Skin is excoriated and sore and can have secondary infection.
- Treat with systemic antiparasitic (such as mebendazole) and a local barrier cream.
- Emphasize the need for improved hand washing to prevent reinfection.

Eczema and psoriasis
- May present on the vulva as part of a generalized condition.
- *Vulval ulceration:* differential diagnosis:
  - aphthous ulcers
  - Behçet's disease
  - Lipschütz ulcer
  - herpes simplex (in a young child, consider the possibility of abuse).

Warts
- In sexually active teenagers human papilloma virus (HPV) 6 and 11 are most common.
- In children common cutaneous warts (HPV 2) are found.
- Most will resolve untreated within 5yrs (destructive treatments may be poorly tolerated in children, but may be useful).

⚠ Sexual abuse should be considered in children with anogenital warts, but vertical transmission can present up to 3yrs of age and transmission can occur from existing warts on the child's fingers.

Gynaecological disorders: in adolescence

Following menarche there is a continuing change in pituitary-ovarian activity. Regular ovulatory cycles usually establish within 2–3yrs. If irregular cycles or menorrhagia persist after this time, then there may be an underlying disorder.

Menstrual disorders (📖 see Chapter 15, p.501)

⚠ Do not assume that heavy, painful periods, irregular menses, or pelvic pain are a physiological part of adolescence.

Amenorrhoea
- 1° with no 2° sexual characteristics should be investigated by 14yrs.
- 1° with 2° sexual characteristics by 16yrs (See 📖 Menstrual disorders: amenorrhoea, p. 506).
- 2° = no periods for at least 6mths.
- Eating disorders are common in this age group and, if missed, anorexia nervosa can have life-threatening complications.

⚠ Don't forget pregnancy—talk to the patient privately.

Oligomenorrhoea
Normal puberty is associated with an increase in insulin resistance.
- If associated hirsutism or excessive weight gain, consider PCOS.
- Weight loss should be strongly advised if overweight.
- Long-term risks of insulin resistance and endometrial hyperplasia are harder to get across to adolescents.
- Management can be with the COCP and advice regarding weight loss.

Norethisterone can be taken (21 days with 1wk break). ⚠ It is important to explain this will not work as a contraceptive.

Menorrhagia
- Try to get them to quantify loss in terms of pad soakage.
- The COCP is very useful in this age group.
- Tranexamic acid is also effective.

Ovarian cysts

Consider all types occurring in adults but with varying frequency
(see 📖 Benign ovarian tumours: diagnosis, p. 690).
- Simple unilateral, unilocular cysts are the most commonly found cysts
  in children and adolescents (most resolve spontaneously).
- Complex/solid ovarian tumours are most likely to be germ cell in
  origin, most commonly benign cystic teratomas.

⚠ 10% of ovarian tumours in children are malignant.

▶ Epithelial tumours account for less than 20% of ovarian cysts in children
and adolescents.

▶ 3–5% of ovarian tumours in children are sex-cord tumours.

▶ Preservation of reproductive function should always be considered
in children and adolescents undergoing treatment for ovarian masses
whether benign or malignant.

Pelvic pain in adolescence

Acute pelvic pain

See 📖 Acute pelvic pain, p. 564.
- Adolescents may be more prone to torsion of the ovary or fallopian
  tube than older women and this should always be considered.
- Consider acute pelvic inflammatory disease.

⚠ Don't forget to consider pregnancy.

Chronic pelvic pain

- 1° dysmenorrhoea occurs in >80% of adolescents.
  - associated with an early menarche and menorrhagia
  - has a significant effect on schooling, sleep, exercise, and family life
  - treat with NSAIDS and the COCP
  - pain unresponsive to NSAIDS/COCP should be investigated with
    transabdominal pelvic ultrasound +/– diagnostic laparoscopy
  - consider Mirena® intrauterine system (IUS) (may need insertion
    under GA).
- Endometriosis often presents atypically in adolescents and symptoms
  may be non-cyclical.
- Rare müllerian anomalies (e.g. obstructed rudimentary horn) may
  present with cyclical pelvic pain of increasing severity and predispose
  to endometriosis: if suspected, get an MRI.

⚠ Chronic pelvic pain is commonly reported in individuals who have
suffered sexual abuse. Be aware of any signs of ongoing abuse.

⚠ Extremely rare. All should be managed in a tertiary referral centre
with links to the UK Children's Cancer Study Group (UKCCSG).

Gynaecological cancers: in childhood

The most common is an ovarian germ cell tumour with the second being a vaginal embryonal rhabdomyosarcoma (sarcoma botryiodes).

Ovarian cancer in children
- Incidence 1.7/million in children under 15yrs, 21/million in girls aged 15–19yrs.
- >80% are germ cell tumours (most are dysgerminomas).
- Others include epithelial tumours (especially in the teens) and sex-cord stromal tumours (usually <10yrs).
- Present most commonly with pain, and ovarian mass on pelvic USS.
- Hormone-producing tumours may present with vaginal bleeding and/or precocious puberty.
- Check hormonal profile and tumour markers (see 📖 Ovarian cancer: presentation and investigation, p. 722), for details of investigations and management).
- In childhood 1° treatment is surgery with chemotherapy if required (as childhood ovarian cancer is so rare the majority will be entered into trials).
- Prognosis is good for germ cell tumours: 5yr survival >85% for all stages.

Non-ovarian cancers in children
- Most common is vaginal embryonal rhabdomyosarcoma, but this is still extremely rare, with incidence of approximately 0.5/million girls.
- Most present before the age of 5yrs with vaginal bleeding, discharge, and classically a polypoid mass in the vagina.
- Examination under anaesthetic, biopsy, cystoscopy, and rectal examination are required for diagnosis.
- Multi-agent chemotherapy is the mainstay of treatment.
- 5yr survival is approximately 82% overall.
- Clear cell adenocarcinomas of the cervix and vagina are now incredibly rare, as diethylstilbestrol (DES) (a synthetic oestrogen) has not been used in pregnancy since the 1970s.

Fertility implications of childhood cancer

- Childhood cancer has a cumulative risk of ~1:650 by age 15yrs.
- Most common are leukaemias.
- Advances in the treatment means there is an overall survival rate in excess of 70%, leading to increasing numbers of young adults affected by the reproductive consequences.

Late effects of cancer therapy

Ovary

- Premature ovarian failure can be caused by radiotherapy or chemotherapy.
- A prepubertal ovary is more resistant to damage (↑ reserve of primordial follicles).
- Can present as delayed puberty, 2° amenorrhoea, or premature menopause depending on:
  - age at time of treatment
  - dose of radiotherapy
  - chemotherapeutic agents used (some have no effect on ovarian function).

Uterus

Abdominal, pelvic, or total body irradiation (TBI) can damage uterine function causing reduced uterine volume, decreased elasticity of uterine musculature, and impaired vascularization. Successful pregnancies have been reported following radiotherapy, but there is risk of miscarriage, premature delivery, and intrauterine growth restriction. Chemotherapy does not seem to affect uterine function.

Hypothalamus/pituitary

Cranial irradiation or TBI can lead to hypogonadotrophic hypogonadism. With high-dose cranial irradiation progressive compromise occurs, 60% having gonadotrophin deficiency 4yrs after treatment. Even with low-dose cranial irradiation the presence of regular periods does not equate with fertility.

▶ Early referral is essential for these women if they present with subfertility.

Further malignancy

Up to 4% of childhood cancer survivors will develop a second 1° malignancy within 25yrs of the initial cancer. This is thought to be the carcinogenic (stochastic) effect of radiotherapy and certain alkylating agents.

Fertility preservation in cancer

⚠ Urgent referral to a specialist-assisted reproduction centre for advice before commencing cancer therapy is essential.

Rapid advances are being made in this field. Current techniques offered are:

- *Oophoropexy:* laparoscopic translocation of the ovaries away from the field of radiation to minimize exposure.
- *Ovarian stimulation and cryopreservation of mature oocytes or embryos:* generally not suitable for paediatric patients.
- *Harvesting and cryopreservation of ovarian tissue prior to treatment:* achieving fertility by *in vitro* maturation of oocytes followed by assisted reproductive techniques.

Normal menstruation and its disorders

Physiology of the menstrual cycle

The menstrual cycle involves the coordinated hormonal control of the endometrium allowing pregnancy or regular shedding (periods). Peptide hormones from the hypothalamus and pituitary direct the ovary to produce steroid hormones (HPO axis), which in turn control the endometrium (see Fig. 15.1). The process is complex and aspects of its initiation, control, and cessation are not fully understood. The average ages of menarche and menopause are 12.8 (falling) + 51, respectively. Day 1 of a cycle is the first day of fresh bleeding and this should always be clarified on history of LMP.

Follicular phase

- Pulsatile release of hypothalamic GnRH → anterior pituitary to produce FSH.
- FSH promotes ovarian follicular development → recruitment of a dominant follicle containing oocyte.
- Follicular granulosa cells produce oestrogen → endometrial proliferation.
- ↑ Oestrogen levels → −ve feedback on the hypothalamo-pituitary (HP) axis (via follicular inhibin) to stop further FSH production.

Ovulation

Increasing dominant follicle oestrogen (positive feedback via follicular activin) → altered hypothalamic GnRH pulsatility → pituitary production of LH—LH surge 36h before ovulation.

Luteal phase

- The follicle collapses down to become the corpus luteum (CL) ('yellow body'), which produces oestrogen and progesterone (from theca cells).
- Progesterone and oestrogen act on an oestrogen-primed endometrium to induce secretory changes → thickening and ↑ vascularity.
- The corpus luteum has a fixed lifespan of 14 days (programmed cell death) before undergoing involution → corpus albicans ('white body').
- If implantation occurs, hCG (luteotrophic) 'rescue' of the CL allows continued production of progesterone to support the endometrium.
- In the absence of pregnancy, CL degeneration → a rapid fall in progesterone and oestrogen, initiating menstruation.

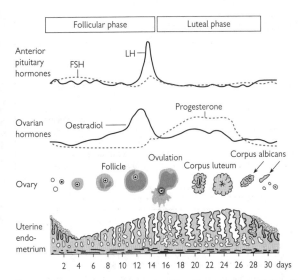

Fig. 15.1 The menstrual cycle. Reproduced from Sanders S, Dawson J, Datta S, et al. (eds) (2005). *Oxford Handbook for the Foundation Programme*. Oxford: OUP. By permission of Oxford University Press.

Menstrual phase

- Rapid ↓ in steroids → shedding of the unused endometrium.
- Inflammatory mediators (PGs, ILs, and tumour necrosis factor (TNF)) → vasospasm (approx. 24h) in spiral end arteries → hypoxia and endometrial devitalization.
- Vasodilatation and spiral artery collapse → loss of the layer and bleeding from vessels.
- Endometrium lost down to basalis layer (1/3 of loss reabsorbed).
- Complex vascular changes controlled by above secondary messengers, also → natural haemostatic mechanisms including platelet plugs, coagulation cascade, and fibrinolysis.
- All steroid hormones now at basal level, negative feedback is lifted, and GnRH–FSH production can begin a new cycle.

Normal cycle or pathological?

- Ovulatory cycles vary, but are usually 21–32 days with a basically regular pattern.
- Ovulatory cycles that vary do so due to the follicular phase (luteal phase fixed).
- Shorter or longer cycles usually result from oligo-ovulation/anovulation.
- After menarche, cycles often irregular for months or for several years until maturation of the HPO axis reliably triggers ovulation.
- Peri-menopausal periods are commonly irregular (usually ↑ cycle length) due to ovarian resistance to gonadotrophins and anovulatory cycles.
- ⚠ Do NOT blame erratic, chaotic, or constant bleeding in women >45yrs on 'the menopausal change'—it needs further investigation to exclude genital tract cancer.
- Nearly all women will experience some menstrual irregularity in timing or flow at some stage—many cases are transient.

Bleeding and pain: what is normal?

- Bleeding can be for 1–7 days with an average of 3–5 days.
- Reported amount of blood loss is highly variable.
- Periods described as 'heavy' should always be viewed as such.
- Pain is 'normal' (vasospasm and ischaemia), but is highly variable.

⚠ Pain interfering with normal functioning needs to be addressed.

⚠ Bleeding between periods (IMB), after intercourse (PCB), or totally erratic/constant bleeding is *always* abnormal.

Menstrual disorders: amenorrhoea

- 1° amenorrhoea is lack of menstruation by age 16 in the presence of 2° sexual characteristics or 14 in their absence.
- 2° amenorrhoea is an absence of menstruation for 6mths.

Diagnosis

History

Emphasis on:
- Sexual activity, risk of pregnancy, and type of contraceptive used.
- Galactorrhoea or androgenic symptoms (weight gain, acne, hirsutism).
- Menopausal symptoms (night sweats, hot flushes).
- Previous genital tract surgery (intrauterine instrumentation or LLETZ).
- Issues with eating or excessive exercise.
- Drug use (especially dopamine antagonists for psychiatric conditions).

Examination

- BMI <17/>30, hirsutism, 2° sexual characteristics (Tanner staging).
- Stigmata of endocrinopathies (including thyroid) or Turner's syndrome.
- Evidence of virilization (deep voice, male pattern balding, cliteromegaly).
- *Abdominal:* may show masses due to tumours or genital tract obstruction.
- *Pelvic:* imperforate hymen, blind ending vaginal septum, absence of cervix and uterus.

Management

Must be guided by the diagnosis and fertility wishes. Options include:
- Treat any underlying causes including attaining normal BMI.
- Cabergoline or surgery for hyperprolactinaemia.
- Cyclical withdrawal bleeds (COCP for PCOS).
- HRT for POF.
- Relief of genital tract obstruction: cervical dilation, hysteroscopic resection, incision of hymen.
- Specific treatment for endocrinopathies and tumours.

▶ Major congenital abnormalities, AIS, etc. should be managed by multi-disciplinary teams in specialist centres.

Common causes of amenorrhoea

Physiological causes

⚠ Pregnancy must always be excluded.
- Lactation.
- Menopause.

Iatrogenic causes

- *Progestagenic contraceptives:* Depo-Provera®, Mirena IUS®, Nexplanon®, POP.
- Therapeutic progestagens, continuous COCP use, GnRH analogues, rarely danazol.

Investigations for amenorrhoea

- ⚠ Pregnancy test.
- *FSH/LH:* ↑ in premature ovarian failure (POF), ↓ hypothalamic causes (not useful in PCOS).
- Testosterone and sex hormone-binding globulin (SHBG) are most useful for PCOS.
- Prolactin should always be tested.
- TFTs.
- Pelvic ultrasound:
  - can define anatomical structures, congenital abnormalities, Asherman's syndrome, haematometra, and PCOS morphology
  - can indicate physiological activity or endometrial atrophy in POF.
- Karyotype if uterus absent or suspicion of Turner's syndrome.
- Specific tests for endocrinopathies where there is clinical suspicion.

Pathological causes of amenorrhoea

- *Hypothalamic:*
  - functional—stress, anorexia, excessive exercise, pseudocyesis
  - non-functional— space-occupying lesion (SOL), surgery, radiotherapy, Kallman's syndrome (1° GnRH deficiency).
- *Anterior pituitary:*
  - micro- or macroadenoma (prolactinoma) or other SOL
  - surgery
  - Sheehan's syndrome (post-partum pituitary failure).
- *Ovarian:*
  - PCOS
  - POF
  - resistant ovary syndrome
  - ovarian dysgenesis, especially due to Turner's syndrome (45XO).
- *Genital tract outflow obstruction:*
  - imperforate hymen
  - transverse vaginal septum
  - cervical stenosis
  - Asherman's syndrome (iatrogenic intrauterine adhesions).
- *Agenesis of uterus and müllerian duct structures:* sporadic or associated with AIS.
- *Endocrinopathies:*
  - hyperprolactinaemia
  - Cushing's syndrome
  - severe hypo/hyperthyroidism
  - CAH.

Oestrogen—or androgen—secreting tumours: usually ovarian or adrenal, e.g. granulosa-thecal cell tumours and gynandroblastoma.

Menstrual disorders: oligomenorrhoea

When cycles are longer than 32 days they usually represent anovulation or intermittent ovulation. Transient oligomenorrhoea is common ('stress' or emotionally related causes are often cited) and usually self-limiting.

Causes of oligomenorrhoea

Similar to many of the causes of 2° amenorrhoea:

- PCOS is the commonest cause (see ▣ Polycystic ovarian syndrome, p. 570).
- Borderline low BMI.
- Obesity without PCOS.
- Ovarian resistance leading to anovulation, e.g. incipient POF, is rare, but important,
- Milder degrees of hyperprolactinaemia need to be excluded as well as mild thyroid disease.

Management of oligomenorrhoea

What does the patient want? Regular periods or fertility?

- Provide reassurance.
- Treat any underlying causes as for amenorrhoea.
- It is not uncommon for no cause to be found, but serious pathology must be excluded.
- Attain normal BMI (weight loss or gain as appropriate).
- Provide regular cycles:
  - COCP or cyclical progestagens
  - for PCOS a minimum of 3 periods/yr is recommended to ↓ the risk of endometrial hyperplasia due to unopposed oestrogen.
- Full fertility screening should be performed if ovulation induction is required.

Menstrual disorders: dysmenorrhoea

- 1° *dysmenorrhoea*: the pain has no obvious organic cause.
- 2° *dysmenorrhoea*: the pain is due to an underlying condition.

Pain is highly subjective and varies greatly between women. However, if a woman describes her periods as unacceptably painful, then they are!

Diagnosis

History

- *Timing and severity of pain (including degree of functional loss)*: commonly premenstrual pain ↑ in the first 1–2 days of bleeding, then eases.
- Pelvic pain and deep dyspareunia (may signify pelvic pathology).
- Previous history of PID or STIs.
- Previous abdominal or genital tract surgery (may cause adhesions).

Examination

- Abdominal exam to exclude pelvic masses.
- Pelvic exam; cervical excitation, adnexal tenderness, mobility, and masses.

Investigations

- STI screen (including *Chlamydia* swab).
- USS, endometriomata, PID sequelae, fibroids, congenital abnormalities.
- Laparoscopy is usually reserved for women with USS abnormalities, medical treatment failures, or those with concomitant subfertility.

▶ When no disease is identified then ovulation suppression by tricycling COCP or GnRH analogues for up to 6–12mths will limit the number of 'periods' and therefore pain. This is an empirical trial of hormonal therapy.

▶ Pain clinic, psychological support, and self-help groups may be of benefit to some women who wish to maintain their fertility, especially when they have other pelvic pain symptoms.

1° dysmenorrhoea

Pain in the menstrual cycle is a feature of ovulatory cycles and is due to uterine vasospasm and ischaemia, nervous sensitization due to PGs and other inflammatory mediators, and uterine contractions. A maternal or sibling history of dysmenorrhoea is very common and the problem usually starts soon after menarche. Theories accounting for 1° dysmenorrhoea include:

- Abnormal PG ratios or sensitivity.
- Neuropathic dysregulation.
- Venous pelvic congestion.
- Psychological causes.

2° dysmenorrhoea

Underlying causes include:

- Endometriosis.
- Adenomyosis.
- PID.
- Pelvic adhesions.
- Fibroids (though not always causal).
- Cervical stenosis (iatrogenic post-LLETZ or instrumentation).
- Asherman's syndrome.
- Congenital abnormalities causing genital tract obstruction, e.g. non-communicating cornua.

Management of dysmenorrhoea

- Appropriate reassurance and analgesia may be all that is required.
- *Symptom control:*
  - mefenamic acid 500mg tds with each period is effective
  - COCP to abolish ovulation
  - data on Mirena IUS® demonstrate benefit
  - paracetamol, hot-water bottles, etc., may be helpful for some
  - TENS, vitamin B1, and magnesium may be of benefit to some women.
- Treat any underlying causes:
  - Endometriosis—COCP, progestagens, GnRH analogues
  - antibiotics for PID
  - relief of obstruction (usually surgical).
- *Therapeutic laparoscopy—for above indications:* gold standard for diagnosis + management of endometriosis/adhesions/complicated PID.
- Hysterectomy is now rare for this indication alone.
- Laparoscopic uterine nerve ablation (LUNA) is not currently recommended.

Dysfunctional uterine bleeding: scope of the problem

Dysfunctional uterine bleeding (DUB) is a diagnosis of exclusion and is defined as any abnormal uterine bleeding in the absence of pregnancy, genital tract pathology, or systemic disease.

- Menorrhagia is the commonest symptom and DUB will ultimately be the cause in 50–60% of women with this symptom.
- Menorrhagia is responsible for 15–20% of gynaecological referrals to hospital and an even higher proportion of GP gynae consultations.

⚠ Objective measures of blood loss >80mL are clinically meaningless and should not be used outside research. If periods are reported as unacceptably heavy, then they are!

Aetiology

The exact causes of DUB are unknown. Proposed mechanisms at the endometrial level include:
- Abnormal PG ratios (+ other inflammatory mediators) favouring vasodilatation and platelet non-aggregation.
- Excessive fibrinolysis.
- Defects in expression/function of matrix metalloproteinases (MMPs), vascular growth factors, and endothelins.
- Aberrant steroid receptor function.
- Defects in the endomyometrial junctional zone.

The medical treatments tend to reflect the underlying pathologies (see 📖 Dysfunctional uterine bleeding (DUB): diagnosis and investigations, p. 514).

DUB at a glance

- Menorrhagia is the commonest gynaecological symptom you will see, and most of these women will have DUB.
- DUB is an umbrella term and only diagnosed after exclusion of pathology.
- Women under 45 can safely be treated without investigation in the absence of erratic bleeding.
- TVS is the first-line investigation if the woman is >45yrs with failed medical therapy to identify endometrial polyps + fibroids (i.e. focal pathology).
- In the presence of erratic bleeding in women >45yrs an endometrial biopsy is required.
- The majority of women will respond to medical therapy, especially tranexamic ± mefenamic acid.
- The Mirena IUS® is an excellent treatment that significantly reduces the number of women requiring surgery.
- Surgery should only be used in women who have completed their family and have had failed adequate medical therapy.
- *Endometrial ablation:* microwave endometrial ablation (MEA), balloon ablation, or Novasure are easy to perform and should be offered before hysterectomy.
- Hysterectomy has higher morbidity and cost, but is a guaranteed cure, and long-term satisfaction rates are high.

Dysfunctional uterine bleeding: diagnosis and investigations

Diagnosis

Symptoms

- Heavy and/or prolonged vaginal bleeding (with clots and flooding): irregular, heavy periods usually occur at the extremes of reproductive life (post-menarche and peri-menopausal).
- May be associated with dysmenorrhoea.
- Systemic symptoms of anaemia and disruption of life due to bleeding.
- A smear history and contraceptive use are vital information.

⚠ Totally erratic bleeding, IMB, or PCB should prompt a search for cervical or endometrial pathology.

Clinical signs

- Anaemia.
- Abdomino-pelvic examination is usually normal. If the uterus is significantly enlarged, fibroids are likely.

Differential diagnosis for DUB

- Submucous fibroids.
- Adenomyosis.
- Endometrial polyps, hyperplasia, or cancer.
- Very rarely, hypothyroidism or coagulation defects.

Investigations

⚠ Pregnancy should always be considered and excluded.
- FBC (Hb + MCV).
- Ferritin, TFTs, and clotting screens are *not* routine investigations—only consider if clinically indicated.
- Cervical smears are not done opportunistically if smear history normal.
- STI screen including *Chlamydia*.
- The risk of endometrial pathology in women <45yrs is very small so no further investigation required—treat and await clinical response.
- If >45yrs, with risk factors for endometrial disease, or no clinical response:
  - TVS USS—is good for identifying fibroids and polyps, and measuring endometrial thickness. The risk of endometrial pathology with a normal TVS USS is small, but it may be less accurate during menstruation
  - pipelle endometrial biopsy to exclude hyperplasia or cancer
  - hysteroscopy and biopsy (preferably outpatient) may be appropriate as above or if there is no response to initial medical treatment
  - hysteroscopy is mandatory with erratic bleeding in a woman >45yrs if USS reveals focal pathology, e.g. polyp, or is unable to assess the whole endometrium, biopsy is inadequate, or bleeding is persistent or repeated.

Dysfunctional uterine bleeding: medical management

Regular DUB

Mirena IUS®

- Releases measured doses of levonorgestrel into the endometrial cavity for 5yrs inducing an atrophic endometrium. Blood loss ↓ by up to 90% and ~30% will be amenorrhoeic at 12mths.
- Provides contraception.
- *Side effects:* insertional issues, irregular PV bleeding for first 4–6mths (usually abates); progestagenic side effects are rare due to minimal systemic absorption.

▶ This IUS has resulted in a major ↓ in number of hysterectomies.

- *Antifibrinolytics:* tranexamic acid 1g tds days 1–4 (40% ↓ in loss):
  - safe, non-hormonal, non-contraceptive.
  - side effects—leg cramps, minor GI upset. Caution in cardiac disease.
- *NSAIDS:* mefenamic acid 500mg tds days 1–5 (20–30% ↓ in loss and significant ↓ in dysmenorrhoea):
  - safe, non-hormonal/contraceptive.
  - side effects—GI upset including ulceration, renal impairment. Caution if asthmatic, CV disease, renal impairment, peptic ulcer.
- *COCP:* 20–30% ↓ loss and improvement in dysmenorrhoea:
  - provides contraception
  - for cautions and side effects see ☐ Combined oral contraceptive pill: overview, p. 622
- *Oral progestagens:* are generally of no benefit in regular menorrhagia other than—short term continuous treatment to stop bleeding.

Irregular DUB

- *Mirena IUS®:* as above.
- Tranexamic and mefenamic acid are useful to ↓ loss during periods.
- COCP will also regulate an irregular cycle (safe up to the menopause if no other cardiovascular risk factors).
- Cyclical (days 5–26) Norethisterone 5mg tds or medroxyprogesterone acetate 5–10mg tds:
  - regulates cycle, but little evidence to suggest ↓ in loss
  - side effects—bloating, headache.

Where first-line therapy has failed, further medical treatment may be used in very anaemic women, bleeding continuously, having their life disrupted, or who have cautions or contraindications to surgery.

- GnRH analogues can achieve amenorrhoea quickly by inducing a medical menopausal state: side effects—vasomotor symptoms and use limited to 6–12mths maximum due to bone loss.
- *High-dose progestagens:* medroxyprogesterone acetate 10mg tds continuously will induce amenorrhoea, but may be time-limited due to side effects as before.

▶ Danazol and ethamsylate are no longer indicated.

Choice of management for DUB

This will depend on:
- Treatment being directed to symptom relief and improved QoL.
- A woman's wishes for treatment being of prime importance.
- Her reproductive wishes and contraceptive needs.
- Whether her periods are regular or irregular.

▶ Many women may just need reassurance that there is no serious cause.

▶ Women may continue medical treatments for as long as they are beneficial.

▶ Anaemia should be corrected by treating the underlying cause of bleeding and using ferrous sulphate (or equivalent) to replace lost iron stores.

Further patient information

NICE. (2010). *Heavy menstrual bleeding: understanding NICE guidance*. NICE guideline CG44.
   ℘ www.nice.org.uk/CG044publicinfo

Dysfunctional uterine bleeding: surgical management

Surgery should be reserved for the minority of women who fail to respond to medical management.

⚠ Women have to be certain their families are complete before surgery.

Endometrial ablation

Destruction of the endometrium down to the basalis layer is effective for most women and should be offered to all for consideration.

Methods include:
- Microwave (MEA).
- Thermal balloon (Thermachoice).
- Novasure (electrical impedance).

▶ Hysteroscopic resection, or rollerball ablation, are now used much less often due to ↑ operative complications.

⚠ Endometrial ablation is less effective if the endometrial cavity is >10cm.

Typical endometrial ablation results in normal size cavities:
- 80–90% of women are significantly improved.
- 30% will become amenorrhoeic.
- 20% will need a second procedure by 5yrs.
- The newer procedures above are generally very safe and straight-forward; however, there is a small risk of bleeding, infection, uterine perforation, and failed procedure.
- They are generally carried out under GA, but may occasionally be done under cervical block.

Hysterectomy

- Hysterectomy is the only guaranteed cure for DUB, but RCTs have shown higher morbidity, longer recovery, and financial costs compared to endometrial ablation.
- Complications include haemorrhage; infection; and bladder, ureteric, or bowel injury (<1%). Death is extremely rare.
- Long-term satisfaction rates for hysterectomy are generally very high and regardless of method most women report improved sexual function—as one patient put it, 'I actually have sex now I'm not bleeding all the time'.

Current evidence regarding method of hysterectomy

- Vaginal hysterectomy is the route of choice over abdominal, where possible, as recovery, post-operative pain, and cost are reduced.
- Laparoscopic-assisted vaginal hysterectomy (LAVH) takes longer than abdominal or vaginal, and has higher rates of urinary tract injury. No evidence supports routine use of this method.
- Subtotal hysterectomy is quicker and has a lower risk of bladder injury, but the possible improved sexual satisfaction rates are as yet unproven. There is a small risk of continuing light menstruation if residual endometrial cells are left, and women will continue to require smear tests.

Premenstrual syndrome: overview

Any definition of premenstrual syndrome should include:
- Distressing psychological, physical, and/or behavioural symptoms.
- Occurrence during the luteal phase of the menstrual cycle (or cyclically after hysterectomy with ovarian conservation).
- Significant regression of symptoms with onset of or during the period.

In the general population 15% of women are asymptomatic, 50% have mild premenstrual syndrome (PMS) symptoms, 30% moderate, and 5–10% severe.

Aetiology

Probable multiple aetiologies, but cyclical ovarian activity is likely to be the central component (ovarian 'trigger', such as ovulation, may initiate a cascade of events). A central increased responsiveness to a combination of steroids, chemical messengers (E2/serotonin, progesterone/GABA), and psychological sensitivity may play a part.

Diagnosis

- Most women self-diagnose.
- A detailed history can suggest a diagnosis of PMS, but only prospective assessment with a symptom diary can establish its true nature.
- A variety of symptom charts are available from the National Association of Premenstrual Syndrome.
- Moderate/severe PMS involves disruption of work and interpersonal relationships, or interference with normal activities.
- DSM-IV diagnostic criteria (USA) for premenstrual dysphoric disorder are considered equivalent to severe PMS.

▶ It is important to exclude organic disease and significant psychiatric illness. Perimenopausal women may have increasing premenstrual symptoms as well as menopausal symptoms.

DSM-IV criteria for premenstrual dysphoric disorder

At least 5 symptoms present for most of the late luteal phase with remission within a few days of onset of menses and absence of symptoms in the week post menses. At least one symptom must be from the following first four:

- Markedly depressed mood, feelings of hopelessness, or self-deprecation.
- Marked anxiety, tension (being 'on edge').
- Marked affective lability (e.g. feeling suddenly sad or tearful).
- Persistent and marked anger/irritability/increased conflicts.
- Decreased interest in usual activities (school, friends, hobbies).
- Subjective sense of difficulty in concentrating.
- Lethargy, easy fatiguability/lack of energy.
- Marked change in appetite, overeating, or specific food cravings.
- Hypersomnia or insomnia.
- Subjective sense of being overwhelmed or out of control.
- Other physical symptoms, such as breast tenderness or swelling, headaches, joint or muscle pain, a sense of 'bloating', weight gain.

Further reading

National Association of Premenstrual Syndrome. ℘ www.pms.org.uk

Premenstrual syndrome: management

Hormonal

Progesterone and progestogens

A meta-analysis suggests no benefit of progesterone pessaries, suppositories, depot injections, or oral formulations.

Ovulation suppression agents

• *COCP:* appears useful for some women. However, some women have PMS-type progestagenic side effects or symptoms during the pill-free interval. Yasmin® contains drospirenone with a better side effect profile, and newer pills with a 2–4-day break or with no pill-free interval may be more therapeutic.

• *Danazol:* 4 RCTs report benefit for PMS, but there are significant masculinizing side effects. Treatment in luteal phase only is effective for breast tenderness.

• *Oestrogen:* transdermal oestrogen or implants at doses sufficient to suppress ovulation are not currently licensed, but they are a well established and accepted treatment of PMS. Estradiol patch 100 micrograms twice weekly with a progestogen (cyclical basis). Implants generally makes them unsuitable for those who may wish to conceive.

• *GnRH analogues ± addback HRT:* are of proven benefit for moderate to severe PMS, but with a licence for 6mths treatment only due to bone loss. Usually given with addback tibolone (fewer side effects and bone loss). 'GnRH test' useful for those considering hysterectomy and bilateral salpingo-oophrectomy (BSO) for severe symptoms.

Non-hormonal

• *SSRIs/selective noradrenalin reuptake inhibitors:* a meta-analysis confirms benefit for continuous and luteal phase only treatment. No current licence in the UK so careful documentation is required as some women are reluctant to accept antidepressants. Side effects may be problematic, but are reduced by luteal phase only dosing.

• *Antidepressants:* tricyclics and anxiolytics have benefits for selected patients as indicated in at least 9 studies.

Surgery

Two trials have confirmed a benefit of removal of the ovarian trigger with the uterus to avoid the need for combined HRT as definitive treatment for severe PMS. However, it is generally recommended that a 'GnRH test' is performed to ensure that a benefit will be realized and/or another indication for hysterectomy is present.

Self-help techniques for managing PMS

Dietary alteration
Possible benefit with less fat, sugar, salt, caffeine, and alcohol, frequent starchy meals, more fibre, fruit, and vegetables, and 4-hourly small snacks.

Dietary supplements
- *Vitamin B6:* possible benefit for PMS symptoms and depressive symptoms.
- *Vitamin E:* studies small, but promising.
- *Calcium:* two studies (1200–1600mg) revealed some improvement in symptoms.
- *Magnesium:* appears most beneficial for premenstrual anxiety.
- *Evening primrose oil:* of value for mastalgia only.

Exercise
Moderate regular aerobic exercise promoting cardiovascular work is beneficial (three controlled studies).

Stress reduction
Relaxation techniques, yoga, meditation, breathing techniques, and encouragement of healthier lifestyle may also help.

Cognitive behavioural therapy
Several studies have indicated a long-term benefit for women with PMS.

Complementary and alternative therapies used in PMS
- *Acupuncture:* several RCTs show positive data for dysmenorrhoea.
- *Homeopathy:* in a pilot study ($n = 20$), improvement in 90% compared to placebo.
- *Progesterone and wild yam:* no benefit demonstrated in many studies.
- *Phytoestrogens:* possible benefit for PMS symptoms (may be difficult to incorporate into a western diet).
- *Herbal remedies:*
  - two good trials confirm benefit of *Vitex agnus castus* (20mg od)
  - St John's wort may also be of value due to its action as an SSRI; further studies awaited.
- *Mind–body:* aromatherapy, reflexology, photic stimulation, and magnotherapy may show some benefit, but data are sparse.

Further reading
🖰 www.bms.org.uk
🖰 www.pms.org.uk

Early pregnancy problems

Termination of pregnancy: overview

Around 200 000 TOPs are performed annually in England, Wales, and Scotland. Over 98% of these are undertaken because of risk to the mental or physical health of the woman or her children (see Box 16.1). At least 1/3 of British women will have had a TOP by the time they reach 45yrs of age.

Box 16.1 UK law

Legislation varies throughout the world, with terminations remaining illegal in some countries. The Abortion Act of 1967 legalized abortion in the UK and identified 5 categories:

- *A*: continuance of the pregnancy would involve risk to life of pregnant woman greater than if pregnancy were terminated.
- *B*: termination is necessary to prevent grave permanent injury to physical or mental health of pregnant woman.
- *C*: pregnancy has not exceeded 24th week and continuance of the pregnancy would involve risk, greater than if pregnancy were terminated, of injury to physical or mental health of pregnant woman.
- *D*: pregnancy has not exceeded 24th week and continuance of pregnancy would involve risk, greater than if pregnancy were terminated, of injury to physical or mental health of any existing child(ren) of family of pregnant woman.
- *E*: there is a substantial risk that if the child were born it would suffer from such physical or mental abnormalities as to be seriously handicapped.

▶ Clauses A, B, and E have no time limit. Clauses C and D have a legal limit of 24wks.

Do doctors have an obligation to participate in TOPs?

According to the General Medical Council (GMC):

- Doctors must ensure their personal beliefs do not prejudice patient care.
- Doctors have the right to refuse to participate in TOPs on grounds of conscientious objection. If so, they must always refer the patient to another doctor who will help.

What about patients under 16?

Patients under 16yrs should be encouraged to involve their parents, but provided they are considered to be Fraser competent, they can give their own consent.

Termination of pregnancy: methods

Method of TOP depends on gestation of pregnancy and the woman's choice. Procedures offered also vary from one centre to another (usually determined by local resources).

Surgical

- *<7wks:* conventional suction termination should be avoided.
- *7–13wks:* conventional suction termination is appropriate, although, in some settings, the skill and experience of the practitioner may make medical TOP more appropriate at gestations >12wks.
- *>13wks:* dilatation and evacuation following cervical preparation; requires skilled practitioners (with necessary instruments and sufficiently large case load to maintain skills). The greater gestation, the higher the risk of bleeding, incomplete evacuation, and perforation.
- Cervical preparation is highly beneficial:
  - it reduces difficulties with cervical dilation
  - particularly if patient is <18yrs or gestation is >10wks.
- Possible regimes include:
  - misoprostol 400 micrograms PV 3h prior to surgery, or
  - gemeprost 1mg PV 3h prior to surgery, or
  - mifepristone 600mg PO 36–48h prior to surgery.

Outpatient suction devices under LA are being explored for <9wks; data from overseas suggest they are safe in experienced hands, but more information is required including cost-effectiveness and patient acceptability.

Medical

- *<9wks:* using mifepristone priming plus a prostaglandin regime is the most effective method of TOP in gestations <9wks.
- *9–13wks:* medical TOP is an appropriate, safe, and effective alternative to surgery (incomplete procedure rates increase after 9wks).
- *13–24wks:* medical TOP as above is also appropriate, safe, and effective in this group. Feticide should be considered in advanced gestations (>20wks).

Medications used in TOP

- *Mifepristone:* antiprogesterone (given 24–48h prior), which results in uterine contractions, bleeding from the placental bed, and sensitization of uterus to prostaglandins. Its use has been shown to reduce the treatment to delivery interval in medical TOP.
- *Misoprostol:* prostaglandin E1 analogue, used off-licence in medical TOP and for cervical preparation prior to surgical TOP. It stimulates uterine contractions.
- *Gemeprost:* prostaglandin E1 analogue. It is licensed for softening and dilatation of the cervix before surgical TOP in the first trimester and for therapeutic TOP in the second trimester. See Complications of TOP, p.529 for side-effects.

Termination of pregnancy: management

Considerations before termination of pregnancy

- *Counselling/support:* women should receive verbal advice and written information. Patients who may require additional support or counselling (evidence of coercion, poor social support, or psychiatric history) should be identified and additional care offered.
- *Blood tests:*
  - Hb
  - blood group and antibodies
  - if clinically indicated, HIV, HBV, HCV, haemoglobinopathies.
- *USS:* considered good practice for all TOPs as it will give accurate gestation and identify already non-viable pregnancies and occasional ectopic pregnancies.
- *Prevention of infection:* strategy for minimizing risk of post-abortion infection is important. May include screening for lower genital tract infections, such as Chlamydia (with treatment and contact tracing if +ve).

Prophylactic antibiotic regimes used for TOP

- Metronidazole 1g PR at time of TOP, plus doxycycline 100mg PO bd for 7 days, commencing on day of TOP.
- Metronidazole 1g PR at time of TOP, plus azithromycin 1g PO on day of TOP.

Following TOP

- Anti-D should be given to all Rh −ve women undergoing medical or surgical TOP (250IU ≤20wks; 500IU >20wks).
- Provide written patient information, which should include:
  - symptoms that may be experienced following TOP
  - symptoms requiring further medical attention
  - contact numbers.
- Follow-up within 2wks of TOP.
- Refer for further counselling if required.
- Discuss and prescribe/provide ongoing contraception.

Complications of TOP

- Significant bleeding (1:1000).
- Genital tract infection (5–10%).
- Uterine perforation (surgical TOP: 1–4:1000).
- Uterine rupture (mid-trimester medical TOP: <1:1000).
- Cervical trauma (surgical TOP: 1:100).
- Failed TOP (surgical: 2.3:1000; medical: 1–14:1000).
- Retained products of conception (1:100).
- Nausea, vomiting, diarrhoea due to PGs: occasional, but transient.
- Psychological sequelae: short-term anxiety and depressed mood.
- Long-term regret and concern about future fertility has been shown to be common.

Further reading

Bpas abortion care. ℘ www.bpas.org, Tel 0845 7304030

Family Planning Association. ℘ www.fpa.org.uk, Tel 0845 3101334

Marie Stopes International UK. ℘ www.mariestopes.org.uk, Tel 0845 3008090

RCOG. (2011). *The care of women requesting induced abortion.* RCOG Evidence-based clinical guideline 7. ℘ http://www.rcog.org.uk/files/rcog-corp/Abortion%20guideline_web_1.pdf

Bleeding in early pregnancy and miscarriage

Bleeding in early pregnancy may be associated with:
- Miscarriage.
- Ectopic pregnancy.
- Gestational trophoblastic disease.
- Rarely gynaecological lower tract pathology (e.g. Chlamydia, cervical cancer, or a polyp).

Miscarriage
- Miscarriage is common, occurring in at least 15–20% of pregnancies (Table 16.1).
- Possibly up to 40% of all conceptions.
- Defined as the expulsion of a pregnancy, embryo, or fetus at a stage of pregnancy when it is incapable of independent survival:
  - includes all pregnancy losses before 24wks
  - the vast majority are before 12wks.

Early pregnancy assessment units
- TVS and serum hCG estimations are invaluable in the diagnosis of early pregnancy problems.
- These should be readily available in dedicated early pregnancy assessment units (EPAUs).
- TVS provides the definitive diagnosis if a miscarriage is not clinically apparent.
- These units allow for timely assessment, with easy access from the community, improved continuity of care, and fewer admissions.
- Work on the psychological impact of early pregnancy problems demonstrates a major improvement in care with good EPAU care.

Anti-D prophylaxis
Anti-D should be given to all non-sensitized Rh −ve patients in the following circumstances:
- <12wks (250IU IM):
  - uterine evacuation (medical and surgical)
  - ectopic pregnancies.
- >12wks: all women with bleeding (250IU IM before 20wks and 500IU IM after 20wks).

See 📖 Rhesus isoimmunization (immune hydrops), p. 135.

Table 16.1 Classification, diagnosis, and management of miscarriage

	Clinical	USS findings	Management
Threatened miscarriage	Bleeding ± abdominal pain Closed cervix	Intrauterine gestation sac. Fetal pole. Fetal heart activity	Anti-D if >12wks or heavy bleeding or pain
Complete miscarriage	Bleeding and pain cease Closed cervix	Empty uterus Endometrial thickness <15 mm	Anti-D if >12wks Serum hCG to exclude ectopic if any doubt Review if bleeding persists >2wks and consider endometritis or retained products of conception
Incomplete miscarriage	Bleeding ± pain Possible open cervix	Heterogenous tissues ± gestation sac. Any endometrial thickness	Expectant generally preferable/medical/ surgical Anti-D if >12wks or heavy bleeding or pain or medical/surgical management
Missed miscarriage/ early fetal demise	± Bleeding ± pain ± loss of pregnancy symptoms Closed cervix	Fetal pole >7*mm with no fetal heart activity Mean gestation sac diameter >25*mm with no fetal pole or yolk sac	Expectant/medical/ surgical Anti-D if >12wks or medical/surgical management
Inevitable miscarriage	Bleeding ± pain Open cervix	Intrauterine gestation sac ± fetal pole ± fetal heart activity	Expectant/medical/ surgical Anti-D if >12wks or heavy bleeding or pain or medical/surgical management
Pregnancy of uncertain viability	± Bleeding ± pain Closed cervix	Intrauterine gestation sac <25*mm with no fetal pole or yolk sac. Fetal echo with CRL <7*mm with no fetal heart activity	Rescan in 1wk Anti-D if heavy bleeding or pain
Pregnancy of unknown location (PUL)	± Bleeding ± pain Closed cervix	Positive pregnancy test Empty uterus. No sign of extrauterine pregnancy	Serial serum hCG assay (48h apart) + initial serum progesterone level to exclude ectopic pregnancy/failing PUL Anti-D if heavy bleeding

* Until further research establishes definitive, safe parameters these should be used and all patients should have a second scan prior to an evacuation procedure.

Miscarriage: management

Expectant management
- Appropriate in those women who are not bleeding heavily.
- It is highly effective for women with an incomplete miscarriage.
- In women with an intact sac, resolution may take several weeks and may be less effective.
- A repeat TVS should be offered at 2wks to ensure complete miscarriage—can be repeated after another 2wks if a woman wishes to continue with conservative management.
- Patients should be offered surgical evacuation at a later date if expectant management is unsuccessful.

Medical management
- Prostaglandin analogues (usually misoprostol) are used, administered orally or vaginally, usually with antiprogesterone priming (mifepristone) 24–48h prior.
- Bleeding may continue for up to 3wks after medical uterine evacuation, but completion rates up to 80–90% can be expected under 9wks gestation.
- ⚠ Women should be warned that passage of pregnancy tissue may be associated with pain and heavy bleeding (though unusual for the majority) and 24h telephone advice and facilities for emergency admission should be available.

Surgical management of miscarriage (SMM)
- An ERPC should be performed in patients who have excessive or persistent bleeding or request surgical management.
- Suction curettage should be used.

Complications of SMM
- Infection.
- Haemorrhage.
- Uterine perforation (and rarely intraperitoneal injury).
- Retained products of conception.
- Intrauterine adhesions.
- Cervical tears.
- Intra-abdominal trauma.

⚠ Uterine and cervical trauma may be minimized by administering prostaglandin (misoprostol or gemeprost) before the procedure.

RCOG (2006). *The management of early pregnancy loss.* RCOG Guideline 25. ⏵ http://www.rcog.org.uk/womens-health/clinical-guidance/management-early-pregnancy-loss-green-top-25

Psychological sequelae
- Miscarriage is usually very distressing.
- Offer appropriate support and counselling, and written information.

Postmiscarriage counselling: patient's FAQs

What did I do to cause it?

Nothing. It was not stress at work, carrying heavy shopping, having sex, or any other reason women commonly worry about. Sadly, miscarriages happen in up to about 40% of pregnancies.

If I had had a scan earlier could you have stopped it happening?

No, we might have found out it was happening sooner, but we could not have stopped it. There is no effective treatment available to stop a 1st-trimester miscarriage.

How bad will the pain be if I opt for expectant management?

It will be like severe period pain, which comes to a peak when tissue is being passed, then settles down shortly afterwards. Ibuprofen, paracetamol, or codeine should help and may be taken. If pain is very bad contact hospital for advice.

What is heavy bleeding?

Soaking more than 3 heavy sanitary pads in under 1h or passing a clot larger than the palm of your hand. If you bleed heavily you should seek medical attention urgently.

How long will I bleed for?

It should gradually get less and less but may be up to 3wks after the miscarriage before the bleeding stops completely.

Do I need bed rest afterwards?

No, not necessarily, but obviously it can be physically and emotionally draining so a few days off work may help. You can return to normal activities as soon as you feel ready.

How long will the pregnancy test remain positive?

hCG is excreted by the kidneys and it can take up to 3wks after a miscarriage for it all to be removed from the bloodstream and a pregnancy test to record as –ve.

How long before we can try again?

There is no good evidence that the outcome of a subsequent pregnancy is affected by how soon you conceive after a miscarriage. As long as you have had either a period or a –ve pregnancy test since you miscarried, you can try again as soon as you feel physically and emotionally ready.

Does this make me more likely to have another miscarriage?

There are a very small number of women who will have recurrent miscarriages, but for the vast majority, next time they get pregnant they will face the same odds; 40% risk of miscarriage and 60% chance of a baby.

Association of Early Pregnancy Units. ℘ www.earlypregnancy.org.uk

Miscarriage Association. ℘ www.miscarriageassociation.org.uk

Ectopic pregnancy: diagnosis

⚠ ALL women of reproductive age are pregnant until proved otherwise and it is ectopic until clearly demonstrated to be intrauterine.
- **Definition:** implantation of a conceptus outside the uterine cavity.
- **Incidence:** 1–2:100 pregnancies and increasing.
  - 98% are tubal; the remainder are abdominal, ovarian, cervical, or rarely in CS scars
  - due to early presentation, with the advent of EPAUs.
- **Symptoms** (see Box 16.2):
  - often asymptomatic, e.g. unsure dates
  - amenorrhoea (usually 6–8wks)
  - pain (lower abdominal, often mild and vague, classically unilateral)
  - vaginal bleeding (usually small amount, often brown)
  - diarrhoea and vomiting should never be ignored
  - dizziness and light-headedness
  - shoulder tip pain (diaphragmatic irritation—haemoperitoneum)
  - collapse (if ruptured).
- **Signs:**
  - often have no specific signs
  - uterus usually normal size
  - cervical excitation and adnexal tenderness occasionally
  - adnexal mass very rarely
  - peritonism (due to intra-abdominal blood if ectopic ruptured).

⚠ There is no evidence that examining patients may lead to rupturing the ectopic. More important to examine them so you do not miss significant abdominal or pelvic tenderness.

⚠⚠ Includes: threatened or complete miscarriage, bleeding corpus luteal cyst, ovarian cyst accident, and pelvic inflammation.

Investigations

- *TVS/USS:* to establish the location of the pregnancy, the presence of adnexal masses or free fluid: a good EPAU will positively identify EP on TVS in 90% of cases, rather than the absence of an intrauterine gestation.
- *Serum progesterone:* helpful to distinguish whether a pregnancy is failing: <20nmol/L is highly suggestive of this, whether ectopic pregnancy (EP) or intrauterine pregnancy (IUP).
- *Serum hCG:* repeated 48h later:
  - the rate of rise is important
  - a rise of ≥66% suggests an IUP
  - a suboptimal rise is suspicious, but *not* diagnostic of an EP.
- *Laparoscopy:* gold standard, but should only be necessary for clinical reasons or in a minority where a diagnosis cannot be made (remember TVS/USS should pick up 90%!)

⚠ At serum hCG ≥1500IU, an IUP should be seen with TVS/USS. However, there is considerable variation in normal IUPs and this is a guide only—care is needed to avoid harming an early IUP. The rate of change is more important than any one value (see Box 16.3).

Box 16.2 ⚠ Symptoms of ectopic pregnancy

- Tend to have a poor positive predictive value to help discriminate between intra- and extrauterine pregnancy.
- The majority of women with an ectopic pregnancy will be clinically well and stable with minimal symptoms and signs.

All women with a positive pregnancy test should therefore be considered to have an ectopic pregnancy until proved otherwise.

Box 16.3 Risk factors for ectopic pregnancy

May be present in 25–50% of patients (therefore majority will have *no* obvious risk factors):

- History of infertility or assisted conception.
- History of PID.
- Endometriosis.
- Pelvic or tubal surgery.
- Previous ectopic (recurrence risk 10–20%).
- IUCD *in situ*.
- Assisted conception, especially IVF.
- Smoking.

Ectopic pregnancy: management

Expectant and medical management are safe options even with a diagnosed EP if there are strict selection criteria:

- Clinically stable.
- Asymptomatic or minimal symptoms.
- hCG, initially <3000IU (can be tried >3000IU but less successful).
- EP <3cm and no fetal cardiac activity on TV USS.
- No haemoperitoneum on TV USS.
- Fully understand symptoms and implications of EP.
- Language should not be a barrier to understanding or communicating the problem to a third party (such as phoning an ambulance).
- Live in close proximity to the hospital and have support at home.
- You deem the patient will not default on follow-up.

Expectant

- With a falling hCG level and fulfilling the above criteria.
- Requires serum hCG initially every 48h until repeated fall in level; then weekly until <15IU.
- With a plateauing hCG, as long as they remain clinically well it is perfectly acceptable to wait as the hCG will usually decline if given time as the pregnancy fails—hCG measurement is as above.
- With slow rising hCG in asymptomatic patient, a decision for expectant management should only be made by a senior early pregnancy unit (EPU) clinician.

Medical

- Methotrexate is given intramuscularly as a single dose of 50mg/m^2.
- hCG levels should be measured at 4 and 7 days, and another dose of methotrexate given (up to 25% of cases) if the ↓ in hCG is <15% on days 4–7.

▶ Women should be given clear, written information about adverse effects and the possible need for further treatment.

▶ They should use reliable contraception for 3mths after, as methotrexate is teratogenic.

Surgical

Laparoscopy is preferable to laparotomy as it has shorter operating times and hospital stays, ↓ analgesia requirements, and ↓ blood loss.

⚠ In haemodynamically unstable patients, laparotomy is more appropriate, as it is quicker.

Salpingectomy is preferable to salpingotomy when the contralateral tube and ovary appear normal. There is no difference in subsequent intrauterine pregnancy rates, but salpingectomy is associated with lower rates of persistent trophoblast and recurrent ectopic pregnancy.

⚠ In the presence of visible contralateral tubal disease, laparoscopic salpingotomy is appropriate if safe or possible.

❶ Remember Anti-D in Rh −ve patients.

⚠ **Treatment of the haemodynamically unstable patient**

Resuscitation
- Two large-bore IV lines and IV fluids (colloids or crystalloids).
- Cross-match 6U blood.
- Call senior help and anaesthetic assistance urgently.

Surgery
- Laparotomy with salpingectomy once the patient has been resuscitated.

RCOG (2004). *Tubal pregnancy management*. RCOG Guideline 21. ℘ http://www.rcog.org.uk/files/rcog-corp/GTG21_230611.pdf

Side effects of methotrexate
- Conjunctivitis.
- Stomatitis.
- Gastrointestinal upset.

⚠ Some women will experience abdominal pain, which can be difficult to differentiate from the pain of a rupturing ectopic.

Expectant management of ectopic pregnancy

⚠ All women managed expectantly or medically should be counselled about importance of compliance with follow-up and should be within easy access of the hospital.

⚠ There is no level of hCG at which rupture cannot occur even when it is falling—symptoms and the clinical parameters are always more important than blood tests and scans!

Less common sites for ectopic pregnancy
- Cervical, ovarian, CS scar, and interstitial pregnancies need expert input as there are no universally agreed ways to treat them.
- Generally, preference is for medical treatment, with surgical reserved for clinical need. Case series report high rates of success with medical management as long as the patient is asymptomatic and stable.
- Consider referral to a regional EPAU as these units have the best experience of these rare entities.

Pregnancy of unknown location

Definition Where there is no sign of an intrauterine pregnancy, ectopic pregnancy, or retained products of conception in the presence of a positive pregnancy test or serum hCG >5IU/L.

- This is the first diagnosis in ~10% of EPAU attenders.
- The possible outcomes can be:
  - early IUP
  - failing PUL
  - ectopic pregnancy (10% of PULs)
  - persisting PUL
  - complete miscarriage
  - very, very rarely another source (hCG secreting tumours).

⚠ Even if the history is highly suggestive of a complete miscarriage having occurred, classify as a PUL until you have evidence of an IUP.

⚠ 5–10% of 'complete miscarriages' diagnosed on history alone with an empty uterus, on scan, will in fact be ectopic pregnancies!

Presentation
- Asymptomatic.
- PV bleeding.
- Abdominal pain.

Management
- The symptoms and clinical parameters of the patient are the most important factors as for ectopic pregnancy.
- Women with significant pain, tenderness, or a haemoperitoneum usually need laparoscopy.
- If patient is well and stable then give serum progesterone and hCG at the first visit, and repeat hCG after 48h.

Interpreting hCG and progesterone results in PUL

If progesterone <20nmol/L
- Likely failing pregnancy.
- Repeat hCG in further 7 days.

If hCG ≥66% rise from 0–48h
- Likely IUP.
- Rescan in 10–14 days.

If rise in serial hCG <66% or plateauing
- Possible ectopic.
- Close monitoring with serial hCG and TVS until diagnosis made or hCG <15IU/L.

If hCG plateauing or fluctuating
- Persistent PUL after 3 consecutive samples with no diagnosis.
- Conservative management if asymptomatic or methotrexate.

If initial hCG >1500IU/L
- Probable ectopic pregnancy.
- Consider all management options depending upon clinical need.

⚠ All the same principles and criteria of expectant and medical management of ectopic pregnancies apply equally to PULs.

Understanding βhCG

βhCG is a bi-peptide secreted by the trophoblast. It is almost identical to LH, varying by one amino acid in its β subunit, hence its ability to sustain the corpus luteum. It is detectable very early and modern urinary pregnancy tests detect as little as 25IU.

What is the pattern of hCG in pregnancy?

In normal IUPs hCG rises quickly and is of main clinical use between 4 and 8wks when it rises in a predictable manner.

- hCG should rise by >/= 66% every 48h during this period.
- >8 wks it will be raised but is highly variable and fluctuates.

⚠ There is no absolutely reliable 'discriminatory zone' above which you definitely see an IUP on TVS; quoted levels of 1500IU are a guide only.

⚠ Remember also:
- 90+% of ectopics should be visible on TVS at some point.
- On a single hCG you do not know if the level is ↑ or ↓.
- In an asymptomatic patient there is no rush to act.
- ? Multiple pregnancy (↑ hCG but no IUP seen).

hCGs at different gestations

- hCG levels for any given gestation vary too much to be clinically useful: it is the relative change that matters.
- When hCG levels are very high it is suggestive of molar pregnancy.

▶ Molar pregnancies are diagnosed with TVS and confirmed by histology, *not* with hCG levels, but hCG is a vital marker for subsequent monitoring and follow-up especially after chemotherapy in gestational trophoblastic disease.

Interpreting changes in hCG

For PULs
- *hCG >/– 66% rise over 48h:* probable early IUP.
- *<66% hCG rise:* possible ectopic pregnancy or failing PUL.
- *hCG falling:* indicative of a failing pregnancy regardless of location.
- *hCG static:* there is still active trophoblast somewhere (production = excretion): consider most probable source given clinical picture.
- ▶ Caution: check whether it was actually 48h between tests.
- ▶ Remember you are treating the patient *not* the hCG. Always use hCG as a part of the whole clinical picture.

▶ Remember, clinical symptoms are *always* more important than any hCG levels or scan findings (See 📖 Ectopic pregnancy: management, p. 536).

Serum hCG levels

Valid use

- For aiding diagnosis (ectopic, early intrauterine, failing pregnancy).
- Monitoring of PUL.
- Conservative and medical management of ectopic pregnancy and persistent PULs.
- Follow-up of ectopic pregnancy postsalpingotomy/significant haemoperitoneum to exclude persistent trophoblast.
- Follow-up of women with trophoblastic disease.

▶ Remember, hCG assays are a guide to diagnosis only when a pregnancy cannot be seen on TV USS.

Inappropriate use

- Known IUPs
- Management in women with significant symptoms—treat them clinically!
- Women who have received hCG support in assisted conception.
- Known multiple pregnancy.

▶ '3 strikes and you're out'! If you do not have a diagnosis and/or management plan after 3 hCGs you need to ask for advice. *Do not* bring them back in 48h for another hCG—*get help instead!*

Recurrent miscarriage: overview

> **Definition** Three or more consecutive, spontaneous miscarriages occurring in the first trimester with the same biological father, which may or may not follow a successful birth.

Incidence is 1–2% and half of these are unexplained.

Risk factors
Advanced maternal age and increasing number of miscarriages are two independent risk factors.

Causes

Antiphospholipid syndrome (APS)

Most important treatable cause and present in 15% of women with recurrent miscarriages. APS is defined as the presence of anticardiolipin antibodies or lupus anticoagulant antibodies on two separate occasions with any criteria listed below:
- 3 or more consecutive fetal losses before the 10th week.
- 1 fetal loss 10wks gestation or older.
- 1 or more births of a morphologically normal fetus at ≤34wks associated with severe pre-eclampsia or placental insufficiency.

Genetic

In 3–5% of couples, one partner carries a balanced reciprocal or Robertsonian translocation. The carrier is phenotypically normal, but 50–75% of their gametes will be unbalanced.

Fetal chromosomal abnormalities

Can be incompatible with life. As number of pregnancies ↑, prevalence of chromosomal abnormality ↓ and chance of recurring maternal cause ↑.

Anatomical abnormalities

Frequency of congenital uterine abnormalities (uterine septae and bicornuate uterus) in the general population is unknown. Minor variations (e.g. arcuate) are 2–3%. In women with recurrent loss prevalence is estimated to be between 2 and 8%.

Fibroids

Present in up to 30% of women, but their effect on reproductive outcome is controversial. Submucosal and intramural are thought to be more causative, though little data support this assertion.

Thrombophilic disorders

Pregnancy is a hypercoaguable state. Gene mutations in factor V Leiden and factor II prothrombin G20210A have been associated with recurrent miscarriage. Protein C and protein S deficiency similarly have a weak association.

Infection

Inconsistent link to bacterial vaginosis with 1st trimester losses. Recurrent 2nd trimester loss has a stronger association.

Endocrine disorders

Well-controlled diabetes and thyroid disease is not a risk factor nor is hypersecretion of LH in PCOS.

Cervical weakness

History of late miscarriage preceded by painless cervical dilatation is a cause of recurrent mid-trimester loss but does not appear to have an association with 1st trimester miscarriage.

Immune dysfunction

Excessive uterine natural killer (NK) cell activity is currently purely hypothetical and no link between peripheral and uterine NK activity has been proven.

Recurrent miscarriage: management

Investigations
- Parental blood for karyotyping.
- Cytogenetic analysis of products of conception (at time of miscarriage).
- Pelvic USS.
- Thrombophilia screening.
- Lupus anticoagulant: (Dilute Russell Viper Venom Test (dRVVT)/ APTT).
- Anticardiolipin antibodies (aCL IgG and IgM).
- Screening for bacterial vaginosis during early pregnancy in women with 2nd trimester miscarriage is inappropriate.
- Cervical weakness is diagnosed on history alone and may be over-diagnosed as there is no objective testing in the non-pregnant state.

▶ There is insufficient evidence for asymptomatic women to be routinely tested for thyroid disease, thyroid antibodies, diabetes, and hyperprolactinaemia.

▶ TORCH (toxoplasmosis, rubella, cytomegalovirus, herpes simplex, and HIV) screening is unhelpful.

▶ NK cell assays should not be taken outside of a research setting.

Management
At least 35% of couples with recurrent miscarriage will have lost pregnancies by chance and fall into the unexplained group. They have 75% chance of a successful pregnancy next time with no therapeutic intervention if offered supportive care alone in the setting of a dedicated EPAU.
- Empirical treatment in the unexplained miscarriage group is unnecessary and should be avoided.
- Patient with recurrent miscarriage should be seen in a dedicated clinic and be offered supportive care in early pregnancy.
- Surgical intervention for intrauterine abnormalities (uterine septum) or uterine fibroids may be beneficial in highly selective cases—a full discussion of the potential risks and benefits is vital.
- In women with APS, future live birth rate is significantly improved from 40% with low dose aspirin (75mg) alone to 70% with combination therapy of aspirin and heparin. These should be commenced as soon as the viability of fetus is confirmed in first trimester up to late 3rd trimester.
- Cervical cerclage may be offered to an extremely select group after meticulous consideration of the diagnosis.
- Genetic referral for parental karyotype abnormalities or fetal chromosomal abnormality.
- Proven bacterial vaginosis in mid-trimester loss in previous pregnancy may indicate regular vaginal swabs along with rotating prophylactic antibiotics like clindamycin and amoxicillin up to 3rd trimester.

Other strategies that have been tried for recurrent miscarriage

Lifestyle factors that have not been proven to effect the outcome of a pregnancy include:
• Bed rest.
• Smoking cessation.
• Reducing alcohol intake.
• Losing weight.

Steroids do not improve the live birth rate of women with recurrent miscarriage associated with APS or proposed immune dysfunction and may ↑ significant maternal and fetal morbidity. They should not be used without another indication.

Other treatments that have been suggested for recurrent miscarriage, but which are not backed by clinical evidence, include;
• Oestrogen or progesterone supplementation.
• Paternal white cell immunization.
• Intravenous immunoglobulin.
• Trophoblastic membrane infusion.
• hCG.
• Vitamin supplementation.

Hyperemesis gravidarum

Vomiting in pregnancy is common (>50% of women). Hyperemesis gravidarum is excessive vomiting and is rare, with an incidence of 1/1000. Women with multiple or molar pregnancies may be at ↑ risk, due to ↑ hCG; however, the majority will have a normal singleton pregnancy.

Diagnosis

Symptoms and signs

1st trimester: persistent and intractable vomiting (inability to keep food or fluid down), weight loss, muscle wasting, dehydration, ptyalism (inability to swallow saliva), hypovolaemia, electrolyte imbalance, behaviour disorders, haematemesis (Mallory–Weiss tears).

Complications

Maternal risks

Liver and renal failure in severe cases.

⚠ Hyponatraemia and rapid reversal of hyponatraemia leading to central pontine myelinosis.

⚠ Thiamine deficiency may lead to Wernicke's encephalopathy.

Fetal risks

Growth restriction (IUGR) is theoretically possible.

⚠ Fetal death may ensue in cases with Wernicke's encephalopathy.

Treatment

- Admit if not tolerating oral fluid.
- *IV fluids (NaCl or Hartmann's:* avoid glucose-containing fluids as they can precipitate Wernicke's encephalopathy).
- *Daily U&E:* replace K^+ if necessary.
- Keep nil by mouth (NBM) for 24h, then introduce light diet as tolerated.
- *Antiemetics:* if no response to IV fluid and electrolyte replacement consider promethazine or cyclizine 50mg/8h PO/IM/IV as first line.
- *Prochlorperazine:* 12.5mg IM/IV tds or 5mg PO tds and/or metoclopramide 10mg/8h PO/IM/IV are usually used as second line.
- *Thiamine:* thiamine hydrochloride 25–50mg PO tds or thiamine 100mg IV infusion weekly).
- *Ondansetron or granisetron:* may be used third line. They are not licensed for pregnancy, but data are generally reassuring.
- If vomiting remains unresponsive consider a trial of corticosteroids (prednisolone 40–50mg PO daily in divided doses or hydrocortisone 100mg/12h IV). Data on steroids for this are slight and probably biased by the fact that they are used when things are usually settling spontaneously.
- In the event of intractable hyperemesis gravidarum, TOP may be the only last option or, indeed, requested by woman and/or partner.

Investigations for suspected hyperemesis gravidarum
- Urinalysis to detect ketones in urine.
- MSU to exclude UTI.
- FBC (↑ haematocrit (hct)).
- U&E (↓ K^+, ↓ Na^+, metabolic hyp. chloraemic alkalosis).
- LFT (↑ transaminases, ↓ albumin).
- USS for reassurance and to exclude multiple and molar pregnancies.

▶ There is no role for TFTs as they are often transiently abnormal.

Genital tract infections and pelvic pain

Vaginal discharge

Normal (physiological) discharge occurs in women of reproductive age and varies with the menstrual cycle and hormonal changes.

Causes of increased vaginal discharge

Physiological
- Oestrogen related—puberty, pregnancy, COCP.
- Cycle related—maximal mid-cycle and premenstrual.
- Sexual excitement and intercourse.

Pathological
Infection
- Non-sexually transmitted (BV, candida).
- Sexually transmitted (TV, chlamydia, gonorrhoea).

Non-infective
- Foreign body (retained tampon, condom, or post-partum swab).
- Malignancy (any part of the genital tract).
- Atrophic vaginitis (often blood-stained).
- Cervical ectropion or endocervical polyp.
- Fistulae (urinary or faecal).
- Allergic reactions.

History
- Characteristics of discharge (onset, duration, odour, colour) (Table 17.1).
- Associated symptoms (itching, burning, dysuria, superficial dyspareunia).
- Relationship of discharge to menstrual cycle.
- Precipitating factors (pregnancy, contraceptive pill, sexual excitement).
- Sexual history (risk factors for sexually transmitted infections).
- Medical history (diabetes, immune-compromised).
- Non-infectious causes (foreign body, ectopy, malignancy, dermatological conditions).
- Hygiene practices (douches, bath products, talcum powder).
- Allergies.

Examination
- External genital inspection for vulvitis, obvious discharge, ulcers, or other lesions.
- Speculum: appearance of vagina, cervix, foreign bodies, amount, colour and consistency of discharge.
- Bimanual examination (masses, adnexal tenderness, cervical motion tenderness).

Investigations
- Endocervical or vulvovaginal swabs for gonorrhoea and chlamydia.
- High vaginal swab (Amies transport medium).
- Vaginal pH measurement.
- Saline wet mount and Gram staining (readily available in a genitourinary medicine (GUM) clinic, but not usually in gynaecology outpatients.)
- Colposcopy (if abnormal cervical appearance).

Table 17.1 Typical characteristics of common causes for vaginal discharge

	Colour	Consistency	Odour	Vulval itching	Treatment
Physiological	Clear/white	Mucoid	None	None	Reassure
Candida infection	White	Curd-like	None	Itching	Antifungal
Trichomonal infection	Green/grey	Frothy	Offensive	Itching	Metronidazole
Gonococcal infection	Greenish	Watery	None	None	Antibiotics
Bacterial vaginosis (BV)	White/grey	Watery	Offensive	None	Metronidazole
Malignancy	Bloody	Watery	Offensive	None	According to disease
Foreign body	Grey or bloody	Purulent	Offensive	None	Remove object
Atrophic vaginitis	Clear/blood-stained	Watery	None	None	Topical oestrogen
Cervical ectropion	Clear	Watery	None	None	Cryotherapy

Clinical Effectiveness Unit (2012). *Management of vaginal discharge in non-genitourinary medicine settings.* © http://www.bashh.org/documents/4264

Sexually transmitted infections

- Impact disproportionately on adolescents and young adults.
- Partner notification and treatment vital.
- Best treated at specialist GUM clinic to provide counselling and support, as well as assistance with contact tracing.
- Confidentiality paramount:
  - GUM notes are kept separately from hospital notes
  - the patient's GP is not routinely informed of the patient's attendance.

▶ This is a requirement defined by statute in the Venereal Diseases Act of 1917.

▶ Assessment of competency should be undertaken if under 16yrs old (Fraser competence).

Risk factors for STIs
- Multiple partners (two or more in the last year).
- Concurrent partners.
- Recent partner change (in past 3mths).
- Non-use of barrier protection.
- STI in partner.
- Other STI.
- Younger age (particularly aged ≤25yrs).
- Involvement in the commercial sex industry.

History
- *Symptoms*: lumps, bumps, ulcers, rash, itching, IMB or PCB, low abdominal pain, dyspareunia, sudden/distinct change in discharge.
- Past history of STIs/GUM clinic attendance/last HIV –ve test.
- All sexual partners in past 12mths.
- Risk factors for blood-borne viruses:
  - patient or partner from area of high HIV prevalence
  - IV drug use
  - bisexual male partners.

Testing for sexually transmitted infections—incubation period
- Tests should be done at the time of presentation.
- Incubation period before tests for STIs become positive can give false negative after a single episode of sex.
  - for bacterial STIs this is 10–14 days
  - for HIV and syphilis it may be up to 3mths.

Chlamydia

Epidemiology
- *Chlamydia trachomatis:* obligate intracellular parasite.
- Commonest bacterial STI in the UK.
- Over 215 000 new cases (127 000 female) diagnosed in the UK in 2010—HPA.
- An important cause of tubal infertility.

Symptoms Dysuria, vaginal discharge, or irregular bleeding (IMB or PCB), but 70% of cases are asymptomatic.

Complications of Chlamydia infection
- Pelvic inflammatory disease (10–40% of infections result in PID).
- Perihepatitis (Fitz–Hugh–Curtis syndrome).
- Reiter's syndrome (more common in men):
  - arthritis
  - urethritis
  - conjunctivitis.
- Tubal infertility.
- Risk of ectopic pregnancy.

Diagnosis Vulvovaginal (which can be self-taken) or endocervical swab for nucleic acid amplification test (NAAT). Requires specific medium.

Treatment
- Azithromycin 1g single dose or doxycycline 100mg bd for 7 days— both have similar efficacy of >95%.
- Contact tracing and treatment of partners.

Screening for Chlamydia
During 2010/11 the National Chlamydia Screening Programme (NCSP) carried out 1.4 million chlamydia tests in England, ensuring 25% coverage of 15–24yr-olds. The Department of Health (DH) estimated that the NCSP may have produced a 20% drop in chlamydia prevalence in under 25s.
ॐ http://www.chlamydiascreening.nhs.uk/ps/index.html

Implications in pregnancy
Association with preterm rupture of membranes and premature delivery. The risks to the baby are of:
- Neonatal conjunctivitis (30% within the first 2wks).
- Neonatal pneumonia (15% within the first 4mths).

▶ Treat pregnant woman with erythromycin 500mg bd for 10–14 days (73–95% effective).

Herpes simplex

Epidemiology

- DNA virus—herpes simplex type 1 (orolabial/genital) and type 2 (genital only).
- Third most common STI in England in 2010.
- Nearly 30 000 primary attacks were diagnosed in England 2010.

Symptoms

Primary HSV infection is usually the most severe and often results in:
- Prodrome (tingling/itching of skin in affected area).
- Flu-like illness +/− inguinal lymphadenopathy.
- Vulvitis and pain (may cause urinary retention).
- Small, characteristic vesicles on the vulva, but can be atypical with fissures, erosions, erythema of skin.

Recurrent attacks are thought to result from reactivation of latent virus in the sacral ganglia, and are normally shorter and less severe. They can be triggered by many factors including:
- Stress.
- Sexual intercourse.
- Menstruation.

> **Complications of HSV infection (usually of primary infection)**
> - Meningitis.
> - Sacral radiculopathy—causing urinary retention and constipation.
> - Transverse myelitis.
> - Disseminated infection.

Diagnosis

- Usually from appearance of the typical rash.
- PCR testing of vesicular fluid (most sensitive—gold standard).
- Culture of vesicular fluid.
- Serum antibody tests are of no use for diagnosing primary herpes.

Treatment

- No cure for genital herpes. Symptomatic relief with simple analgesia, saline bathing, and topical anaesthetic.
- Oral aciclovir (200mg 5x day for 5 days or similar), double dose/length if immunosuppressed.
- Topical aciclovir is not beneficial.
- Condoms/abstinence whilst prodromal/symptomatic (unless history of HSV in both partners) may reduce transmission rates.
- Suppressive antiviral treatment—considered if >6 recurrences/year.

Implications in pregnancy

See 📖 Herpes simplex, p. 166.

Gonorrhoea

Epidemiology
- *Neisseria gonorrhoeae*: intracellular Gram −ve diplococcus.
- Fourth most common STI in the UK.
- >18 000 cases were reported in 2010 in the UK.
- >35% of strains are resistant to ciprofloxacin, 70% to tetracyclines.

Symptoms
Usually asymptomatic, often diagnosed when screening on contact tracing.
Can present with vaginal discharge, low abdominal pain, IMB or PCB.

Diagnosis
- Endocervical or vulvovaginal swab with NAAT. Urethral, pharyngeal, and rectal swabs if contact with gonorrhoea.
- If diagnosed on NAAT, culture for sensitivity testing should be taken from all sites prior to antibiotic treatment.

> ### Complications of gonococcus infection
> - PID (~10% of infections result in PID).
> - Bartholin's or Skene's abscess.
> - Disseminated gonorrhoea may cause:
>   - fever
>   - pustular rash
>   - migratory polyarthralgia
>   - septic arthritis.
> - Tubal infertility.
> - Risk of ectopic pregnancy.

Treatment
- Ceftriaxone 500mg IM stat, plus azithromycin 1g PO stat.
- Spectinomycin 2g IM, plus azithromycin 1g PO stat (if severe penicillin allergy).
- Contact tracing and treatment of partners.
- The same antibiotics are recommended for treating gonorrhoea in pregnancy.

Implications in pregnancy
- Gonorrhoea associated with:
  - preterm rupture of membranes and premature delivery
  - chorioamnionitis.
- The risks to the baby are of ophthalmia neonatarum (40–50%).

Further reading
British Association for Sexual Health and HIV ℘ http://www.bashh.org/

Syphilis

Epidemiology
- *Treponema pallidum*—spirochaete.
- Relatively rare STI in the UK; however, a 12-fold rise 1997–2007.
- Doubling of congenital syphilis from 1999–2007.
- Nearly 3000 cases were diagnosed in 2010 in the UK.

Symptoms
Primary syphilis
- 10–90 days postinfection.
- Painless, genital ulcer (chancre)—may pass unnoticed on the cervix.
- Inguinal lymphadenopathy.

Secondary syphilis
- Occurs within the first 2yrs of infection.
- Generalized polymorphic rash affecting palms and soles.
- Generalized lymphadenopathy.
- Genital condyloma lata.
- Anterior uveitis.

Tertiary syphilis
- Presents in up to 40% of people infected for at least 2yrs, but may take 40+yrs to develop.
- *Neurosyphilis:* tabes dorsalis and dementia.
- *Cardiovascular syphilis:* commonly affecting the aortic root.
- *Gummata:* inflammatory plaques or nodules.

Diagnosis
- Specific treponemal enzyme immunoassay (EIA) for screening (IgG + IgM).
- 1° lesion smear may show spirochaetes on dark field microscopy.
- Quantitative cardiolipin (non-treponemal) tests, i.e. rapid plasma reagin (RPR)/VDRL are useful in assessing need for and response to treatment.

Treatment
- *Depends on penicillin allergy:*
  - benzathine benzylpenicillin 2.4 MU single dose IM (used in pregnancy)
  - doxycycline 100mg bd PO for 14 days (contraindicated in pregnancy),
  - erythromycin 500mg qds PO for 14 days (used in pregnancy).
- Treatment courses are longer in tertiary syphilis.
- Contact tracing (potentially over several years).

Implications in pregnancy
- Preterm delivery.
- Stillbirth.
- Congenital syphilis.
- Miscarriage

See Syphilis, 🕮 p. 175.

Trichomonas

Epidemiology
- *Trichomonas vaginalis*—flagellated protozoan.
- Nearly 5000 reported cases in England in 2010.
- Found in vaginal, urethral, and para-urethral glands.
- Cervix may have a 'strawberry' appearance from punctate haemorrhages (2%).

Symptoms
Asymptomatic in 10–50%, but may present with:
- Frothy, greenish, offensive smelling vaginal discharge.
- Vulval itching and soreness.
- Dysuria.

Diagnosis
- Direct observation of the organism by a wet smear (normal saline) or acridine orange stained slide from the posterior vaginal fornix (sensitivity 40–70% cases).
- Culture media are available and will diagnose up to 80% cases.
- NAATs have been developed and sensitivities and specificities approaching 100% have been reported.

Complications
There is some evidence that trichomonal infection may enhance HIV transmission.

Treatment
- Metronidazole 2g orally in a single dose.
- Metronidazole 400–500mg bd for 5–7 days.
- Contact tracing and treatment of partners.

Implications in pregnancy
- Trichomonas is associated with:
  - preterm delivery
  - low birth weight.
- Trichomonas may be acquired perinatally, occurring in 5% of babies born to infected mothers.

Human papillomavirus

Epidemiology
- DNA virus, many subtypes.
- Subtypes 6 and 11 cause genital warts (condylomata acuminata).
- 25% of people presenting with warts have other concurrent STIs.
- Commonest viral STI in England.
- >75000 new cases of genital warts diagnosed in England in 2010.
- Subtypes 16 and 18 associated with CIN and cervical neoplasia.

Symptoms Majority asymptomatic. Painless lumps anywhere in the genitoanal area. Perianal warts are common in the absence of anal intercourse.

Diagnosis Usually identified by clinical appearance. Non-wart HPV infection often diagnosed by characteristic appearance on cervical cytology (smear tests) or colposcopy (whitening on topical application of acetic acid).

Complications
HPV 16 and 18 associated with high-grade CIN and cervical neoplasia. Smoking and immunosuppression both affect viral clearance thereby increasing the risk.

Treatment for genital warts
Removal of the visible wart. High rate of recurrence due to the latent virus in the surrounding epithelial cells.

Clinic treatment
- Cryotherapy.
- Trichloroacetic acid.
- Electrosurgery/scissors excision/curettage/laser.

Home treatment (both contraindicated if pregnancy risk)
- *Podophyllotoxin cream or solution:* this is self-applied and must be used for about 4–6wks.
- *Imiquimod cream:* this is also a self-applied immune response modifier. It may need to be used for up to 16wks.

Implications in pregnancy
- Genital warts tend to grow rapidly in pregnancy, but usually regress after delivery.
- Very rarely, babies exposed perinatally may develop laryngeal or genital warts.
- Not an indication for CS.

Routine vaccination
- From 2008 the DH has recommended HPV vaccination for all girls aged 12–13.
- Initially the selected vaccine was active against HPV 16 and 18, but in 2012 was changed to include HPV 6 and 11 as well.

Bacterial vaginosis

Epidemiology
- BV is caused by an overgrowth of mixed anaerobes, including *Gardnerella* and *Mycoplasma hominis*, which replace the usually dominant vaginal lactobacilli.
- Commonest cause of abnormal vaginal discharge in women of childbearing age.
- Prevalence 5–15% white women, 45–55% black African-American women.
- Not sexually transmitted.
- About 12% of women will experience BV at some point in their lives, but what triggers it remains unclear.

Symptoms
May be asymptomatic, but usually presents with a profuse, whitish grey, offensive smelling vaginal discharge. The characteristic 'fishy' smell is due to the presence of amines released by bacterial proteolysis and is often distressing to the woman.

Diagnosis
(Amsel criteria—3 out of 4 required for diagnosis.)
- Homogenous grey-white discharge.
- Increased vaginal pH >5.5.
- Characteristic fishy smell.
- 'Clue cells' present on microscopy (squamous epithelial cells with bacteria adherent on their walls).

Complications
Increased risk of pelvic infection after gynaecological surgery.

Treatment
May resolve spontaneously and if successfully treated has a high recurrence rate. However, most women prefer it to be treated.
- Metronidazole 400mg orally bd for 5 days; *or*
- Metronidazole 2g (single dose).
- Clindamycin 2% cream vaginally at night for 7 days.

Lifestyle factors—avoidance of vaginal douching/overwashing which can destroy natural vaginal flora.

Implications in pregnancy
Associated with an increased risk of:
- Mid-trimester miscarriage.
- Preterm rupture of membranes.
- Preterm delivery.

Candidiasis (thrush)

Epidemiology
- Yeast-like fungus (90% *Candida albicans*, remainder other species, e.g. *C. glabrata*).
- About 75% of women will experience at least one episode, and 10–20% are asymptomatic chronic carriers (increasing to 40% during pregnancy).
- Predisposing factors are those that alter the vaginal micro-flora and include:
  - immunosuppression
  - antibiotics
  - pregnancy
  - diabetes mellitus
  - anaemia.

Symptoms
May be asymptomatic, but usually presents with:
- Vulval itching and soreness.
- Thick, curd-like, white vaginal discharge.
- Dysuria.
- Superficial dyspareunia.

Diagnosis
- Characteristic appearance of:
  - vulval and vaginal erythema
  - vulval fissuring
  - typical white plaques adherent to the vaginal wall.
- Culture from HVS or LVS.
- Microscopic detection of spores and pseudohyphae on wet slides.

Complications
Unlikely to cause any significant complications unless the woman is severely immunocompromised.

Treatment
- As so many women are chronic carriers, candidiasis should only be treated if it is symptomatic.
- Clotrimazole 500mg pessary +/− topical clotrimazole cream; *or*
- Fluconazole 150mg (single dose)—contraindicated in pregnancy.

Other simple measures may help to decrease recurrent attacks, e.g.:
- Wearing cotton underwear.
- Avoiding chemical irritants, e.g. soap and bath salts.

Implications in pregnancy
- It is very common in pregnancy with no apparent adverse effects.
- Topical imidazoles are not systemically absorbed and are therefore safe at all gestations.

Pelvic inflammatory disease: overview

Definition PID is infection of the upper genital tract.

Incidence
The exact prevalence is hard to ascertain as many cases may go undetected, but is thought to be in the region of 1–3% of sexually active young women.

Causes
- Most commonly caused by ascending infection from the endocervix, but may also occur from descending infection from organs such as the appendix.
- There are multiple causative organisms:
  - 25% of cases estimated to be caused by *Chlamydia trachomatis* and *Neisseria gonorrhoeae*
  - anaerobes and endogenous agents, either aerobic or facultative, may be responsible for the remainder.

History and examination
- A full gynaecological history including sexual history.
- An abdominal examination to elicit the site and severity of the pain.
- Speculum and vaginal examination to assess for adnexal masses, vaginal discharge, or cervical excitation.

Risk factors for PID
- Age <25.
- Previous STIs.
- New sexual partner/multiple sexual partners.
- Uterine instrumentation such as surgical termination of pregnancy and intrauterine contraceptive devices.
- Post-partum endometritis.

Protective factors
These include the use of barrier contraception, the levonorgestrel (LNG) (Mirena® IUS) and the COCP.

Pelvic inflammatory disease: diagnosis and treatment

Signs and symptoms

PID may be relatively asymptomatic, the diagnosis only being made retro-spectively during investigation of subfertility. Symptoms may include some or all of the following:
- Pelvic pain (may be unilateral), constant or intermittent.
- Deep dyspareunia.
- Vaginal discharge (usually due to concurrent vaginal infection).
- Irregular and/or more painful menses.
- IMB/PCB.
- Fever (unusual in mild/chronic PID).

Signs (at least one of which should be present when making a PID diag-nosis) are:
- Cervical motion pain (cervical excitation).
- Adnexal tenderness (commonly bilateral, but may be unilateral).
- Elevated temperature (unusual in mild/chronic infection).

Investigations
- Tests for gonorrhoea and chlamydia.
- WCC and CRP may be elevated.
- USS may be indicated if a tubo-ovarian abscess is suspected.
- Laparoscopy is the gold standard test; however, it is invasive and only used where diagnosis is uncertain.

Complications of PID
- Tubo-ovarian abscess.
- Fitz-Hugh–Curtis syndrome.
- Recurrent PID.
- Ectopic pregnancy.
- Infertility.

Treatment
Early empirical treatment is recommended. Multiple antibiotic regimes are required to cover all potential causative organisms (see 📖 Pelvic inflam-matory disease: diagnosis and treatment, p. 563).
- Most patients can be treated in an outpatient setting.
- Review after 72h to ensure adequate response.
- Contact tracing and treatment of partners is essential.
- Inpatient treatment may be required if symptoms are severe, fail to respond, or abscess is suspected.
- If there is USS evidence of a tubo-ovarian abscess, drainage may be required either by ultrasonic guided aspiration or at laparoscopy.

Outpatient management of PID

- IM ceftriaxone 500mg stat plus oral doxycycline 100mg bd 14 days plus oral metronizadole 400mg bd 14 days; or
- Ofloxacin orally 400mg bd 14 days plus metronidazole 400mg bd 14 days (avoid if high risk of gonococcal disease).

⚠ Doxycycline and metronidazole are commonly used in clinical practice, but there are no clinical trials to support their effectiveness

Inpatient management of PID

- IV ceftriaxone 2g od plus IV doxycycline 100mg bd, followed by oral doxycycline 100mg bd 14 days plus oral metronidazole 400mg bd 14 days; or
- IV clindamycin 900mg tds + IV gentamicin 2mg/kg loading dose followed by 1.5mg/kg tds, followed by either oral clindamycin 450mg qds for a total of 14 days or oral doxycycline 100mg bd + oral metronidazole 400mg bd for a total of 14 days; or
- IV ofloxacin 400mg bd + IV metronidazole 500mg tds for a total of 14 days.

Further reading

RCOG. (2008). *Management of acute pelvic inflammatory disease*. RCOG guideline 32. ⅋ http://www.rcog.org.uk/womens-health/clinical-guidance/management-acute-pelvic-inflamma-tory-disease-32

Acute pelvic pain

⚠ Acute pelvic pain in a woman of reproductive age with a +ve pregnancy test is an ectopic pregnancy until proven otherwise.

History

- *Pain:* site, nature, radiation, aggravating/relieving factors.
- LMP.
- Contraception.
- Recent unprotected sexual intercourse (UPSI).
- Risk factors for an ectopic pregnancy (see 📖 Ectopic pregnancy: diagnosis, p. 534).
- Vaginal discharge or bleeding.
- Bowel symptoms.
- Urinary symptoms.
- Precipitating factors (physical and psychological).

Examination

- *Is she haemodynamically stable?* Risk of bleeding from ectopic.
- *Abdomen:* does she have an acute abdomen? masses?
- *Pelvic:* are discharge, cervical excitation, adnexal tenderness, masses present?

Investigations

- Urinary/serum hCG.
- MSU.
- Triple swabs (high vaginal, cervical, and endocervical Chlamydia).
- FBC, Group and Save (cross-match if ectopic suspected), CRP.
- Pelvic USS—transvaginal or abdominal as appropriate.
- Abdominal X-ray (+/− contrast), CT, MRI as appropriate.
- Diagnostic laparoscopy.

Treatment

- Resuscitate if necessary.
- Analgesia.
- Specific treatment will depend on cause of pain.
- Avoid unnecessary laparoscopy, especially in a woman with a history of chronic pain.

Gynaecological causes of acute pelvic pain

- *Early pregnancy complications:*
  - ectopic pregnancy (see 📖 Ectopic pregnancy: diagnosis, p. 534)
  - miscarriage (see 📖 Miscarriage: management, p. 532)
  - ovarian hyperstimulation syndrome (see 📖 Ovarian hyperstimulation syndrome, p. 604).
- PID (see 📖 Pelvic inflammatory disease: overview p. 561).
- *Ovarian cyst accident:*
  - torsion
  - haemorrhage
  - rupture.
- *Adnexal pathology:*
  - torsion of fallopian tube/parafimbrial cyst
  - salpingo-ovarian abscess.
- Mittelschmerz (German: Mittel = middle, Schmerz = pain).
- Pregnancy complications (see 📖 Abdominal pain in pregnancy: pregnancy related (<24wks), p. 90):
  - fibroid degeneration
  - ovarian cyst accident
  - ligament stretch.
- Primary dysmenorrhoea (see 📖 Menstrual disorders: dysmenorrhea, p. 510).
- Haematometra/haematocolpos.
- Non-gynaecological causes.
- Acute exacerbation of chronic pelvic pain.

Non-gynaecological causes of acute pelvic pain

Gastrointestinal

- Appendicitis.
- Irritable bowel syndrome (IBS).
- IBD.
- Mesenteric adenitis.
- Diverticulitis.
- Strangulation of a hernia.

Urological

- UTI.
- Renal/bladder calculi.

Chronic pelvic pain: gynaecological causes

> **Definition** Intermittent or constant pelvic pain in the lower abdomen or pelvis of at least 6mths' duration, not occurring exclusively with menstruation or intercourse and not associated with pregnancy.
> Chronic pelvic pain (CPP) is a symptom, not a diagnosis.

Prevalence
- Annual prevalence in women aged 15–73 is 38/1000 (asthma: 37/1000, back pain: 41/1000).
- Many women do not receive a diagnosis even after many years and multiple investigations.

Causes
Endometriosis
See 📖 Endometriosis: overview, p. 582.

Adenomyosis
- Characterized by the presence of ectopic endometrial tissue in the myometrium.
- Often occurs after pregnancy, particularly after CS or TOP (breaches the integrity of the endometrial/myometrial junction).
- Initially causes cyclical pelvic pain and menorrhagia, but can worsen until pain is present daily.

Adhesions
Trapped ovary syndrome
After hysterectomy the ovary becomes trapped within dense adhesions at the pelvic side wall.

Pelvic venous congestion
- Dilated pelvic veins, believed to cause a cyclical dragging pain.
- Worst premenstrually and after prolonged periods of standing and walking.
- Dyspareunia is also often present.

Further reading
RCOG. (2012). *Chronic pelvic pain: initial management.* RCOG Guideline 41. ⅋ http://www.rcog.org.uk/womens-health/clinical-guidance/initial-management-chronic-pelvic-pain-green-top-41

Chronic pelvic pain: non-gynaecological causes

Gastrointestinal causes

- *Irritable bowel syndrome (IBS):* common, occurring in ~20% of women of reproductive age.
- *Constipation:* common cause of pelvic pain that is easily treated.

⚠ Opiate analgesics should not be prescribed for CPP without a laxative.

- *Hernia:* abdominal or pelvic hernias may cause pain.

Urological causes

Interstitial cystitis (IC)
- Inflammatory disorder causing pain and urinary frequency.
- Diagnosed on cystoscopy.
- Pain is often relieved by voiding.

Urethral syndrome
- Associated with frequency/dysuria in absence of infective cystitis.
- Aetiology is not known, possibly due to a chronic low grade infection of the paraurethral glands ('female prostatitis').

Calculi
- May occasionally trigger a chronic pain cycle.

Musculoskeletal causes

Fibromyalgia
- Widespread pain especially in the shoulders, neck, and pelvic girdle.
- Characterized by tender points and a reduced pain threshold.
- Often shows cyclical exacerbations.

Neurological causes

Nerve entrapments
- Trapped in fascia or narrow foramen or in scar tissue after surgery.
- Classically results in pain and/or dysfunction in nerve distribution.

Neuropathic pain
- Results from actual damage to the nerve (surgery, infection, or inflammation).
- Classically described as shooting, stabbing, or burning.

Psychological associations with CPP

- A number of studies have shown that women with CPP have increased number of −ve cognitive and emotional traits, although it is not known whether these are cause or consequence of pain.
- History of abuse (physical, sexual, and psychological) also associated with CPP, but may not be revealed at the first consultation.

Chronic pelvic pain: diagnosis and treatment

History
As for acute pelvic pain, but also including:
- A detailed history of the pain, including events surrounding its onset, site, nature, radiation, time course, exacerbating and relieving factors, and any cyclicity.
- A sexual history and future fertility wishes should be explored (it may be possible to discuss abuse at this point).

Examination
- As for acute pelvic pain.
- Speculum may not be appropriate if history of vaginismus or pain 2° to difficult smear or abuse.

Investigations Be careful not to overinvestigate initially.

Therapeutic trial of GnRH analogues

With clearly cyclical pain, a trial of a GnRH analogue (GnRHa) can be a useful diagnostic tool:
- Women requesting hysterectomy with bilateral salpingo-oopherectomy can be reassured that it may be a successful treatment if their pain is relieved with a GnRHa.
- If their pain persists on GnRHa treatment, they should be counselled that hysterectomy is unlikely to remove their pain and other causes for it should be explored.

Treatment

Analgesia
- Pre-emptive analgesia may prevent emergency admissions.
- Opiates may be required for severe, acute exacerbations, but if needed regularly, referral to a dedicated pain clinic should be made.
- Neuropathic treatments such as amitriptyline, gabapentin, and pregabalin can be useful.

Hormonal treatments
The COCP, progestagens, and GnRH analogues can be effective. If pain is improved with a GnRHa then this can be combined safely with low-dose HRT for at least 2yrs.

Complementary therapy
A variety of complementary therapies can produce good results and should be encouraged if the woman suggests them. Support groups can also give reassurance.

Surgery
This has a limited role to play, but hysterectomy can be helpful, as above.

Chapter 18

Subfertility and reproductive medicine

Polycystic ovarian syndrome: overview

Background
- PCOS is the most common endocrine disorder in women.
- Responsible for 80% of all cases of anovulatory subfertility.
- Estimated prevalence is 6–10% of women of childbearing age.
- USS evidence of polycystic ovaries is seen in 20–30% of women.

Rotterdam criteria for diagnosing PCOS
Requires the presence of two out of the following three variables and exclusion of other disorders:
- Irregular or absent ovulations (cycle >42 days).
- Clinical or biochemical signs of hyperandrogenism:
  - acne
  - hirsutism
  - alopecia.
- Polycystic ovaries on pelvic USS: ≥12 antral follicles on one ovary.
- Ovarian volume >10mL.

Aetiology
The pathogenesis of PCOS is not fully known. There is hypersecretion of LH in ~60% of PCOS patients (LH stimulates androgen secretion from ovarian thecal cells). Elevated LH:FSH ratio is often seen, but is not needed for diagnosis. The following factors have been implicated:
- Genetic (familial clustering).
- Insulin resistance with compensatory hyperinsulinaemia (defect on insulin receptor).
- Hyperandrogenism (elevated ovarian androgen secretion).
- Obesity:
  - BMI >30 in 35–60% of women with PCOS
  - central obesity
  - worsens insulin resistance.

Investigations
- *Basal (day 2–5):* LH, FSH, TFTs, prolactin, and testosterone.
- If hyperandrogenisim:
  - dehydroepiandrosterone sulphate (DHEAS)
  - androstenedione
  - SHBG.
- Exclude other causes of 2° amenorrhoea.
- Pelvic USS.

Examination
- BMI.
- Signs of endocrinopathy, hirsutism, acne, alopecia, acanthosis nigricans.

Long-term health consequences of PCOS

- Obesity, insulin resistance, and metabolic abnormalities including dyslipidaemia are all risk factors for ischaemic heart disease, though long-term studies in PCOS are not proven.
- Type II diabetes is a known risk of obesity and insulin resistance, and pregnant women with PCOS are at increased risk of gestational diabetes (📖 Gestational diabetes, p. 240).
- Long periods of 2° amenorrhoea, with resultant unopposed oestrogen, are a risk factor for endometrial hyperplasia and, if untreated, endometrial carcinoma.

Polycystic ovarian syndrome: management

The options should focus on the main concern of the woman.

Lifestyle modification

This is the cornerstone to managing PCOS in overweight women. Even a modest weight loss (5%) can improve symptoms. Moreover, weight loss through exercise and diet has been proven effective in restoring ovulatory cycles and achieving pregnancy. Weight loss through diet and exercise should be encouraged, and patients should feel supported.

Improving menstrual regularity

- Weight loss.
- COCP.
- Metformin.

Controlling symptoms of hyperandrogenism

- Cosmetic (depilatory cream, electrolysis, shaving, plucking).
- Antiandrogens such as eflornithine facial cream, finasteride, or spironolactone:
  - can be used to help with acne and hirsutism
  - can take 6–9mths to improve hair growth
  - avoid pregnancy (feminizes a male fetus).
- COCP:
  - reduces serum androgen levels by increasing SHBG levels
  - co-cyprindiol combines ethinylestradiol and cyproterone acetate, providing a regular monthly withdrawal bleed and beneficial antiandrogenic effects.

Subfertility

- Weight loss alone may achieve spontaneous ovulation.
- Ovulation induction with antioestrogens or gonadotrophins.
- Laparoscopic ovarian diathermy.
- IVF if ovulation cannot be achieved or does not succeed in pregnancy.

See 📖 Female subfertility: management, Ovulation induction, p. 596.

⚠ Women with PCOS who undergo IVF are at increased risk of ovarian hyperstimulation syndrome (see 📖 Ovarian hyperstimulation syndrome, p. 604).

Insulin sensitizers

Metformin has been most widely used (not licensed for this in the UK):
- Metformin combined with ovulation induction with clomifene citrate
  ↑ ovulation and pregnancy rates, but may not significantly improve live birth rate.
- Does not significantly improve hirsutism, acne, or weight loss, despite lowering androgen levels and improving insulin sensitivity.

Psychological issues

PCOS can be difficult to manage and patients may require additional motivation. Symptoms can be distressing and result in low self-esteem. It is therefore important to manage patients sensitively, and to adopt a holistic approach, incorporating all members of the multidisciplinary team.

Hirsutism and virilization: overview

Background

Vellus hair (prepubertal, unpigmented, downy hair) is irreversibly transformed into *terminal hair* (pigmented, coarse) through either increased free androgen or increased sensitivity of 5-α reductase (conversion of testosterone to the more potent dihydrotestosterone) in the skin. In women testosterone originates either directly from the ovaries (25%) and adrenal glands (25%) or from peripheral conversion of androstenedione or dihydroepiandrostenedione (-sulphate), which are produced in the ovaries and adrenal glands (50%). Testosterone is bound to SHBG (80%) and albumin (19%). In women, only 1% is free (active). LH stimulates ovarian theca cells and ACTH the adrenal glands to synthesize androgen.

Hirsutism

- *Hirsutism:* presence of excessive facial and body hair in women.
- Caused by ↑ of systemic or local androgen, resulting in a male hair growth pattern.
- Incidence of hirsutism is estimated to be around 10% in developed countries.
- Most commonly found in patients with PCOS, together with acne, alopecia, and acanthosis nigricans.
- Even mild forms of hirsutism are often felt unacceptable by the patient and may cause mental trauma.
- Should also not be confused with hypertrichosis, which is a very rare, androgen-independent disorder:
  - hypertrichosis can involve vellus, lanugo, and terminal hair occupying the entire body surface including the face ('werewolf appearance')
  - congenital forms have been described (usually more severe)
  - can be caused by drugs (phenytoin, ciclosporin, glucocorticoids), hypothyroidism, and anorexia nervosa.

Virilization

- Can be distinguished from hirsutism by the presence of:
  - clitoromegaly
  - balding
  - deepening of the voice
  - male body habitus.
- Is relatively rare and usually secondary to androgen-producing tumours or CAH.

Causes of hirsutism
Ovary
- Polycystic ovarian syndrome 95%.
- Androgen-secreting tumours <1%.
- Luteoma <1%.

Adrenal gland
- CAH <1%.
- Cushing's syndrome <1%.
- Androgen-secreting tumours <1%.
- Acromegaly 1%.

External causes
- Iatrogenic hirsutism <1%.
- Drugs with androgenic effects (anabolic steroids, danazol, testosterone) <1%.

Reasons for increased androgen levels
Reduced SHBG levels
- Hyperinsulinaemia.
- Liver disease.
- Androgens.
- Hyperprolactinaemia.
- Hypothyroidism.

Increased production
- Tumours.
- Enzyme defects (including CAH).
- Cushing's syndrome.
- Hyperinsulinaemia.
- Increased LH levels stimulate theca cells.

External androgen sources
- Androgens.
- Progestagens with androgenic potential.

Increased 5-α reductase sensitivity
Insulin growth factor-1 in patients with insulin resistance or hyperinsulinaemia.

Hirsutism and virilization: clinical appearance and investigations

Women mostly present with coarse and pigmented (terminal) hair on the face (upper lip, chin), chest, abdomen, back, and thighs. Ethnic differences in the severity of hair growth are common. Fair-skinned white women show less hair growth, while Mediterranean women have the greatest amount of terminal hair. Genetic differences in the activity of 5-α reductase seem to correlate with the severity of disease. Hirsutism is often accompanied by seborrhoea, acne, and male pattern alopecia.

History

- *Age:*
  - children with non-classical CAH
  - pregnant women with luteoma.
- *Rate of onset of symptoms:* rapid onset of severe symptoms may indicate an androgen-producing tumour.
- *Menstrual cycle:* oligo- or amenorrhoea.
- *Genetic factors:*
  - PCOS
  - enzyme deficiencies
  - type II diabetes.
- *Drugs:*
  - COCPs with androgen effects
  - drug abuse (body builders).
- *General health and other symptoms:*
  - Cushing's
  - acromegaly
  - liver disease.

Physical examination

- Exclude hypertrichosis.
- Signs of virilization should prompt a search for an androgen-producing tumour.
- BP:
  - ↑ with Cushing's and acromegaly
  - ↓ in hypothyroidism and CAH.
- Look for acanthosis nigricans:
  - marker of insulin resistance and hyperinsulinaemia
  - skin grey-brown, velvety appearance mainly in the neck, axillae, vulva, and groin.

Ferriman–Gallwey score to grade hirsutism

Nine locations are evaluated and each receives a score between 0 (no growth) and 4 (complete hair cover):

- Upper lip.
- Chin.
- Chest.
- Upper abdomen.
- Lower abdomen.
- Upper back.
- Lower back.
- Upper arms.
- Thighs.

A score >8 is considered androgen excess.

❧ This score is subjective, difficult to compare between different ethnic groups, and has a reduced validity in pretreated women. It is therefore usually reserved for clinical studies.

Investigations for hirsutism

- *Testosterone*: measure of ovarian and adrenal activity.
- *DHEAS*: measure of adrenal activity.
- *OGTT*: in women with indication of hyperinsulinaemia/insulin resistance.
- *17-OHP*: to rule out CAH, if indicated.

▶ TVS/USS to visualize polycystic ovaries is not necessary to diagnose PCOS in a woman with hirsutism and oligo-/amenorrhoea. However, TVS/USS should always be done, first, to exclude any ovarian tumours and, second, to help in confirming the diagnosis.

▶ Investigations to rule out rare causes of hirsutism such as Cushing's syndrome and acromegaly should be undertaken if clinically indicated.

Hirsutism: first-line treatment

Treatment is aimed at the underlying cause (especially important for the non-ovarian causes such as Cushing's or CAH).

- Lifestyle changes aiming at weight reduction in women with PCOS.
- *COCP*:
  - treatment of choice in women not trying to conceive
  - *progestational component*—LH suppression; 5-α reductase inhibition)
  - *oestrogenic component*—SHBG ↑
  - COCP with ethinylestrodid + drospirenone
  - ethinylestradiol + cyproterone acetate (co-cyprindiol) licensed in the UK for facial hirsutism (not for contraception!).
- *Medroxyprogesterone acetate*:
  - if COCP is contraindicated
  - LH suppression (less than COCP)
  - SHBG ↓ (counterproductive)
  - testosterone clearance ↑ (induction of liver enzymes)
  - overall, similar results to COCP.

▶ Discontinue treatment after 1–2yrs to observe if ovulatory cycles occur. Suppression of testosterone will last for 6–12mths after discontinuation in anovulatory patients.

Cosmetic approaches

- Hair removal will only be permanent if dermal papilla is destroyed.
- Non-permanent approaches, such as shaving and waxing, do not worsen hirsutism.

Permanent measures

Laser

- 694–1064nm.
- Uses melanin in hair bulb as chromophore.
- Heat causes papillar destruction.
- Works best on fair-skinned women with dark hair.
- Dark-skinned patients at higher risk of dermal damage (scarring and discomfort as more energy is needed).

Electrolysis

- Fine probe inserted into skin.
- Short-wave radio frequency causes heat, thereby destroying dermal papilla.
- Only permanent measure approved by the Food and Drug Administration (FDA).

Non-permanent measures

- Local chemical depilatories (not for face).
- Bleaching.
- Waxing.
- Tweezing.
- Mechanical epilators.

Hirsutism: second-line treatment

- *Spironolactone* (50–200mg daily, ↓ to 25–50mg qds after a few weeks):
  - aldosterone antagonist (diuretic)
  - inhibits ovarian/adrenal androgens
  - competes for androgen receptor in skin
  - inhibits 5-α reductase in skin
  - slow onset (at least 6mths)
  - hyperkalaemia possible (watch renal function)
  - add contraceptive as may cause feminization of male fetus.
- *Cyproterone acetate* (2mg plus 35 micrograms ethinylestradiol in co-cyprindiol):
  - progestational agent with antiandrogenic potency
  - inhibits LH secretion and binds competitively to androgen receptor
  - best after 3mths of treatment
  - *side effects*—fatigue, oedema, weight gain, libido loss, mastalgia.
- *Finasteride* (5mg daily):
  - inhibits 5-α reductase (type II >type I; type I in skin, therefore limited potency for hirsutism and alopecia)
  - few side effects
  - best after 6mths
  - *teratogenic*—contraception needed.
- *Flutamide* (250mg daily):
  - non-steroidal antiandrogen
  - best after 6mths, also for treatment of alopecia
  - hepatotoxicity (monitor liver enzymes regularly)
  - add contraceptive as may cause feminization of male fetus.
- *Eflornithine hydrochloride* (cream topically bd):
  - inhibits ornithine decarboxylase, responsible for hair growth
  - reduces speed of hair growth and hair becomes less coarse
  - works within 8wks, but quick recurrence after cessation
  - may worsen acne (obstructing pilosebaceous glands)
  - recommended for postmenopausal hair growth on upper lip.
- *GnRH agonists* (depot prescriptions):
  - suppress gonadotrophins, thereby suppressing ovarian androgens
  - should be combined with add-back HRT
  - expensive and equally effective as other approaches.

Last resort treatment

- *Ketoconazole* (400mg daily):
  - antifungal agent
  - reduces androgen levels by inducing hepatic cytochrome p450 metabolic pathways
  - hepatotoxicity (monitor liver enzymes regularly)
  - loss of scalp hair
  - abdominal pain.

△ Most of the drugs mentioned are not licensed for this indication. Cyproterone acetate/ethinylestradiol, and eflornithine are the exceptions.

Hirsutism and the menopause

About 17% of patients are menopausal, mainly with facial hirsutism.

Treatment
- Eflornithine cream.
- Spironolactone.
- Cyproterone acetate with HRT (not ethinylestradiol).
- Estradiol + drospirenone HRT.

Endometriosis: overview

Endometriosis is the presence of endometrial-like tissue outside the uterine cavity. It is oestrogen dependent, and therefore mostly affects women during their reproductive years. If the ectopic endometrial tissue is within the myometrium itself it is called *adenomyosis*.

Aetiology

The exact aetiology remains unknown, various theories exist, but none accounts for all aspects of endometriosis.

- *Retrograde menstruation with adherence, invasion, and growth of the tissue (Sampson):* most popular theory; however, >90% show menstrual blood in pelvis at time of menstruation.
- Metaplasia of mesothelial cells (Meyer).
- Systemic and lymphatic spread (Halban).
- Impaired immunity (Dmowski).

Incidence of endometriosis
- *General female population:* 10–12% (estimated).
- *Infertility investigation:* 20–50%.
- *Sterilization:* 6%.
- *Chronic pelvic pain investigation:* 20–50%.
- *Dysmenorrhea:* 40–60%.

Typical presentation of endometriosis (often combination)
- Infertility.
- Pain (often chronic pelvic pain):
  - cyclic or constant (ectopic endometrial tissue undergoes same cycle, causing repeated inflammation, which may result in the formation of adhesions)
  - severe dysmenorrhoea (can be due to adenomyosis)
  - dyspareunia (deep; indicates possible involvement of uterosacral ligaments)
  - dysuria (involvement of bladder or peritoneum or invasion into bladder)
  - dyschezia and cyclic pararectal bleeding (for rectovaginal nodules with invasion of rectal mucosa)
  - chronic fatigue.

⚠ Pain symptoms are often non-specific, resulting in the delay of the diagnosis by up to 12yrs.

► In 2–50% of cases there are no symptoms!

Location of endometriosis

Common sites

- Pelvis (most common):
  - pouch of Douglas
  - uterosacral ligaments
  - ovarian fossae
  - bladder
  - peritoneum.

Rare sites

- Lungs.
- Brain.
- Muscle.
- Eye.

▶ Endometriosis has been described in girls prior to menarche, and in men.

Appearance of endometriosis

- *Peritoneal endometriotic lesions:* appear as minuscule (powder burn) to 1–2cm lesions (red, bluish, brown, black, white; vesicular, cystic, petechial).
- *Ovarian endometriotic cysts:*
  - endometriomas can be >10cm in size
  - usually filled with brownish fluid ('chocolate cysts'; old blood and tissue)
  - often associated with local fibrosis and adhesions.
- *Deep infiltrating endometriosis:* rectovaginal nodules can frequently result in fibrosis of surrounding tissue. Often have solid appearance.

Further reading

RCOG. (2006). Endometriosis, investigation and management. Green-top guideline 24. Available at: ℘ http://www.rcog.org.uk/womens-health/clinical-guidance/investigation-and-management-endometriosis-green-top-24
Women's Health Specialist Library. ℘ www.womenshealthresearch.org/

Endometriosis: diagnosis

History
- Menstrual cycle.
- Nature of the pain:
  - site
  - relationship to cycle (mid cycle/dysmenorrhoea)
  - deep dypareunia.
- Haematuria or rectal bleeding during menstruation.

Examination
- Bimanual pelvic examination for:
  - adnexal masses (endometriomas) or tenderness
  - nodules/tenderness in the posterior vaginal fornix or uterosacral ligaments
  - fixed retroverted uterus
  - rectovaginal nodules.
- Speculum examination of vagina and cervix (rarely, lesions may be visible).

Investigations
- Transvaginal USS:
  - endometriomas
  - possibly for endometriosis of urinary bladder or rectum.
- Laparoscopy with biopsy for histological verification:
  - especially important for deep infiltrating lesions
  - positive is confirmative, negative does not rule it out
  - endometriomas >3cm should to be resected to rule out malignancy (rare).
- Laparoscopy should not be performed within 3mths of hormonal treatment (leads to underdiagnosis).
- Indications for laparoscopy:
  - NSAID-resistant lower abdominal pain/dysmenorrhoea
  - pain resulting in days off work/school or hospitalization
  - pain and infertility investigation.
- It is good practice to document the extent of disease (photos or DVD).
- MRI, intravenous urography (IVU), or barium enema (to assess extent of rectovaginal, bladder, ureteric, or bowel involvement).
- Serum CA125 is sometimes elevated with severe endometriosis, but there is no evidence that it is a useful screening test for this condition.

Grading of endometriosis

The current system (Revised American Society of Reproductive Medicine classification, rASRM 1996) classifies the extent of endometriosis on a point system, taking into account:

Location

- Peritoneal.
- Ovarian.
- Pouch of Douglas.

Size

- <1cm.
- 1–3cm.
- >3cm.

Depth of infiltration

- Superficial.
- Deep.

Adhesions

- Filmy or dense.
- Extent of enclosure (<1/3; 1/3–2/3, >2/3).
- Colour and form.

The points are added up and the stage of endometriosis is graded accordingly:

- *Stage I:* Minimal endometriosis (1–5 points).
- *Stage II:* Mild endometriosis (6–15 points).
- *Stage III:* Moderate endometriosis (16–40 points).
- *Stage IV:* Severe endometriosis (>40 points).

This system of values is highly controversial because of its subjectivity. The severity of disease has not been shown to have any correlation with the severity of pain. It may be of value in infertility prognosis and management.

Endometriosis: treatment

The approach should be determined by:
- Reason for treatment (pain or fertility).
- Side effect profile.
- Cost-effectiveness of each drug.

▶ All drugs are equally effective in relieving pain and are associated with up to 50% recurrence after approximately 12–24mths after stopping.

▶ It is acceptable to treat women empirically with progestagens or COCP without a laparascopic diagnosis. Combined hormonal contraceptives, ideally administered continuously, should be considered as first-line agents. NSAIDs are effective and may be used with hormonal drugs.

▶ Severe cases of endometriosis should be referred to a centre with expertise in advanced laparoscopic surgery.

Treatments for pain

Medical treatment
See Table 18.1.

Surgical treatment
- No RCTs have compared medical with surgical treatment.
- Surgical management indicated once medical treatment has failed.
- There are no data supporting preoperative hormonal treatment.
- Postoperative 6mths treatment with GnRH analogues is effective in delaying recurrence at 12 and 24mths (not the case with COCP).
- Coagulation, excision, or ablation are recommended surgical techniques and should be done by laparoscopy.
- As a last resort hysterectomy may be considered in patients with severe, treatment refractory dysmenorrhoea: if performed, bilateral oophorectomy should be considered with add-back HRT.

Treatments for subfertility

Medical treatment
No medical treatment can improve fertility in endometriosis patients.

Surgical treatment
- Spontaneous pregnancy rate after surgical removal of endometriotic lesions is probably ↑ in minimal/mild endometriosis.
- Unclear efficacy for moderate/severe disease as no RCTs exist.
- Endometriomas (≥3cm) should be removed: best by cystectomy rather than drainage to ↓ recurrence rates.

▶ Fertility-sparing surgery should be the goal, to increase chance of spontaneous conception. However, in moderate to severe disease, IVF may be the treatment of choice.

Table 18.1 Medical treatment for pain from endometriosis

Drug	Applications/ duration	Effect	Side effects
COCP	Continuous >> cyclic Long term	Ovarian suppression	Headaches Nausea DV Stroke
Medroxy-progesterone acetate or other progestagens	Orally or IM/SC injection (depot) Long term	Ovarian suppression	Weight gain Bloating Acne Irregular bleeding Depression
GnRH analogues	2nd line therapy SC/IM injection or nasal spray Short or long term Should never be used without add-back HRT	Ovarian suppression	Loss of bone density (reversible) Hot flushes Vaginal dryness Headaches Depression
Levonorgestrel-releasing IUD	Intrauterine Long term (change every 5yrs if age <40)	Endometrial suppression; sometimes ovarian suppression	Irregular bleeding Spontaneous expulsion
Danazol	Oral 6mths (longest experience)	Ovarian suppression	Acne Hirsutism Irreversible voice changes
Aromatase inhibitors	Oral Probably 6mths (still experimental and not licensed)	Local oestrogen suppression in endometrial lesions	Ovarian cysts Loss of bone density (reversible)

Gonadotrophin-releasing hormone in health and disease

Biochemistry

- GnRH is a decapeptide synthesized in the hypothalamus.
- Released in a pulsatile manner in both males and females.
- Acts on G-protein coupled receptors in the anterior pituitary.
- Has a short half-life ($t_{1/2}$) of 2–4min.

Physiological functions

The frequency and amplitude of the GnRH pulses are more important than absolute hormonal levels. During the fetal and neonatal periods GnRH is involved in normal development. The amplitude of pulsatile release is then decreased during childhood until puberty. It is not known what factor(s) trigger the increased frequency and amplitude of secretion seen during puberty, but this results in the release of gonadotrophins (high-frequency pulses of LH and low-frequency pulses of FSH) from the anterior pituitary gland and subsequently sex steroids from the ovary. A complex system of positive and negative feedback loops between GnRH, LH, FSH, progesterone, and oestrogen regulate the normal menstrual cycle (see 📖 Physiology of the menstrual cycle, p. 502).

Congenital GnRH deficiency

- Congenital hypothalamic hypogonadism is usually only diagnosed in females when a delay in puberty is noted, as female infants are phenotypically normal.
- When associated with an absence of the sense of smell (anosmia) it is known as *Kallman's syndrome*.
- It can be difficult to distinguish hypothalamic hypogonadism from delayed puberty; however, in the former, pubic hair is present as adrenarche occurs normally and children are usually of normal height for their age.

Acquired GnRH deficiency

Acquired GnRH deficiency can be due to:
- Damage to the hypothalamus by:
  - trauma
  - tumour.
- Disruption of the hypothalamic–pituitary axis can occur 2° to:
  - intense physical training
  - anorexia nervosa.

GnRH as a treatment

- Pulsatile intravenous infusions of GnRH can be used to induce puberty and ovulation with a congenital deficiency.
- If deficiency is acquired, it is more usual to use oestrogen and progesterone on a long-term basis, or LH/FSH to induce ovulation.

Gonadotrophin-releasing hormone agonists and antagonists

The short half-life of natural GnRH restricts its pharmacological use to IV pulsatile use. However, longer-acting GnRH analogues (agonists) or receptor antagonists can be used to induce a temporary, reversible menopausal state as a treatment for a number of conditions.

GnRH analogues

- A number of different GnRH analogues exist, including:
  - goserelin acetate
  - leuprorelin acetate
  - nafarelin
- *Administration:*
  - SC injection (daily, monthly, or 3-monthly)
  - intranasally
  - intravaginally.
- They produce a prolonged activation of the GnRH receptor, resulting in an initial ↑ in FSH and LH secretion: this may cause a worsening of symptoms ('initial flare').
- Continued activation of the receptor leads to ↓ LH/FSH secretion:
  - serum oestradiol levels are suppressed by approximately 21 days
  - remain at similar levels to postmenopausal women with continued dosing.
- Indications and adverse effects are shown in Boxes 18.1 and 18.2.
- Adequate barrier contraception should be used during treatment as there is a theoretical risk of teratogenicity and miscarriage.

Bone mineral density (BMD)

- Up to 6% BMD may be lost after the first 6mths treatment.
- If treatment is to be continued for longer than 3mths, the use of 'addback' HRT is recommended: combined GnRH agonist and HRT add-back has been shown to be safe for a period of up to 5–10yrs.
- Resumption of menstruation and return of fertility occur soon after stopping treatment.

GnRH antagonists

GnRH antagonists, such as cetrorelix, bind to receptors without activation and therefore do not cause an initial worsening of symptoms. They are currently licensed for assisted conception protocols and are used experimentally in endometriosis treatments. However, their effect on BMD and other side effects are similar to agonists.

Box 18.1 Indications for GnRH analogue treatment

- *Pre-surgery:*
  - endometrial thinning prior to ablation/resection
  - fibroid shrinkage prior to myomectomy/hysterectomy.
- Endometriosis.
- Adenomyosis.
- Assisted reproduction: pituitary down-regulation prior to superovulation.
- Diagnostic tool in chronic pelvic pain (see 📖 Chronic pelvic pain, p. 568).
- Breast cancer.
- Prostate cancer.

Box 18.2 Adverse effects of GnRH agonists/antagonists

- Hot flushes.
- Mood swings.
- Vaginal dryness.
- Abnormal vaginal bleeding.
- Decreased libido.
- Breast swelling/tenderness.
- ↑ low density lipoprotein (LDL), ↓ high density lipoprotein (HDL).
- Insomnia.
- Headaches.
- Loss of bone mineral density.
- Alterations in eyesight.
- Initial flare (agonists only).
- Bruising at injection site.

Female subfertility: overview

- Very common, with 1 in 6 couples seeking specialist help.
- ~84% will achieve a pregnancy in 1yr of regular UPSI: this ↑ to 92% after 2yrs.
- Referral for specialist advice should be considered after at least 1yr of trying, though in certain situations prompt investigations and referral may be recommended:
  - female age >35yrs
  - known fertility problems
  - anovulatory cycles
  - severe endometriosis
  - previous PID
  - malignancy.
- Treat couples on an individual basis. There is not necessarily a right answer as to when investigations and treatment should start.
- The management of subfertility aims to correct any specific problem that may or may not be diagnosed.

Causes of subfertility
- Ovulation disorder: 21%.
- Tubal factor: 15–20%.
- Male factor: 25%.
- Unexplained: 28%.
- Endometriosis: 6–8%.

Causes of anovulation
Primary ovarian failure
- Premature ovarian failure.
- *Genetic:* Turner's syndrome (45XO; hypergonadotrophic hypogonadism).
- Autoimmune.
- *Iatrogenic:*
  - surgery
  - chemotherapy.

Secondary ovarian disorders
- PCOS.
- Excessive weight loss or exercise.
- Hypopituitarism:
  - tumour
  - trauma
  - surgery.
- Kallman's syndrome (anosmia; hypogonadotrophic hypogonadism).
- Hyperprolactinaemia.

Female subfertility: diagnosis

History

It is vitally important to take a relevant and careful history in a sensitive manner, however embarrassing this may be for you. Couples are often seen together and sometimes it can be difficult to ask about sensitive issues; if necessary, each partner can be seen alone, though this is not ideal. Also ask if a cervical smear is needed and about breast examinations.

- Age.
- Duration of subfertility.
- Menstrual cycle regularity and LMP (pregnancy test?).
- Pelvic pain (dysmenorrhoea; dyspareunia).
- Cervical smear history.
- Previous pregnancies.
- History of ectopic pregnancy.
- Previous tubal or pelvic surgery.
- Previous or current STIs.
- Previous PID.
- Coital frequency.
- Any relevant medical or surgical history.
- Drug history (any prescription drugs that may be contraindicated in pregnancy and ask about recreational drug use).
- Smoking.
- Number of units alcohol/week.
- Folic acid.

Clinical examination

General examination

- BMI
- *Signs of endocrine disorder:* hyperandrogenism (acne, hair growth, alopecia), acanthosis nigricans (see 🕮 Polycystic ovarian syndrome: overview, p. 570); thyroid disease (hypo- and hyperthyroidism); visual field defects (? prolactinoma).

Pelvic examination

- Exclude obvious pelvic pathology (adnexal masses, uterine fibroids, endometriosis (painful, fixed uterus), vaginismus).
- Cervical smear.
- Chlamydia screening.

Investigations

Primary care

- Chlamydia screening.
- Baseline (day 2–5) hormone profile including FSH (high in POF; low in hypopituitarism), LH, TSH, prolactin, testosterone.
- Rubella status.
- Mid-luteal progesterone level (to confirm ovulation >30nmol/L).
- Semen analysis (see 🕮 Male subfertility, p. 598).

Secondary care

This assessment should ideally take place within a specialist clinic with appropriately trained multidisciplinary staff. The history should be confirmed with the couple and any missing details checked.

Assessment of tubal patency

Hysterosalpingography (HSG)

- Easily done.
- Good sensitivity and specificity.
- Can be uncomfortable.
- May have false +ve results (suggesting tubal blockage due to spasm).

Laparoscopy and dye test

- Day-case procedure that can be combined with a hysteroscopy to assess the uterine cavity if necessary.
- 'Gold standard'.
- Pelvic pathology (endometriosis, peritubular adhesions) can be diagnosed and treated.
- Requires general anaesthetic.
- Carries surgical risks.

Hysterosalpingo-contrast-sonograph (HyCoSy)

- Ultrasound with galactose-containing contrast medium.
- Similar sensitivity to HSG.
- No radiation exposure.

Female subfertility: management

Management depends on duration and possible cause of subfertility. Couples should be informed of their options and given relevant evidence-based advice so they can make an informed choice.

Lifestyle modification
- Healthy diet.
- Stop smoking/recreational drugs.
- Reduce alcohol consumption.
- Regular exercise.
- Folic acid.
- Avoid timed intercourse (every 2–3 days).
- Avoid ovulation induction kits/basal temperature measurements (no evidence of success, and stressful).

Ovulation induction
- PCOS is the most common cause of secondary amenorrhoea and is responsible for 75–80% of anovulatory subfertility. Correction of the specific problem such as hyperprolactinaemia or excessive weight may be enough.
- Weight loss/gain as appropriate.
- Antioestrogens (e.g. clomifene 50mg days 2–6):
    - ↑ endogenous FSH levels via negative feedback to pituitary
    - 8–10% multiple pregnancy
    - side effects (hot flushes, mood labiality)
    - clomifene limited to 12 cycles maximum (? possible link to ovarian cancer)
    - needs ultrasound monitoring (abandon cycle if overresponse).
- Gonadotrophins or pulsatile GnRH:
    - used for low oestrogen/normal FSH or clomifene-resistant PCOS
    - injections
    - expensive
    - multiple pregnancy risk
    - ultrasound monitoring (abandon cycle if overresponse)
    - more easily titrated.
- Laparoscopic ovarian diathermy:
    - aims to restore ovulation in patients with PCOS
    - effect lasts 12–18mths if successful.
- Insulin sensitizers (metformin 500mg tds):
    - used in women with PCOS
    - may achieve spontaneous ovulation
    - can be combined with clomifene to increase efficacy
    - recent conflicting data
    - not licensed
    - weight loss is more effective.
- Surgery:
    - preferably laparoscopic
    - treat endometriosis (laser/diathermy/excision)
    - tubal surgery (microsurgery/adhesiolysis).
- Assisted reproduction (IUI, IVF, oocyte donation).

Psychological issues

Subfertility and its management can be very distressing. Some treatments have side effects and are not guaranteed to be successful. The stress of this and disappointment of failed treatment needs to be addressed. Couples should be offered counselling before and after treatment, along with information regarding patient support groups.

Further reading

℞ www.nice.org.uk
℞ www.rcog.org.uk

Male subfertility

Accounts for 20–25% of cases of subfertile couples. Investigation should start in primary care after 1yr, or earlier if history of genital surgery, cancer treatment, or previous subfertility. Trend of declining sperm concentration is not affecting global fecundity but there is increasing 'testicular dysgenesis syndrome' with an increase in cryptorchidism, testicular cancer, and hypospadias. Normal male fertility is dependent on normal spermatogenesis, erectile function, and ejaculation.

Normal semen analysis (WHO criteria 2009)

- Volume >1.5mL.
- Concentration >15 × 10^6/mL.
- Progressive motility >32%.
- Total motility >40%.

Azoospermia
No sperm in ejaculate.

Oligozoospermia
Reduced number of sperm in ejaculate.

Investigations

- *FSH:* elevated in testicular failure.
- *Karyotype:* exclude 47XXY.
- *Cystic fibrosis screen:* congenital bilateral absence of the vas deferens (CBAVD).

Management

- Treat any underlying medical conditions.
- Address lifestyle issues (↓ alcohol, stop smoking).
- *Review medications:*
  - antispermatogenic (alcohol, anabolic steroids, sulfasalazine)
  - antiandrogenic (cimetidine, spironolactone)
  - erectile/ejaculatory dysfunction (α or β blockers, antidepressants, diuretics, metoclopramide).
- *Medical treatments:*
  - gonadotrophins in hypogonadotrophic hypogonadism
  - sympathomimetics (e.g. imipramine) in retrograde ejaculation.
- *Surgical:*
  - relieve obstruction
  - vasectomy reversal.

⚠ Surgical treatment of varicocele does not improve pregnancy rate and is therefore not indicated.

- *Sperm retrieval:*
  - from postorgasmic urine in retrograde ejaculation
  - surgical sperm retrieval from testis with 50% chance of obtaining sperm (greater if FSH is normal).
- *Assisted reproduction:*
  - IUI
  - IVF-ICSI (*in vitro* fertilization and intracytoplasmic sperm injection).
- Donor sperm.
- Adoption.

Pathogenesis of male subfertility

Semen abnormality (85%)
- Idiopathic oligoasthenoteratozoospermia (OATS).
- Testis cancer.
- Drugs (including alcohol, nicotine).
- Genetic.
- Varicocele.

Azoospermia (5%)
- *Pretesticular:* anabolic steroid abuse; idiopathic hypogonadotrophic hypogonadism (HH); Kalmann's, pituitary adenoma.
- *Non-obstructive:* cryptorchidism, orchitis, 47XXY, chemoradiotherapy.
- *Obstructive:* CBAVD, vasectomy, *Chlamydia*, gonorrhoea.

Immunological (5%)
- Antisperm antibodies.
- Idiopathic.
- Infection.
- Unilateral testicular obstruction.

Coital dysfunction (5%)
- Mechanical cause with normal sperm function.
- Ejaculation normal (hypospadias, phimosis, disability).
- Retrograde ejaculation (diabetes, bladder neck surgery, phenothiazines).
- Failure in ejaculation (multiple sclerosis (MS), spinal cord/pelvic injury).

Assisted reproduction: *in vitro* fertilization and intracytoplasmic sperm injection

Assisted reproductive technologies (ART) refer to all fertility treatments in which sperm and oocytes are handled with the aim of achieving pregnancy. It includes IVF, ICSI, preimplantation genetic diagnosis (PGD), PGS, egg donation, and surrogacy.

In vitro fertilization

Indications may include:
- Tubal disease.
- Male factor subfertility.
- Endometriosis.
- Anovulation.
- ↓ Fecundity observed with ↑ maternal age.
- Unexplained infertility for more than 2yrs.
  Success is dependent on many factors including:
- *Duration of subfertility:* ↓ success with ↑ duration.
- *Age:*
  - pregnancy rates are highest between 25 and 35 with a steep decline thereafter
  - elevated basal FSH levels may indicate a poor response to ovarian stimulation
- Previous pregnancy: higher chance of successful IVF outcome.
- Previous failed IVF cycles: ↓ success.
- Presence of hydrosalpinx or intramural fibroid: ↓ success.
- Smoking and ↑ BMI: ↓ success.

Intracytoplasmic sperm injection

- A single sperm is injected into the ooplasm of the oocyte in ICSI.
- Used for men with severely abnormal semen parameters.
- May also be tried when failed fertilization has occurred in IVF cycles.
- Higher fertilization rates are obtained if the selected sperm exhibit some motility, but otherwise there are no strict selection criteria.
- Has greatly ↑ the success of IVF with severe male factor subfertility.
- Sperm may be retrieved from ejaculate or surgically from epididymis or testes.
- Men with severe oligozoospermia should have karyotype and cystic fibrosis screening prior to ICSI.

♠ There are concerns regarding transmission of genetic mutations when using ICSI. Sperms containing oxidatively induced DNA damage are capable of fertilizing oocytes. There is an ↑ incidence of Y chromosome deletions on subfertile men and this may be further propagated by transmission to the offspring born by ICSI, resulting in infertility.

IVF: how it's done

▶ In preparation, the HFEA consents and 'Welfare of the Child' issues must be considered.

- *Down-regulation of the ovaries using GnRH analogues from day 21 (luteal phase) of the previous cycle:* alternatively in antagonist cycles ('short protocol') GnRH antagonists are co-administered with gonadotrophins during ovarian stimulation.
- *Ovarian stimulation with recombinant FSH or human menopausal gonadotrophins:* response is monitored by transvaginal USS.
- Follicular maturation by administration of hCG, when significant mature-size follicles are seen on USS.
- Transvaginal oocyte retrieval by needle-guided aspiration (36h later).
- Sperm sample collected (or thawed if frozen), prepared, and cultured with oocytes overnight.
- Fertilization checks of embryos.
- Embryo transfer by a fine catheter through cervix on day 2–3 (cleavage stage) or day 5 (blastocyst stage):
  - a maximum of 2 embryos are transferred in women under 40 and there is current debate on the move to single embryo transfer given increased neonatal morbidity/mortality and ensuing costs of multiple pregnancy
  - blastocyst transfers increase the success rates of IVF.
- Surplus embryos may be cryopreserved for future frozen embryo replacement cycles.
- Luteal support given in form of progestagens.
- Pregnancy test 2wks later.

Assisted reproduction: other techniques

Preimplantation genetic diagnosis
- Aims to reduce the recurrence of genetic risk in couples known to carry a heritable genetic condition.
- Many couples are fertile, but IVF allows embryo biopsy, single cell diagnosis, and the transfer of unaffected embryos to the woman.
- Biopsies are usually done at cleavage stage, and PCR or FISH used for genetic diagnosis.

Intrauterine insemination
- Couples who may benefit include those with:
  - mild male factor subfertility
  - unexplained subfertility
  - coital difficulties
  - same sex couple.
- Sperm is prepared and placed into the uterus to aid conception.
- The lower threshold for sperm concentration suitability for IUI has been suggested as a total motile count of >10M/mL.
- NICE recommend up to 6 cycles of IUI, but most studies have reported optimal outcome within the first 4 cycles.

 There is no consensus on the role of simultaneous ovarian stimulation, but this should be considered in endometriosis and unexplained infertility when outcome is less favourable.

⚠ If >3 follicles develop the treatment cycle should be cancelled as there is a high rate of multiple pregnancies (>25%).

Egg donation
- May offer a chance of pregnancy for women previously considered to be irreversibly sterile.
- This includes women with:
  - ovarian failure (gonadal dysgenesis, premature, cancer patients 2° to surgery and chemoradiotherapy or menopausal)
  - older women (>45yrs)
  - those with repeated IVF failure.

Donor insemination
- Indicated in men:
  - with azoospermia and failed surgical sperm recovery
  - at high risk of transmitting genetic disorders (e.g. Huntington's disease)
  - at high risk of transmitting infections (HIV).
- Also used for women with no male partner.
- The success of ICSI has ↓ demand for donor insemination.
- Insemination is usually intrauterine: with/without ovarian stimulation and 36–40h after hCG administration.
- Success rates vary from 4% (aged 40–44) to 12% (<34yrs) per cycle.

Special concerns regarding donation of gametes

There are strict criteria for gamete donation, which is regulated by the HFEA.

- Ideally, donors should have no severe medical, psychiatric, or genetic disorders.
- Donors must be counselled.
- Donors must undergo a full infection screen.
- Donors may be known or anonymous to the recipient.
- Egg donors should ideally be <35yrs old.
- Each donor can only be used in up to 10 families within the UK.

⚠ In April 2005 donor anonymity was lifted, meaning that when children born from the use of donor gametes reach the age of 18, they can contact the HFEA for identifying information on the donor.

▶ The supply of donor gametes in the UK is limited. The HFEA may authorize the procurement of gametes from abroad if the supplying clinic fulfils the same quality of standards as the UK.

Surrogacy

IVF surrogacy

- The couple who want the child provide both sets of gametes.
- Following IVF the embryos are transferred to the surrogate.
- This accounts for <0.1% of the total IVF cycles in the UK.
- Indications include women who have congenital absence of the uterus (Rotikansky's syndrome), following hysterectomy, or with severe medical conditions incompatible with pregnancy.

'Natural surrogacy'

- The surrogate is inseminated by the sperm of the male partner of the couple wanting the child.

⚠ Counselling and legal advice is necessary for all parties involved in the surrogacy.

Ovarian hyperstimulation syndrome

Ovarian hyperstimulation syndrome (OHSS) is a complication of ovulation induction or superovulation. Incidence is 0.5–10% and in 1/200
cases it is severe, requiring hospitalization. VEGF is central to underlying
pathophysiology.
- It is characterized by:
  - ovarian enlargement
  - shifting of fluid from the intravascular to the extravascular space.
- Fluid accumulates in the peritoneal and pleural spaces.
- There is intravascular fluid depletion, leading to:
  - haemoconcentration
  - hypercoaguability.
- Risk factors include:
  - polycystic ovaries
  - younger women with low BMI
  - previous OHSS.

Prevention

Management is focused on prediction and active prevention. This may
involve low-dose gonadotrophins, cycle cancellation, 'coasting' during
stimulation, or elective embryo cryopreservation for replacement in a further frozen–thawed cycle.

In vitro maturation may be used in women with polycystic ovaries, with
high antral follicle counts collecting immature eggs, thus avoiding ovarian
stimulation and the risk of OHSS.

Treatment

The treatment is supportive, with the aims of:
- Symptomatic relief.
- Prevention of haemoconcentration and thromboembolism.
- Maintenance of cardiorespiratory function.
  Treatment should consist of:
- Daily assessment of:
  - hydration status (FBC, U&E, LFTs, and albumin)
  - chest and respiratory function (pleural effusions)
  - ascites (girth measurement and weight)
  - legs (for evidence of thrombosis).
- Strict fluid balance with careful maintenance of intravascular volume.
- Thromboprophylaxis:
  - compression stockings
  - consider heparin.
- Paracentesis for symptomatic relief (+/– IV replacement albumin).
- Analgesia and antiemetics.

Sexual dysfunction: overview

Sexual health is a state of physical, emotional, mental, and social well-being in relation to sexuality, not merely the absence of disease or dysfunction. Sexual health necessitates the possibility of having pleasurable and safe sexual experiences, free of coercion, discrimination, and violence. Sexual rights must therefore be respected, protected, and fulfilled.

The prevalence of female sexual dysfunction (FSD) is highly definition-dependent (whether dissatisfaction and disinterest constitute FSD is debated).

Rates are up to 43% in women aged 18–59 compared with 31% in men. Increasing age is inversely proportional to sexual activity. 1/3 of all women over 60 may be sexually active (55% if married). Up to 50% of men will have some degree of erectile dysfunction, which rises to 67% by 70.

Menopause is associated with deterioration of sexual function, with one study suggesting an increase in FSD from 42–88% (45–55yr olds).

Dyspareunia is common and may be present in up to 1/3 of women.

Normal sexual function

Masters and Johnson proposed four components of the sexual response: arousal/excitement, plateau, orgasm, and resolution (based on biological, predominantly male, responses). More recently, intimacy-based models include features of satisfaction, pleasure, and relationship context. Overall the 'normal' for female sexuality is not well characterized and currently FSD is under construction.

Diagnosis

See the woman as she chooses to present herself, with or without a partner, and explore 'why now?' Many present when not in relationships, concerned about their sexual responses.

Presentation may be overt or covert—it is often useful to give the patient time to explore this and always think of the possibility of somatization of problems.

Vital questions in a psychosexual history
- Are you sexually active/do you have a partner?
- Do you have any difficulties?
- Are they a problem for you?
- Do you have pain associated with intercourse?

Examination

'The moment of truth' is a frequent occasion for disclosure of sexual problems manifesting as difficulties with examination, exposure, humiliation, or fantasies of disease or disgust.

Tips on handling consultations

- Be led by the patient.
- The patient is the expert—help her understand her behaviour.
- Reflect your thoughts and feelings.
- Try to understand the relationship between the physical findings, such as prolapse, and the psychological reaction to them.
- Be aware of powerful subconscious defences in the patient, especially with lack of libido and desire disorders.

Consider discussing possible fantasies

- Feeling too small.
- Feeling too big.
- Feeling too loose.
- Vagina with teeth.
- Sharp penis.

Further reading

British Association of Sexual & Marital Therapy. ♫ www.basrt.org.uk
Institute of Psychosexual Medicine. ♫ www.ipm.org.uk
Mary Clegg—devices. ♫ www.maryclegg.com
Vulval Pain Society. ♫ www.vulvalpainsociety.org/

Sexual dysfunction: classification of disorders

Desire disorder

Persistent or recurrent deficiency (or absence) of sexual fantasies/thoughts and/or desire for or receptivity to sexual activity, which causes personal distress (75% of women and 25% of men attending a psychosexual clinic).

The majority of women who have little or no desire are able to derive pleasure from sexual activity. Presentation itself indicates sufficient interest to be hopeful of cure.

Arousal disorder

Persistent or recurrent inability to attain or maintain sufficient sexual excitement, causing personal distress, which may be expressed as a lack of subjective excitement or genital (lubrication/swelling) or other somatic responses. Understanding the sequence of sexual events and the interplay of physical factors (pain, lubrication, environment) helps to deal with the root cause. Lack of sensation is a common presentation of secondary personal or relationship issues.

Orgasmic disorder

Persistent or recurrent difficulty, delay in, or absence of attaining orgasm following sufficient sexual stimulation and arousal, which causes personal distress.

7–10% of women never achieve orgasm with or without a partner. This may not be a concern. Those who can achieve orgasm with masturbation but not with a partner may need to explore their ability to let go or lose control. Up to 25% of women with lifelong anorgasmia have been sexually abused. Women with acquired orgasmic difficulties should explore hormonal status, concomitant medications, and relationship issues. Up to 5% of women with anorgasmia will have an organic cause.

Sexual dysfunction secondary to a general medical condition

Endocrine disorders, psychiatric disorders, and a number of medications will interfere with the sexual response cycle. Treatment of the condition or alteration of therapies may help, but education and explanation may minimize the impact on sexual relationships.

Sexual pain disorders

Dyspareunia

- Dermatological disorders, e.g. psoriasis and lichen sclerosis, infections, such as thrush and recurrent herpes, and atrophic vaginitis are treatable causes of superficial dyspareunia, but may have significant psychological sequelae.
- Poor arousal may be the result or cause of sexual pain: lubricants and topical anaesthetic gels may help break the cycle.
- Deep dyspareunia may be related to a number of medical conditions (endometriosis, PID, adhesions) determined by examination, USS and if necessary laparascopy.

Vaginismus

- Difficulty of the woman to allow vaginal entry of a penis, finger, or object despite the wish to do so.
- This can involve pelvic floor and/or adductor thigh muscle spasm.
- Vaginismus should be regarded as a symptom or sign and not a diagnosis.
- It is generally 2° to another cause—physical, psychological, or both.
- Fear of pain and anticipation of difficulty evolves into avoidance behaviour.
- Check at examination for the presence of anatomical problems, e.g. vaginal septum.

Non-coital sexual pain disorders

- Vulval vestibulitis is the most common pain disorder, but it is frequently difficult to treat.
- Treatment of any skin condition, desensitization, and treatment with topical anaesthetics and lubricants is first-line therapy in conjunction with an exploration of the psychosexual issues.
- Amitriptyline and gabapentin can be considered short term to interrupt the pain cycle.

Sexual dysfunction: treatment

Lifestyle
Address issues including those affecting body image and general well-being, reduction of stress, and dealing with relationship/marital issues.

Education
- Teach people about their bodies and encourage exploration.
- Using 'bibliotherapy' for those needing 'permission' to look at erotic and sexual education material.
- Personal lubricants can be useful for those with arousal difficulties and atrophy (recommend oils or special preparations, but be aware of mineral oil damage to condoms).

Hormonal treatments
- Oestrogen replacement in menopausal women may improve sexuality as well as symptoms of vaginal atrophy: vaginal oestrogens can be used long term.
- Testosterone implants have been used successfully in those who have been oophorectomized and have hypoactive sexual desire disorder (HSDD).
- Testosterone patches are also licensed in the UK.
- Tibolone is licensed for treatment of loss of desire in postmenopausal women.

Complementary therapies
No good evidence for Yohimbine, gingko, khat, or ginseng.

Behavioural therapy
Most sex therapists will use a combination of psychotherapeutic techniques and behavioural interventions. Sensate focus uses a programme of exercises building up in stages:
- Non-genital sensate focus.
- Genital sensate focus.
- Vaginal containment.
- Vaginal containment with movement.

Devices for anorgasmia
- Clitoral stimulators.
- Vibrators.

Vaginal trainers or dilators
May be of use for women with vaginismus and are recommended for those having prolapse procedures and postradiotherapy.

Perineal injections
100mg hydrocortisone, 10mL 0.5% bupivicaine, and 1500U hyaluronidase—may be of value for perineal injuries or for pain trigger points.

Surgery
Rarely necessary—may be for those with a rigid hymen, significant skin webs at the fourchette postsurgery or childbirth, or septae.

Prognostic factors for the success of FSD interventions
- Motivation for treatment (especially in the male partner).
- Quality of the non-sexual relationship.

Sexual dysfunction: male disorders

If you have elicited a problem in a sexually active couple the difficulties of both partners should be gently sought.

Male sexual disorders
- Erectile dysfunction (ED) most common.
- Desire disorders.
- Ejaculatory disorders.

Erectile dysfunction
Routine tests recommended
- Serum glucose.
- Lipids.
- Testosterone (early morning).
- BP.
- Pulse.
- Weight.
- Genitalia.
- Prostate.

⚠ New-onset erectile dysfunction may be a marker for cardiovascular disease.

Treatment options
- Phosphodiesterase inhibitors:
  - sildenafil and vardenafil ↑ erectile function in 60–70%
  - they act in 20–60min and last for up to 8h.
- Tadalafil may be useful for premature ejaculation.
- Apomorphine:
  - dopamine agonist
  - less efficacious (40–50%).
- Androgens: for men with hypogonadism.
- Intracavernous prostaglandin injections.
- Intraurethral prostaglandin pellets.
- Vacuum devices.
- Penile implants.

▶ It is important to remember the psychosexual aspects of sexual difficulties for both partners, as well as concentrating on pharmacological treatments.

Sexual assault

Sexual assault: overview

Sexual offences and rape definitions vary from country to country.

Sexual Offences Act 2003 (UK)
- *Rape:* is defined as non-consensual penetration of mouth, vagina, or anus by a penis.
- *Sexual assaults:* are acts of sexual touching without consent. Sexual assault by penetration involves insertion of object or body parts other than penis into vagina or anus (previously indecent assault).
- Children under 13 cannot legally consent to sexual activity and therefore do not need proof of consent. Mistaken belief of age is not a valid defence.

In assessing a potential victim it is important to establish:
- Whether a sexual act has occurred.
- When it occurred.
- Ability of client to give consent to forensic examination: age, understanding, language, maturity, injury, or intoxication.
- Need for interpreters, 'appropriate adult', or advocate if under age of 16, or with learning difficulties.
- Need of assessment for any acute psychiatric or physical symptoms must always take precedence over forensic examination if needed.
- If reported to the police or victim wants to report it to the police.

⚠ It is crucial that advice is sought from the police or a Sexual Assault Referral Centre (SARC) *before* any examination is undertaken, to preserve possible evidence available.

Presentation

Acute on chronic is also common, particularly with children.

Acute

Victims of acute sexual assault may report to the police directly, or to A&E, GUM, gynaecological, or psychiatric services with covert or overt symptoms. It is crucial to any criminal case that evidence is gathered appropriately and the chain of evidence maintained. 16–58% have genital injuries, but a higher proportion (38–80%) have non-genital injuries. Many have no injuries at all.

⚠ Always consult with the police/SARC if there is any doubt about an individual's presentation.

Delayed

Abuse can present with a number of symptoms (recent or historical). GUM gynaecology, and psychiatry are frequent specialties for disclosure of sexual assault or abuse. There is a significant increase in domestic violence and assault during pregnancy so antenatal services must include screening and referral facilities.

Sexual assault: facts and figures

- The lifetime risk of sexual assault is 1 in 4–6 for women.
- It is estimated that only 1 in 5 adult rapes is reported.
- 1 in 10 victims of sexual assault are men.
- 12% of assaults are by strangers.
- 45% are by acquaintances and 43% by intimate partners.
- 45% involve vaginal rape, 10% anal rape, 15% oral rape, and 25% digital penetration.
- The incidence of child sexual abuse is unknown and possibly only 1 in 20–50 assaults of children are known to supervising authorities.
- The prevalence is far higher than that reflected in numbers reported.

Sexual abuse in children

Concern for children is heightened by:

- Repeated A&E attendances.
- Poor parent–child interactions or behaviour.
- Child known to social services.
- Any injuries to child under 1yr.
- History of domestic abuse.
- Explanation inconsistent with injuries.
- Disclosure of abuse by child.
- Delay in presentation.

⚠ Any concerns should be passed onto the local Safeguarding lead—this may be a nurse, midwife, or paediatrician in your local organization.

Sexual assault: history and examination

History

- *Written consent:* taken before any forensic medical examination. Children <13yrs need an adult with parental responsibility with them to provide written consent. Children 13–16 may consent if considered competent, but should be supported by a responsible adult—ideally one with parental responsibility.
- *Confidentiality issues:* victim may agree to only partial release of information and samples, but is able to change this decision later; forensic samples can be stored for up to 30yrs or 30yrs after their 18th birthday. The SARC would take and store such samples.

Examination

Examination can be performed by the SARC team at the same time as a gynaecological/general examination if necessary (e.g. in A&E or theatre), although it is usually done in the SARC suite. If the victim is <13yrs a paediatrician will normally be in attendance as well as a forensic medical examiner.

The time of the examination and sampling should be noted. The presence of pre-existing conditions such as skin problems or markers of self-harm must also be documented.

> **Key examination points**
> - Demeanour.
> - Intoxication.
> - Height/weight/BP/pulse/temperature.
> - General findings.
> - Injuries (record accurately with diagrams—photographs may be used (involvement of police photographer is preferred):
>   - *non-genital:* none, bruising, petechiae, abrasions, lacerations, incisions, defence injuries
>   - *genital and anal:* none, bruising, abrasions, lacerations, incisions, structure of hymen/remnants in those sexually active (or not)
>   - *oral:* mucosa, teeth, tongue.
> - Clothes may also be important for evidence.

Collecting evidence

- Early evidence kits should be available in all A&E departments or can be brought by the police/forensic examiner. If at all possible evidence should be obtained by someone trained in this procedure, to ensure the highest quality evidence is obtained.
- Evidential samples for sexual offences are likely to be: semen, saliva, vaginal samples, urine, blood, faeces, hair, fibres, vegetation, sanitary pads and/or tampons, toilet paper, clothes, and condoms.

Key samples for reported sexual assault

- *Oral intercourse:* mouth swab/saliva/mouth wash +/– appropriate skin swab.
- *Vaginal intercourse—swabs:* vulval and perineal (both ×2), low vaginal (×2), high vaginal with a Cuscoe's speculum (×2), endocervical (×2), from speculum (×1).
- Lubricant used is also sent.
- *Anal intercourse—swabs:* perianal (×2), rectal (×2), and anal (×2) with proctoscope.
- Buccal swabs are taken for victim DNA.
- Double swabs = 1 dry + 1 wet with saline as these have shown the best return of DNA.
- Fingernail (×2) and hand (×2) swabs and skin (×2 from each site) if stranger assailant.
- *Timescales:* mouth samples for DNA within 48h, skin samples collected within 48h, digital penetration within 12h, penile within 72h, anal within 72h, and vaginal up to 7 days postassault.
- Blood and urine for toxicology should be taken <72h and urine can be useful up to 14 days postassault.

▶ Forensic examination at >7 days for women and >72h for men is unlikely to provide useful DNA evidence; however, it may still be appropriate for documentation of injuries.

Sexual assault: management

Emergency contraception

Should be given if there has been any vaginal contact in women or menstruating girls, irrespective of stage of menstrual cycle. Current recommendations: levonorgestrel 1500 micrograms start within 72h of sexual act (doubled if PEP is used) or IUCD insertion with antibiotic cover within 5 days. Ulipristal can now also be considered within 120h.

Sexually transmitted infections

Risk is estimated at 4–56% depending on the local prevalence and degree of trauma. Consider prophylactic antibiotics particularly if the victim is unlikely to attend for follow-up: 1g azithromycin + 500mg ciprofloxacin (or follow local guidelines). STD screening 2wks after the assault is recommended. Hep B vaccination should be discussed and given where indicated. PEP of HIV should always be considered and discussed (see Box 19.1).

Psychological care

Those at immediate risk of self-harm or suicide must be referred to on-call psychiatric services. Others may be referred to local counselling or support services as well as being given details of emergency out of hours contacts (see 📖 Sexual assault: management, Further reading and useful websites, p. 619). Counselling should aim to contain the trauma of the experience and help the victim bear the 'unbearable'. Those with persistent symptoms after 6mths may have posttraumatic stress disorder and need referral to psychiatric services. Be aware of local services and charities in your area that may provide support to victims of sexual assault and give the victim their details.

Child sexual abuse

It is difficult to know proportions of extra-familial and intra-familial sexual abuse because of underreporting (possibly 2/3 to 1/3, respectively, of reported abuse). Most children do not present acutely and may present because of Social Services or medical concerns regarding chronic physical illness, failure to thrive, or neglect.

⚠ Emergency contraception must be remembered in pubescent girls.
   STIs diagnostic for child sexual abuse are:
• Gonorrhoea (if over 1yr).
• Syphilis and HIV (if congenital infection excluded).
• Chlamydia (if over 3yrs).

Any victim who has children or any young person <16yrs should be automatically referred to social services. All children <13yrs are followed up by the community paediatrician responsible for safeguarding in their area. Those >13yrs can be followed up in the SARC if appropriate.

Principles

- Resuscitation/usual 'ABC' measures are of overriding importance.
- Consideration of collection of evidence.
- Prophylactic antibiotics.
- Postexposure prophylaxis for HIV.
- Emergency contraception.
- Hepatitis B vaccination.
- Analgesia.
- General advice and support.
- Follow-up including counselling.

Risk of transmission of HIV with single exposure (higher if traumatic)

- Receptive vaginal intercourse: 1 in 600–2000.
- Receptive anal intercourse: 1 in 30–150.

Box 19.1 HIV and sexual assault

Risk is dependent on the prevalence in the population and trauma of assault. The prescribing of PEP must be carefully balanced against the side effects and risks of taking them. Consider the higher risk factors: assailant HIV positive or in risk group, anal rape, trauma and bleeding, multiple assailants. If in doubt seek advice from a local HIV physician.

- *PEP*: currently 3 antiretroviral drugs taken ASAP (within 1h if possible) and within 72h. Appropriate follow-up within the week must be arranged for a baseline HIV test, U&E, LFT, FBC because of the toxicity of these drugs. PEP is taken for 1mth and involves several follow-up visits. Full compliance is essential to prevent the emergence of resistant HIV strains. A follow-up HIV test after 6mths is recommended. Counselling is therefore essential prior to prescription of PEP.
- There are no studies of the efficacy of PEP after sexual exposure.

Further reading and useful websites

Brook: helpline and online enquiry service for the under-25s. ℘ www.brook.org.uk. Tel: 020 7284 6040.

Rape Crisis Federation. ℘ www.rapecrisis.org.uk (local numbers available from website).

Rights of Women. ℘ www.rightsofwomen.org.uk. Tel: 020 7251 6577.

Samaritans. ℘ www.samaritans.org.uk. Tel : 08457 90 90 90.

Suzy Lamplugh Trust: for issues of personal safety. ℘ www.suzylamplugh.org.uk. Tel: 020 8392 1839

The Havens: London Sexual Assault Referral Centres. ℘ www.thehavens.co.uk.

Victim Support: for victims of all crimes including sexual assault. ℘ www.victimsupport.org.uk . Tel: 0845 30 30 900.

Contraception

Combined oral contraceptive pill: overview

COCP provides reliable, effective contraception, with a failure rate of 0.2–0.3 per 100 woman-years. Modern COCPs all contain ethinylestradiol (20–35 micrograms) and are classified by type of progestagen they contain. The newer quadriphasic COCP Qlaira® is an exception; it contains estradiol valerate.

Type of progestagen in the COCP
- *2nd generation:*
  - norethisterone
  - levonorgestrel.
- *3rd generation:*
  - desogestrel
  - gestodene (less androgenic)
  - norgestimate (metabolized to levonorgestrel).
- *Yasmin®:* contains drospirenone (antiandrogenic and weak antidiuretic properties).
- *Co-cyprindiol:*
  - contains cyproterone acetate (antiandrogenic)
  - useful in the treatment of hirsutism and acne.

Mode of action
- Ovulation inhibition (−ve feedback on hypothalamus + pituitary).
- Thickened cervical mucus preventing sperm penetration.
- Thin endometrium preventing implantation.

Side effects
- *Breakthrough bleeding:* may occur especially in the first 3mths. Missed pills, STIs, and pregnancy should all be considered.
- *Headache:* try dose of ethinylestradiol or change of progestagen.
- *Weight gain:* no evidence of additional weight gain due to COCP.

Contraindications to the COCP
- Pregnancy.
- Personal history of thromboembolic disease.
- Undiagnosed genital tract bleeding.
- Cardiovascular disorders.
- Migraine with aura.
- Oestrogen dependent tumours.
- Active hepatobiliary disease or liver tumours.
- Hypertension and diabetes.
- ≥35yrs old who smoke (may use 1yr after cessation).
- BMI ≥35.

Advantages and disadvantages of the COCP

Advantages
- ↓ Menstrual blood loss and pain.
- Menstrual cycle can be regulated and controlled.
- ↓ Risks of benign ovarian tumours.
- ↓ Incidence of PID.
- Improvement in skin condition in acne vulgaris.
- Possible ↓ symptoms:
  - premenstrual syndrome
  - endometriosis.
- ↓ Risks of colorectal cancer.
- ↓ Ovarian cancer risk ≥50% during use and for >15yrs after.

Disadvantages
- ↑ Risks (although absolute risk is very low)
  - VTE
  - stroke
  - cardiovascular disease.
- Small ↑ risk of breast cancer: returns to the background risk 10yrs after stopping.
- Very small association with ↑ risk of cervical cancer.

The pill and VTE
The absolute risk of VTE is:
- *Background risk:* 5:100 000 women/yr.
- *2nd generation COCP:* 10–15:100 000 women/yr.
- *3rd generation COCP:* 25:100 000 women/yr.
- *Pregnancy:* 60:100 000 women/yr.

Current CSM advice regarding the COCP and VTE
As long as women are well informed of the small increased risk of thrombosis associated with 3rd generation pills, and do not have any medical contraindications, it should be a matter of user preference and clinical judgement on which COCP is to be prescribed. Combined hormonal contraception is contraindicated where there is a personal history of VTE or a known thrombogenic gene mutation.

Combined oral contraceptive pill: regimes

'Pill-teach'
- Contraception is immediate if the woman starts the pill between days 1 and 5 of her cycle.
- If her first pill is after day 5, other contraception is needed for 7 days.
- Take the pill the same time every day.
- One pill daily for 21 days followed by 7 pill-free days. Some formulations have 7 'dummy pills', rather than the pill-free interval.
- If vomiting or diarrhoea use extra contraception from the onset of illness and continue it for the next 7 days.

Special circumstances
- Post-partum (not breast-feeding): start day 21 after delivery.
- Post-termination: within 7 days of termination.
- Switching from other oral hormonal contraception: start immediately if using other contraception reliably.
- Switching from implant or injectable progestagens: start at any time up to removal of implant or when injection is due.

Drug interactions
- No additional contraception is needed if taking antibiotics unless associated with diarrhoea/vomiting.
- COCP should not be prescribed to lamotrigine users as it decreases the serum drug concentration and therefore increases seizure frequency.
- Patients taking enzyme-inducing medication should be offered alternative contraceptive method due to ↓ efficacy. If it is decided to continue the COCP, the ethinyloestradiol should be increased to 50 micrograms, or the pill-free interval reduced to 4 days.

Missed pills
⚠ Missed pills may lead to failed contraception. The risk of pregnancy is greatest at the beginning and the end of the pack.

Missed pill rules
If 1 pill is missed
- Take the missed pill as soon as possible.
- Continue the rest of the pack as usual.
- No additional contraception is required.

If 2 or more pills are missed
- Take the most recent missed pill as soon as possible.
- Continue the rest of the pack as normal.
- Additional contraceptive cover is required until 7 consecutive pills have been taken.
- *If the missed pills are in day 1–7:* emergency contraception should be considered.
- *If the missed pills are in day 8–14:* emergency contraception not needed.
- *If the missed pills are in day 15–21:* omit the pill free interval.

⚠ Qlaira® has different missed pill rules (see manufacturer's advice).

Other combined hormonal contraceptives
Vaginal ring
- Ethinylestradiol with etonogestrel.
- Remains *in situ* for 21 days, then removed for 7 days to induce a withdrawal bleed.

Transdermal patch
- Ethinylestradiol with norelgestromin.
- Replaced weekly for 21 days, then 7 patch-free days to induce a withdrawal bleed.

▶ Efficacy and side effect profile as for COCP.

Progestagen-only pill

POPs currently marketed contain either levonorgestrel, norethisterone, or etynodiol acetate. The failure rate ranges from 0.3 to 4.0% per 100 woman-years and decreases with age.

▶ Cerazette®, a POP (75 micrograms desogestrel), reliably blocks ovulation, increasing efficacy.

⚠ To be reliable, a POP must be taken at the same time every day.

Mode of action
- Thickened cervical mucus (4h after dose).
- Thin endometrium preventing implantation.
- Inhibition of ovulation (60% old POP, 97% desogestrel).

Indications
Useful in conditions where COCP is contraindicated:
- During lactation—has no effect on quality or quantity of milk.
- Sickle cell disease.
- SLE and other autoimmune diseases.

Side effects
- Menstrual disturbance—regular (40%), irregular (40%), or amenorrhoea (20%).
- Headaches, nausea, mood swings, abdominal bloating, and breast tenderness—usually subside after a few months.

Drug interactions
- Broad spectrum antibiotics do not affect the efficacy of POP.
- Rifampicin and other enzyme-inducing drugs increase the metabolism of POP, leading to a reduction in efficacy.

Contraindications to the POP
- Pregnancy.
- Undiagnosed genital tract bleeding.
- Severe arterial disease.
- Active hepatic disease.
- History of recurrent follicular cysts.

How to take the POP
- Take the pill daily, at the same hour.
- If started on day 1 of the cycle no extra contraception is required.
- If started after day 5, extra contraception should be used for 48h.
- After miscarriage or TOP: start on the day of the miscarriage or TOP.
- After delivery: start on day 21 (whether breast-feeding or not). From COCP to POP: if the first POP is taken the day after the last active COCP, no other contraception is needed.

Missed POP rules
- If >3h late or 27h since last dose:
  - take missed pill as soon as possible
  - take subsequent pill at the usual time
  - use extra contraception for the next 48h.
- If vomit within 2h of ingestion:
  - take another pill now
  - use extra contraception for the next 48h.

⚠ For Cerazette® same rules apply if missed pill is >12h late.

Other forms of contraception

Injectable progestagen

Depo-Provera® (MDPA) (given 12-weekly)
• Useful for women who are unable or unwilling to take a pill.
• Contains 150mg of medroxyprogesterone.

▶ Very effective (failure rate <1 per 100 woman-years).

Side effects
• Menstrual disturbance (regular, irregular, or even amenorrhoea).
• Delayed conception (fertility may not return for 6–12mths).
• Weight gain (probably due to progestagen ↑ appetite).
• Bone loss (small risk of ↓ bone density with prolonged use).

Progestagen-only subdermal implant

Nexplanon® (has replaced Implanon® in the UK):
• Contains etonogestrel.
• Insertion and removal involves a small procedure under local anaesthetic (inserted into the arm).
• It lasts for 3yrs.
• Is radio-opaque.
• Specially designed applicator to minimize incorrect insertion.

▶ Highly effective (failure rate reported as <0.1 per 100 woman-years).

Side effects
Menstrual disturbance—20% amenorrhoea, 50% erratic bleeding.

Copper-bearing IUCD

• Provides long-term reversible contraception.
• Insertion is usually easy.
• May be retained beyond the menopause.

▶ Very effective (failure rate of 0.6–0.8 per 100 woman-years).

Mode of action
• Foreign body reaction in the endometrium prevents implantation.
• Copper content may inhibit spermatozoa motility.

Complications
• Irregular PV bleeding, especially first 3–6mths.
• Risk of infection: screen for Chlamydia prior to insertion.
• IUCD expulsion: most common in the first 3mths after insertion.
• Perforation: poor insertion technique or <4wks post-partum.
• Dysmenorrhoea.

Timing of IUCD insertion
• Insert any time during cycle (as long as pregnancy excluded).
• Post-partum: safe to insert IUCD from 4wks after delivery.
• Following TOP: insert within first 48h after termination.
• Switching from other contraception: any time as long as not pregnant.

Contraindications to copper-bearing IUCD

• Pregnancy.
• Undiagnosed genital tract bleeding.
• Active genital tract infection or PID.
• Uterine anomalies or fibroids distorting cavity.
• Copper allergy.

Levonorgestrel-releasing system (Mirena® IUS)

The LNG-releasing system has a T-shaped rod containing 52mg LNG (20 micrograms released daily). It is a reversible, highly effective contraceptive with a failure rate of 0.18 per 100 woman-years.

Due to its progestagenic content, menstrual blood loss is decreased by >90%, and it is as effective as endometrial ablation in the management of menorrhagia at 1yr.

Mode of action

• It acts on the endometrium, leading to endometrial atrophy and preventing implantation.
• Thickened cervical mucus inhibits sperm penetration.

▶ It is particularly useful when oestrogen is contraindicated.
• May be used in patients with a history of breast cancer: no disease for 5yrs and after consultation with breast surgeon.
• Breast-feeding: can be inserted 4 or more weeks post-partum.

Side effects

• Irregular PV bleeding is common in the first 3–4mths: amenorrhoea in up to 30% by 1yr.
• Hormonal symptoms: nausea, headache, breast tenderness, bloating.

Emergency contraception

Emergency contraception (EC) is licensed for use to protect women from unwanted pregnancy following UPSI or contraceptive failure.

The two main forms are:
- Oral EC—LNG or ulipristal (ellaOne®).
- Copper IUCD EC.

Levonogestrel (LNG EC)
- Consists of a single oral dose of 1.5mg of LNG.
- If taken within 72h of unprotected coitus it is estimated to prevent 85% of expected pregnancies.
- It may be used up to 120h after, but efficacy is uncertain and it is not licensed for use after 72h.
- It may also be used more than once in a cycle if clinically indicated.
- It does not provide contraceptive cover for the remainder of the cycle, another method of contraception must be used.

Side effects
- Nausea is common after ingestion.
- Vomiting only affects 1%.
- If a woman vomits within 2h of ingestion, she should take a further dose as soon as possible.
- Erratic PV bleeding is common in the first 7 days following treatment.

Ulipristal
- Progesterone receptor modulator.
- Licensed for use within 120h of UPSI.
- Can only be used once per cycle.
- Due to mode of action may impair the effectiveness of progestagen-containing contraceptives for the remainder of the cycle and so alternative contraceptive methods are advised.

Copper IUCD
- IUCD acts as an emergency contraceptive by inhibiting fertilization by direct toxicity.
- Affects implantation by inducing an inflammatory reaction in the endometrium.
- The copper content may also inhibit sperm transport.
- IUCD EC can be inserted within 120h following UPSI.
- Failure rates are less than 1%.

The risks and complications for IUCD EC are similar to IUCD use in general. It can be removed after the next menstruation provided that no unprotected coitus has occurred since menstruation, or retained for ongoing contraception.

Female sterilization: preoperative considerations

Sterilization has become increasingly popular since the late 1960s and it is now the most commonly used method of contraception in women over 40yrs of age.

History and examination

- This includes reasons for sterilization, menstrual history, current contraception, obstetric history, previous abdominal surgery, chronic medical conditions, and drug history.
- The patient's BMI should be noted and abdominal examination performed to look for scars from previous surgery or pelvic masses (previous surgery, endometriosis, PID, or fibroids may make the procedure technically difficult).

Counselling

⚠ It is important to establish that the woman is taking the decision of her own free will.

⚠ Alternatives to procedure must be discussed, including long-acting reversible contraceptives (LARCs) and vasectomy.

- Must use effective contraception until her first period following sterilization. The commonest reason for failure is already being pregnant when the procedure is performed or in the same cycle!
- Reassure that there is no increased risk of heavier periods in women >30yrs of age. There is a small association with increased hysterectomy rates, but the reason is unclear.
- Laparoscopy and tubal occlusion with Filshie clips is usually the method of choice and must be explained, including the operative risks.
- Counselling must be supported by printed information leaflets.

> **Consent for female sterilization**
> - Written informed consent must be taken from patient prior to procedure: in case of doubt regarding mental capacity, case should be referred to court for judgement.
> - Patient must fully understand that the procedure is intended to be permanent: success rates with reversal procedures are very small and rarely provided by the NHS.
> - Lifetime risk of failure with tubal occlusion is 1:200:
>   - pregnancies can occur several years after procedure
>   - longest follow-up data available for Filshie clips suggest failure rate after 10yrs of 2–3 per 1000 procedures.
> - In case of failure: ↑ risk of ectopic pregnancy: advise women to seek medical attention if pregnant/have abnormal pain and bleeding.
>
> There is a risk of injury to the blood vessels, bowel, and bladder with laparoscopic surgery: women must be warned about the possibility of a laparotomy, particularly if they have had previous abdominal surgery.

Women at higher risk of regret

Care must be taken when considering sterilization for women from the following groups, as they are more likely to have regret and present requesting reversal:
• Under the age of 30yrs: current RCOG recommendation to avoid.
• Who do not have children.
• Who decide during pregnancy.
• Who have had recent relationship loss.

Female sterilization: the procedure

Preoperative—mandatory checklist
- Document LMP.
- Check current contraception has been used to date.
- Pregnancy test must be performed (a negative test does not exclude the possibility of a luteal phase pregnancy).
- If any doubt exists about certainty of wishes or risk of pregnancy, the procedure should be abandoned.

Intraoperative
- Day case laparoscopic procedure is associated with quicker recovery rates and less morbidity than mini-laparotomy.
- Usually general anaesthesia, but local anaesthesia is an acceptable alternative.
- Laparascopic mechanical occlusion of the tubes by either Filshie clips or rings: diathermy ↑ the risk of ectopic pregnancies and is less easy to reverse.
- When a mini-laparotomy is used, any effective surgical or mechanical method of tubal occlusion can be used (a modified Pomeroy procedure may be preferable for post-partum sterilization or at the time of CS due to lower failure rates).

Postoperative
- The patient must be informed about the method of occlusion used and any procedural complications.
- She must be advised to use effective contraception till her next menstrual period.

Special circumstances
- Tubal occlusion should ideally be performed after an appropriate interval following pregnancy.
- Sterilization post-partum or post-abortion carries a higher risk of regret and possibly increased failure rates.
- In cases of sterilization at the time of CS, counselling and consent should be taken at least 1wk before the procedure.

Newer techniques
Hysteroscopic methods for sterilization are still under evaluation. Essure is the only form of hysteroscopic tubal occlusion licensed for use in the UK at present. It involves placing a metal micro-insert in the fallopian tubes under hysteroscopic guidance. This causes tubal blockage by subsequent fibrosis. A hysterosalpingogram is usually done 3mths after the operation to confirm tubal blockage.

Chapter 21

Menopause

Menopause: overview

All women will go through the menopause and the average age is 52yrs. The menopause is the cessation of the menstrual cycle and is caused by ovarian failure leading to oestrogen deficiency. Worldwide life expectancy is increasing and women live longer than men. A woman's average life expectancy at birth in the UK is currently 81yrs and is estimated to reach 85yrs by 2031. Thus UK women can expect more than 30yrs of post-menopausal life. This population expansion will lead to an increasing importance of the health problems that affect post-menopausal women.

Definitions

- *Menopause* is the permanent cessation of menstruation that results from loss of ovarian follicular activity. Natural menopause is recognized to have occurred after 12 consecutive months of amenorrhoea for which no other obvious pathological or physiological cause is present.
- *Peri-menopause* includes the period beginning with the first clinical, biological, and endocrinological features of the approaching menopause, such as vasomotor symptoms and menstrual irregularity, and ends 12mths after the last menstrual period.
- *Pre-menopause* is a term often used to refer either to the 1–2yrs immediately before the menopause or to the whole of the reproductive period before the menopause. Currently, this term is recommended to be used in the latter sense.
- *Post-menopause* should be defined from the final menstrual period regardless of whether the menopause was induced or spontaneous.
- *Menopausal transition* is the period of time before the final menstrual period, when variability in the menstrual cycle usually is increased.
- *Climacteric* is the phase encompassing the transition from the reproductive state to the non-reproductive state. The menopause itself thus is a specific event that occurs during the climacteric, just as the menarche is a specific event that occurs during puberty.

Menopause: short-term consequences

Vasomotor symptoms

Hot flushes and night sweats are the commonest symptoms of the menopause, and, although they may begin before periods stop, the prevalence of flushes is highest in the first year after the final menstrual period. Although they usually are present for less than 5yrs, some women will continue to flush into their 70s.

Sexual dysfunction

Changes in sexual behaviour and activity are common. The term *female sexual dysfunction* (FSD) is now used. The percentage of women with sexual dysfunction rises from 42% to 88% during the early to late menopausal transition. The underlying reasons for FSD are commonly multifactorial. For example, vaginal dryness, which results from declining levels of oestrogen, can cause dyspareunia. Low androgen levels have been implicated in low sexual desire though the evidence is conflicting. Non-hormonal factors, such as conflict between partners and life stress or depression, are important contributors to a woman's level of interest in sexual activity. In addition, male sexual problems should not be overlooked.

Sexual problems are classified into various types:
- Loss of sexual desire.
- Loss of sexual arousal.
- Problems with orgasm.
- Sexual pain such as painful sex or dyspareunia.

Psychological symptoms

Psychological symptoms associated with the menopause include:
- Depressed mood.
- Anxiety.
- Irritability and mood swings.
- Lethargy and lack of energy.

However, most women do not experience major changes in mood at the menopause and psychological problems are likely to be associated with past problems and current life stresses.

Menopause: long-term consequences

Osteoporosis

Osteoporosis affects 1 in 3 women and 1 in 12 men. It is as 'a skeletal disorder characterized by compromised bone strength predisposing to an increased risk of fracture' (Table 21.1). Bone strength reflects the integration of two main features: bone density and bone quality. Bone density is expressed as grams of mineral per area or volume and, in any given individual, is determined by peak bone mass and amount of bone loss. BMD scan is used to measure the thickness of the bone in the hip and lumbar spine. Bone quality refers to architecture, turnover, damage accumulation (for example, microfractures), and mineralization. A fracture occurs when a failure-inducing force, which may or may not involve trauma, is applied to osteoporotic bone. Thus, osteoporosis is a significant risk factor for fracture. Fractures are the clinical consequences of osteoporosis.

The most common sites of osteoporotic fractures are:
• Lower end of radius (wrist or Colles' fracture).
• Proximal femur (hip).
• Vertebrae.

Cardiovascular disease

Myocardial infarction and stroke are the primary clinical endpoints. Cardiovascular disease (CVD) is the most common cause of death in women over 60. Oophorectomized women are at 2–3-fold higher risk of coronary heart disease (CrHD) than age-matched pre-menopausal women.

Urogenital atrophy

The lower urinary and genital tracts have a common embryological origin and are approximated closely in adult women. Oestrogen receptors and progesterone receptors are present in the vagina, urethra, bladder, and pelvic floor musculature. Oestrogen deficiency after menopause causes atrophic changes within the urogenital tract and is associated with urinary symptoms, such as frequency, urgency, nocturia, incontinence, and recurrent infection. These symptoms may coexist with those of vaginal atrophy, including dyspareunia, itching, burning, and dryness.

Table 21.1 Risk factors for osteoporosis

Risk factor	Example
Genetic	Family history of fracture (particularly a 1st-degree relative with hip fracture)
Constitutional	Low BMI Early menopause (<45yrs of age)
Environmental	Cigarette smoking Alcohol abuse Low calcium intake Sedentary lifestyle
Drugs	Corticosteroids, >5mg prednisolone or equivalent daily Aromatase inhibitors GnRH analogues
Diseases	Rheumatoid arthritis Neuromuscular disease Chronic liver disease Malabsorption syndromes Hyperparathyroidism Hyperthyroidism Hypogonadism

Menopause: history taking and investigations

History

Symptoms, periods, and contraception
- Hot flushes and night sweats.
- Vaginal dryness.
- Other symptoms.
- Date of last menstrual period (could she be pregnant?).
- Frequency, heaviness, and duration of periods.
- Contraception.

Gynaecological history
- Hysterectomy.
- Oophorectomy.

Past medical and surgical history
- Risk factors for osteoporosis (see Table 21.1).
- Confirmed deep vein thrombosis or pulmonary embolism.
- Risk factors for cardiovascular disease (e.g. smoking, hypertension, diabetes).
- Breast cancer, benign breast disease, and date last mammogram (if applicable).
- Does she have migraines?
- Current medications.
- Does she take alternative or complementary therapies?

Family history in close family members
- Breast, ovarian, or bowel cancer.
- Confirmed deep vein thrombosis or pulmonary embolism.
- Cardiovascular disease.
- Osteoporosis.

Investigations
- FSH only helpful if diagnosis is in doubt, such as below age 40 and levels in menopausal range (>30IU/L).
- Luteinizing hormone, oestradiol, and progesterone are of no value in the diagnosis of ovarian failure.
- Thyroid function tests (free T_4 and thyroid-stimulating hormone) as abnormalities of thyroid function can be confused with menopausal symptoms.
- Testosterone levels are of uncertain value.
- BMD if significant risk factors for osteoporosis (Table 21.2).

Consequences of premature menopause

- Women with untreated premature menopause (no oestrogen replacement) are at increased risk of osteoporosis and cardiovascular disease, but at lower risk of breast malignancy.
- Premature menopause can lead to reduced peak bone mass (if <25yrs old) or early bone loss thereafter.

⚠ Mean life expectancy in women with menopause before the age of 40yrs is 2.0yrs shorter than that in women with menopause after the age of 55yrs.

Hormone replacement therapy: overview

More than 50 HRT preparations, which feature different strengths, combinations, and routes of administration, are available. HRT can be given either systemically for hot flushes and osteoporosis or vaginally (or topically) for local symptoms such as vaginal dryness. In non-hysterectomized women HRT consists of an oestrogen combined with a progestagen.

Oestrogens

Oestrogens used in HRT include oestradiol, oestrone, and oestriol, which, although chemically synthesized from soya beans or yams, are molecularly identical to the natural human hormone. Conjugated equine oestrogens containing about 50–65% oestrone sulphate, with the remainder being equine oestrogens (mainly equilin sulphate), are also used.

Progestagens

The progestagens used in HRT are almost all synthetic and derived from plant sources. They are structurally different from progesterone. 17-hydroxyprogesterone and 19-nortestosterone derivatives are the progestagens used most commonly in HRT.

17-Hydroxyprogesterone
- Dydrogesterone.
- Medroxyprogesterone acetate.

19-Nortestosterone derivatives
- Norethisterone.
- Levonorgestrel.

Other hormones used at the menopause
- *Tibolone:* is a synthetic steroid compound that itself is inert, but on absorption is converted to metabolites with oestrogenic, progestagenic, and androgenic actions. It is classified as HRT in the British National Formulary. It is used in post-menopausal women.
- *Testosterone:* patches and implants may be used to improve libido.

Treatment of local symptoms

Some women do not wish to take, or cannot tolerate, systemic HRT and simply require relief of local symptoms, which are usually urogenital. Synthetic or conjugated equine oestrogens should be avoided, as they are well absorbed from the vagina. The options available are low-dose natural oestrogens, such as vaginal estriol by cream or pessary or estradiol by tablet or ring. Treatment is needed in the long term, if not lifelong, as symptoms return on cessation of treatment. With the recommended dose regimens, no adverse endometrial effects should be incurred, and a progestagen need not be added in non-hysterectomized women.

Types of systemic oestrogen-based HRT
- Oestrogen alone in hysterectomized women.
- Oestrogen plus progestagen in non-hysterectomized women.
  - oestrogen and cyclical progestagen in peri-menopausal women
  - continuous combined oestrogen–progestagen ('no bleed' HRT) in post-menopausal women.
- *Routes of administration of oestrogen:*
  - oral
  - transdermal
  - subcutaneous
  - vaginal.
- *Routes of administration of progestagen:*
  - oral
  - transdermal
  - intrauterine (levonorgestrel).

Minimum bone-sparing doses of HRT
- *Estradiol oral:* 1–2mg
- *Estradiol patch:* 25–50 micrograms
- *Estradiol gel:* 1–5g*
- *Estradiol implant:* 50mg every 6mths
- *Conjugated equine estrogens:* 0.3–0.625mg daily

*Depends on preparation: lower doses may be effective.

Side effects of systemic HRT
- Oestrogen-related: fluid retention, bloating, breast tenderness or enlargement, nausea, headaches, leg cramps, and dyspepsia.*
- Progestagen-related: fluid retention, breast tenderness, headaches or migraine, mood swings, depression, acne, lower abdominal pain, and backache.*
- Combined HRT: irregular, breakthrough bleeding (may need investigation).
- All types of HRT: weight gain (but not proved in randomized trials).

* Changing dose, type, and route of administration (tablet to patch) may help.

Hormone replacement therapy: benefits

Two large studies—randomized Women's Health Initiative (WHI) and the observational Million Women Study (MWS)—undertaken in women aged >50 resulted in controversy about use of HRT. There are benefits and risks in its use, and some uncertainty concerning some claims made about HRT.

Benefits of HRT
- ↓ Vasomotor symptoms.
- ↓ Urogenital symptoms and improved sexuality.
- ↓ Risk of osteoporosis.
- ↓ Risk of colorectal cancer.

Relief of vasomotor symptoms
- Oestrogen is effective in treating hot flushes:
  - improvement usually is noted within 4wks
  - maximum therapeutic response usually achieved by 3mths
  - should be continued for at least 1yr or symptoms often recur
  - the most common indication for a prescription of HRT
  - often is used for fewer than 5yrs.
- Oestrogen more effective than SSRIs or clonidine (largely ineffective).

Urogenital symptoms and sexuality
- Urogential symptoms respond well to oestrogen (which may be given vaginally or systemically).
- Improvement may take several months.
- Long-term treatment often is needed, as symptoms can recur.
- Urinary incontinence is not improved by systemic therapy.
- Sexuality may be improved with oestrogen alone, but may need addition of testosterone, especially in young oophorectomized women.

Osteoporosis
- HRT ↓ the risk of spine and hip and other osteoporotic fractures.
- Most epidemiological studies suggest continuous and lifelong use is required for HRT to be an effective method of preventing fracture.
- The efficacy of alternatives such as bisphosphonates in peri-menopausal or early post-menopausal women remains uncertain.
- HRT is significantly cheaper than alternative therapies, such as bisphosphonates, strontium ranelate, and parathyroid hormone.

Colorectal cancer
- HRT ↓ the risk of colorectal cancer by about 1/3.
- Little known about risk when treatment is stopped or in high risk populations.
- Currently, prevention of colonic cancer is not an indication for HRT.

Hormone replacement therapy: risks

Risks of HRT
- ↑ Risk of breast cancer.
- ↑ Risk of endometrial cancer with unopposed oestrogen.
- ↑ Risk of VTE.
- ↑ Risk of gallbladder disease.

Endometrial cancer
- Unopposed oestrogen ↑ the risk of endometrial cancer:
  - the relative risk (RR) is 2.3
  - risk ↑ with prolonged use (RR 9.5 for ≥10yrs)
  - risk remains ↑ for 5 or more years after stopping (RR 2.3).
- This risk is not eliminated completely with the addition of monthly sequential progestagen (especially if used for >5yrs).
- No ↑ risk has been found with continuous combined HRT.

Venous thromboembolism
⚠ HRT more than doubles the risk of VTE, but absolute risk remains small.
- For non-users, over a 5yr period, the incidence of VTE will be:
  - 3:1000 women aged 50–59yrs
  - 8:1000 women aged 60–69yrs.
- The number of additional VTE events in healthy women on HRT ≥5yrs is estimated to be:
  - 4:1000 women aged 50–59yrs
  - 9:1000 women aged 60–69yrs.
- The VTE is more likely in the first year of HRT.
- ↑ Age, obesity, and thrombophilia significantly ↑ risk of VTE.
- Using HRT after VTE has ↑ risk of recurrence in first year of use.
- Transdermal HRT may be associated with a lower risk than oral.

Gallbladder disease
- HRT appears to ↑ the risk of gallbladder disease, but:
- Risk ↑ with age and obesity.
- Women who use HRT may have silent pre-existing disease.

Risk of breast cancer with HRT

- HRT confers a similar degree of risk to late natural menopause:
  - every year the menopause is naturally delayed, the risk ↑ by 2.8%
  - with HRT, the risk ↑ by 2.3% per year.
- The risk is dependent on duration of HRT.
- The effect is not sustained once HRT is stopped: 5yrs after stopping, the risk is the same as for women who have never had HRT.
- The risk of breast cancer with HRT is dependent on the regimen:
  - greatest with combined oestrogen–progestagen HRT
  - less with unopposed oestrogen (but ↑ risk of endometrial cancer).

⚠ Combined HRT probably accounts for an extra 3 breast cancers per 1000 women who start it at the age of 50yrs and use it for 5yrs.

☛ All risk estimates are based on starting HRT at 50; this effect is not seen in women who start it early for premature menopause (therefore duration of exposure to female sex hormones is probably relevant).

☛ The increase in risk of breast cancer found in nulliparous women, those with a high BMI, those who delay their first birth, and those who have a family history may be higher than that conferred by HRT.

Hormone replacement therapy: uncertainties

Uncertainties concerning HRT
- Cardiovascular disease.
- Dementia.
- Ovarian cancer.
- Quality of life.

Cardiovascular disease
- The role of HRT in 1° or 2° prevention is uncertain, and it should not be used primarily for this indication.
- The timing, dose, and possibly type of HRT, however, may be critical in determining cardiovascular effects: women in the WHI who started HRT within 10yrs of the menopause had a lower risk of coronary heart disease than women who started later.

Dementia and cognition
- Oestrogen may delay or ↓ the risk of Alzheimer's disease, but it does not seem to improve established disease.
- It is unclear if there is a critical age to start HRT or an optimal duration of treatment to prevent dementia.

Ovarian cancer
- There is ↑ risk in the very long term (>10yrs) with oestrogen alone.
- This risk is not seen with continuous combined therapy.

🖝 This issue is unresolved and requires further examination. Currently insufficient evidence is available to recommend alterations in HRT prescribing practice.

Quality of life
🖝 Although some studies have shown improvement in both symptomatic and asymptomatic women, others have not. This area is difficult to evaluate because of the different measures used, varying levels of menopausal symptoms, a large placebo effect, and extrinsic factors that may alter women's responses.

Alternative medical treatments to hormone replacement therapy

Publication of the WHI and the MWS studies led to women stopping HRT and considering alternative medical treatments to eleviate menopausal symptoms.

Treatment of vasomotor symptoms

- *SSRIs:* fluoxetine and paroxetine.
- *SNRI:* venlafaxine.
- *Clonidine (α-agonist):* once mainstay treatment, but now shown as having limited effect.

Prevention and treatment of osteoporosis

Agent used to either inhibit bone resorption or stimulate bone formation.

- Calcium and vitamin D.
- Bisphosphonates (inhibits osteoclasts).
- Selective oestrogen reuptake modulators (SERMs).

Urogenital symptoms

- Oestrogen cream, an intra-vaginal sustained-release oestradiol ring, or oestradiol vaginal tablets are the most effective treatment for vaginal atrophy and dyspareunia.
- Patient can be reassured of minimal systemic absorption and no need for added progestagen.
- Alternative treatment to alleviate dyspareunia; vaginal lubricant and bio-adhesive moisturizers (Replens®).

Urogynaecology

Classification of urinary incontinence

Urinary incontinence is the complaint of any involuntary leakage of urine. It can result from a variety of different conditions and it is useful to classify them accordingly.

Stress urinary incontinence
The involuntary leakage of urine on effort or exertion, or on sneezing or coughing. Commonly arises from urethral sphincter weakness.

Urge urinary incontinence
The involuntary leakage of urine accompanied by, or immediately preceded by, a strong desire to pass urine (void). Urgency, with or without urge urinary incontinence, usually with frequency and nocturia is also defined as overactive bladder (OAB) syndrome.

Mixed urinary incontinence
The involuntary leakage of urine associated both with urgency and with exertion, effort, sneezing, or coughing. Usually, one of these is predominant, i.e. either the symptoms of urge incontinence, or those of stress incontinence, are most bothersome.

Overflow incontinence
Occurs when the bladder becomes large and flaccid and has little or no detrusor tone or function. This is usually due to injury or insult, e.g. after surgery or post-partum. The condition is diagnosed when the urinary residual is more than 50% of bladder capacity. The bladder simply leaks when it becomes full.

Continuous urinary incontinence
The complaint of continuous leakage. Classically it is associated with a fistula or congenital abnormality, e.g. ectopic ureter.

Other types of incontinence
- Incontinence arising from urinary tract infections, medications, immobility, or cognitive impairment.
- Situational incontinence, e.g. giggle incontinence.

Urinary symptoms

- *Urinary incontinence:* is the complaint of involuntary urinary leakage, which can be divided, broadly, into stress incontinence and urge incontinence.
- *Daytime frequency:* the number of times a woman voids during waking hours—normally between 4 and 7 voids/day. Increased daytime frequency is when a woman perceives she voids too often.
- *Nocturia:* the complaint of having to wake at night one or more times to void. Up to the age of 70yrs, more than a single void is considered abnormal.
- *Nocturnal enuresis:* urinary incontinence occurring during sleep.
- *Urgency:* sudden compelling desire to pass urine, which is difficult to defer. Urgency is most frequently 2° to detrusor overactivity, although inflammatory bladder conditions such as interstitial cystitis may also present with this.
- *Voiding difficulties* include:
  - hesitancy (difficulty in initiating micturition)
  - straining to void
  - slow or intermittent urinary stream.

These are all suggestive of urethral obstruction, underactive detrusor muscle, or loss of coordination between detrusor construction and urethral relaxation. Intermittency is seen with neurological disease.

- *Post-micturition symptoms* include:
  - feeling of incomplete bladder emptying
  - terminal dribble (a prolonged final part of micturition)
  - post-micturitional dribble (the involuntary loss of urine immediately after passing urine).
- *Absent or reduced bladder sensation:* usually due to denervation caused by spinal cord injuries or pelvic surgery. Leads to infrequent micturition and large-capacity bladder, and is often associated with overflow incontinence.
- *Bladder pain:* felt suprapubically or retropubically. Typically occurs with bladder filling and is relieved by emptying it. Pain is indicative of intravesical pathology, such as interstitial cystitis or malignancy, and warrants further investigation.
- *Urethral pain:* felt in urethra (the woman indicates this as the site of the discomfort).
- *Dysuria:* pain experienced in bladder or urethra on passing urine. Most frequently associated with urinary tract infections.
- *Haematuria:* presence of blood in urine; can be micro- or macroscopic (frank). Always significant and warrants further investigation.

Assessment of the lower urinary tract: history and examination

History

- The onset of urinary symptoms, their duration, and their severity should be recorded (the predominant bother symptom, e.g. urgency, urge incontinence, or stress incontinence, should be identified).
- Different underlying conditions can cause similar urinary symptoms; history alone is often a poor predictor of pathophysiology.
- Check for coexisting medical conditions and optimize their treatment (the onset of diabetes significantly increases urine output and many pharmaceutical agents can alter bladder function).
- Enquire about colorectal symptoms and genitourinary prolapse.

Quality of life assessment

- A good clinical history will enquire how symptoms affect aspects of daily life and social, personal and sexual relationships.
- Disease-specific QoL questionnaires allow in-depth assessment of the impact-specific symptoms on a woman's life: validated questionnaires are available from the International Consultation on Incontinence (⌖ www.iciq.net).

Frequency/volume chart

- The frequency/volume chart (Fig. 22.1) is a simple and practical method of obtaining objective quantification of fluid intake and voiding behaviour.
- Fluid intake, frequency, times of voiding, and leakage episodes (day and night) are recorded for at least 24h (typically 3 days).

Physical examination

General examination

- Weight (BMI), BP, urinalysis.
- Check for signs of systemic disease.
- Mobility and mental state.
- Motivation and manual dexterity.
- Neurological examination, if there are any symptoms that point to a possible neurological cause.

Abdominal examination

- Exclude an abdominal or pelvic mass (⚠ including pregnancy).
- Exclude a full bladder (obstruction/retention).

Pelvic examination

- Condition of the vulval skin (any atrophy, erythema, or oedema).
- Presence and degree of any concurrent uterovaginal prolapse.
- Assessment of urethral and bladder neck descent on straining.
- Assessment of pelvic floor muscle strength (graded 0–5 on a modified Oxford scale; see 📖 Prolapse: clinical assessment, p. 676).

Frequency/Volume Chart

Name: *Mrs Smith* Patient No. *1234567* Week commencing *26 Jan 2006*

Time	Date:26.01.06 Day 1			Date:27.01.06 Day 2			Date:28.01.06 Day 3		
	In	Out	Wet	In	Out	Wet	In	Out	Wet
am									
1		300	X		500	X			
2		300	X						
3					600	X		700	X
4		350	X						
5									
6					600	X		600	X
7		500	X						
8				250	300			500	X
9	250	300		200			250		
10								300	
11							200		
12				200				100	
pm									
1	200	100			100				
2							200	300	
3									
4				200					
5	250	120						200	
6							200		
7				200	100				
8									
9		200			100				
10									
11		100			200		200	200	
12									
Total	650	2270		1050	2500		1050	2800	

Fig. 22.1 A 3-day frequency/volume chart showing severe nocturia.

Information obtainable from a frequency/volume chart

- Functional bladder capacity.
- Volumetric summary of diurnal urinary frequency.
- Volumetric summary of nocturnal urinary frequency.
- Quantification of total fluid intake.
- Distribution of fluid intake throughout the day.
- Total voided volume and diurnal distribution of voiding.
- Evaluation of the severity of urinary incontinence.

Assessment of the lower urinary tract: investigations

Basic investigations

Urinalysis
Reagent strip testing of urine for leucocyte esterase, nitrites, protein, blood, and glucose is a sensitive and cheap screening test.

Urine specimen
Bacteriological analysis of a midstream urine specimen for microscopy, culture, and sensitivity is reserved for those with a positive screening test.

Residual check
A post-void residual check should be carried out (either by USS or by catheterization) to exclude incomplete bladder emptying.

Pad test
This is a simple method of detecting and quantifying urinary leakage based on weight gain of absorbent pads during a set period of time.

▶ It is not helpful in determining the cause of urinary leakage.

Cystourethroscopy
- Allows visualization of all the lower urinary tract: urethra, bladder mucosa, trigone, and ureteric orifices.
- Can be performed using a rigid or flexible cystoscope, with or without anaesthesia.
- Bladder biopsies can be taken to obtain histological diagnosis and exclude malignancy.
- In cases of suspected interstitial cystitis a second-look cystoscopy should be performed after the initial bladder distension, to detect any glomerulations or petechial haemorrhages.

Indications for cystourethroscopy
- Recurrent UTIs.
- Haematuria.
- Bladder pain.
- Suspected urinary tract injury or fistula.
- To exclude bladder tumour or stones.
- If interstitial cystitis is suspected.

Assessment of the lower urinary tract: imaging

Imaging of the lower urinary tract is not justified as a routine investigation in all women presenting with urinary symptoms, but should instead be targeted at specific indications.

- *Ultrasonography:* is widely used to:
  - exclude incomplete bladder emptying
  - check for congenital abnormalities, calculi, tumours
  - detect cortical scarring of the kidneys.
- *Plain abdominal radiograph:* is useful for screening for a variety of conditions, including foreign bodies and calculi.
- *Contrast-enhanced CT:* is the imaging modality of choice for detecting and characterizing renal masses and renal tract calculi, as well as ureteric or bladder lesions.
- *IV urography:* can be used in women with neuropathic bladder or suspected congenital and acquired abnormalities, e.g. uterovaginal fistulae. However, contrast-enhanced CT would provide more accurate and rapid detection.
- *Micturating cystourethrography:* is useful to demonstrate bladder and urethral fistulae, vesicoureteric reflux, and anatomical abnormalities of the lower urinary tract, such as urethral diverticulae.
- *MRI:* remains predominantly a research investigative technique for incontinence and prolapse, because of its cost and availability. It is mainly used for characterization of renal or pelvic masses and tumour staging.

Conditions requiring imaging of urinary tract

- Recurrent UTIs.
- Haematuria.
- Urethral diverticula, which need to be differentiated from paravaginal cysts.
- Suspected ureteric injuries.
- Suspected urethral or vesical fistulae.
- Suspected malignancy or renal stones.

Assessment of the lower urinary tract: urodynamic investigations

Urodynamics

'Urodynamics' describes a combination of tests that look at the ability of the bladder to store and void urine. The tests include uroflowmetry, post-void residual measurement, and cystometry. In addition, urethral pressure profilometry and video-urodynamic investigations may be undertaken.

Uroflowmetry

Simple, non-invasive investigation that can be used to screen for voiding difficulties. The patient voids in privacy on a commode incorporating a urinary flow meter, measures voided volume over time, and plots it on a graph (Fig. 22.2).

Cystometry

- Involves measuring the pressure/volume relationship of the bladder during filling and voiding and is a useful test of bladder function.
- The bladder is filled with saline via a catheter, and the first sensation of filling, first desire to void, and any strong desire to void are recorded (Fig. 22.3).
- Electronic subtraction of the intra-abdominal pressure from the intravesical enables the detrusor pressure to be calculated (Fig. 22.4).
- During filling the patient is asked to cough at regular intervals and to stand, in order to provoke the bladder.
- The presence of detrusor contractions and leakage through the urethra are noted.
- The woman is then asked to void at the end of the test, for pressure/flow analysis.

Video-urodynamics

- Combines fluoroscopic imaging of the bladder neck with cystometry, while filling the bladder with an iodine-based contrast medium.
- Enables detection of detrusor-sphincter dyssynergia, vesico-ureteric reflux, or presence of abnormalities in the renal tract that are commonly seen in women with neurogenic bladder problems.

Ambulatory urodynamic monitoring

- A small recording device is worn and the information is later downloaded to a computer for analysis and review.
- The bladder is filled naturally and the woman should carry out her normal daily activities, including those that provoke symptoms.
- This approach is particularly useful for investigating detrusor over-activity when standard laboratory urodynamics have failed to replicate the symptoms experienced by the woman in her normal environment.

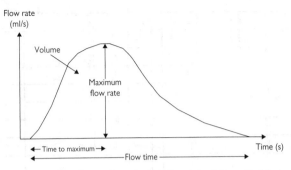

Fig. 22.2 Diagrammatic representation of normal urinary flow rate. *Voided volume*: total volume expelled via the urethra, the area beneath the flow-time curve. *Maximum flow rate*: maximum measured value of the flow rate. *Average flow rate*: volume voided divided by the flow time. *Flow time*: the time over which measurable flow actually occurs.

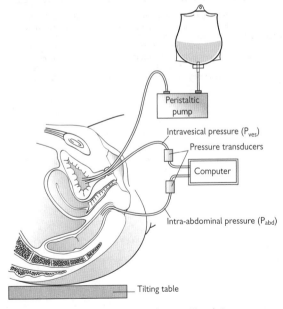

Fig. 22.3 Schematic drawing showing catheter positions during cystometry. Three catheters are required: the first in the bladder to fill it; the second in the bladder to measure vesical pressure; and the third in the rectum to measure abdominal pressure. Reproduced with permission from Cardozo L, Staskin D (2001). *Textbook of female urology and urogynaecology*, published by Taylor and Francis, London.

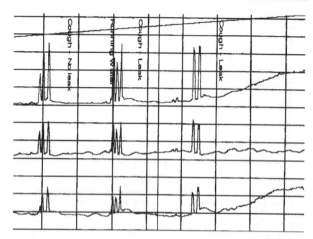

Fig. 22.4 Urodynamic trace showing urodynamic stress incontinence. The upper trace shows intravesical pressure (P_{ves}) and the middle trace shows pressure within the abdomen (P_{abd}), both measured against time. The lower trace, obtained by subtracting intra-abdominal pressure from intravesical pressure ($P_{det} = P_{ves} - P_{abd}$), shows the detrusor pressure. During the test there is no change in detrusor pressure, despite provocation with coughing, and leakage occurs only as a result of the momentary increase in intra-abdominal pressure caused by the coughing.

Stress urinary incontinence: overview

Definitions
- *Stress urinary incontinence (SUI)*: is the complaint of involuntary leakage of urine on effort or exertion, or on sneezing or coughing.
- *Urodynamic stress incontinence (USI)*: is the involuntary leakage of urine during increased intra-abdominal pressure in the absence of detrusor contractions. Unlike SUI, it can only be diagnosed by urodynamic testing (Fig. 22.4).

Incidence
- The commonest urinary complaint for which women seek advice.
- 1 in 10 women will suffer from it at some point in their lives.
- 50% of incontinent women complain of pure stress incontinence.
- 30–40% of incontinent women have mixed symptoms of urge and stress incontinence.

Pathophysiology and aetiology
- SUI occurs when the intravesical pressure exceeds the closing pressure on the urethra.
- Childbirth is the most common causative factor, leading to denervation of the pelvic floor, usually during delivery.
- Oestrogen deficiency at the time of menopause leads to weakening of the pelvic support and thinning of the urothelium.
- Occasionally, weakness of the bladder neck can occur congenitally, or through trauma from radical pelvic surgery or irradiation.

Clinical features
- *Symptoms*: typically a woman will complain of leakage of urine when she coughs, sneezes, runs, jumps, or carries heavy loads. The leakage is usually a small, discrete amount, coinciding with the physical activity.
- *Signs*: prolapse of the urethra and anterior vaginal wall may be present. It may be possible to demonstrate stress incontinence by asking the woman to cough with a fairly full bladder.

Investigations
- *MSU sample*: should be taken to exclude infection or glycosuria.
- *Frequency/volume chart*:
  - typically shows normal frequency and functional bladder capacity
  - slightly ↑ diurnal frequency may be observed, as women may void more frequently to prevent leakage.
- *Urodynamic studies* should be considered when surgery is indicated to:
  - confirm the diagnosis
  - check for any co-existing detrusor overactivity
  - check for voiding dysfunction.

Stress urinary incontinence: conservative management

SUI interferes with a woman's quality of life, but is not a life-threatening condition and therefore conservative measures should always be tried first. They include:

- *Lifestyle interventions:* weight reduction if BMI >30, smoking cessation, treatment of chronic cough and constipation.
- *Pelvic floor muscle training:* for at least 3mths should be considered as the first-line treatment:
  - physiotherapists usually individualize the programme, but 3 sets of 8–12 slow maximal contractions sustained for 6–8s each per day is a common regimen
  - the exercises need to be continued long term.
- *Biofeedback:* refers to the use of a device to convert the effect of pelvic floor contraction into a visual or auditory signal to allow women objective assessment of improvement.
- *Electrical stimulation:* can assist in production of muscle contractions in women who are unable to produce muscle contraction.
- *Vaginal cones:* have been developed as a way of applying graded resistance against which the pelvic floor muscles contract.

Pharmacological management of SUI

Duloxetine: is the only drug licensed for the treatment of moderate to severe SUI.

- It is an SNRI that enhances urethral striated sphincter activity via a centrally mediated pathway.
- However, it is of mediocre efficacy and is associated with significant side effects. It is not recommended for first-line use by NICE.
- Nausea is the most frequently reported side effect (up to 25%).
- Other side effects include dyspepsia, dry mouth, insomnia or drowsiness, and dizziness.

Indications for conservative treatment of stress urinary incontinence

- Mild or easily manageable symptoms.
- Family incomplete.
- Symptoms manifest during pregnancy.
- Surgery contraindicated by co-existing medical conditions.
- Surgery declined by patient.

Stress urinary incontinence: surgical management

Surgery may be considered when conservative measures have failed and the woman's quality of life is compromised. Before attempting surgical repair it is important to be clear about the underlying cause of the incontinence: USI may be successfully treated surgically, but detrusor overactivity may be made worse, and the effects are largely irreversible.

Peri-urethral injections

- Injectable peri-urethral bulking agents have lower immediate success rate (20–40%) and long-term continued decline in continence.
- However, the procedure has low morbidity and can be performed under local anaesthetic in outpatient settings.
- The advent of minimally invasive synthetic slings (e.g. tension-free vaginal tape (TVT)) has largely superseded this surgery.
- Injectables or bulking agents may be appropriate for:
  - frail, older, or unfit women
  - young women who have yet to complete their family.
- The most commonly used peri-urethral bulking agents are:
  - glutaraldehyde cross-linked bovine collagen
  - macroparticulate silicon particles (Macroplastique®, Uroplasty Ltd).

Burch colposuspension

- Largely replaced by TVT, now rarely performed.
- The retropubic space is entered through a low transverse suprapubic incision and two or three sutures placed between the paravaginal fascia and ipsilateral ileopectinal ligament (Cooper's ligament) at the level of the bladder.
- Complications may include: haemorrhage; injuries to the bladder or ureter; voiding difficulties; de-novo detrusor overactivity; enterocele or rectocele formation.
- Overall, meta-analysis of published data suggests that the efficacy of the Burch colposuspension as a primary procedure is 90% and as a repeat procedure is 83% (Table 22.1).

Laparoscopic colposuspension

- Efficacy and complications similar to those of the open procedure.
- The surgery is technically more demanding and requires considerable laparoscopic expertise.

Table 22.1 RMI score and ovarian cancer risk

Risk	RMI score	Risk of cancer
Low	<25	<3%
Moderate	25–250	20%
High	>250	75%

Data from: Davies AP, Jacobs I, Woolas R, et al. The adnexal mass: benign or malignant? Evaluation of a risk of malignancy index. *Br J Obstet Gynaecol* 1993;**100**(10): 927–31.

Tension-free vaginal tape (TVT)

▶ The most commonly performed surgical procedure for USI in the UK.

- A polypropylene tape is placed under the mid-urethra via a small vaginal incision, using local, regional, or general anaesthesia (Fig. 22.5).
- Cystourethroscopy is carried out to ensure no damage to the bladder or urethra.
- The procedure is minimally invasive and most women return to normal activity within 2wks.
- *Complications:*
  - moderately high risk of bladder injuries 5–10%, but these do not seem to have long-term sequelae, if treated appropriately
  - bleeding in retropubic space, infection, and voiding difficulties
  - tape erosion into the vagina and urethra has also been reported.
- The objective cure rate is 82–98% (mean 94%).

Transobturator tape (TOT)

- The polypropylene tape is passed via a transobturator foramen, through the transobturator and adductor muscles.
- The main difference from TVT is that the retropubic space is not entered and the risk of bladder perforation is low.
- Potential disadvantages of transobturator slings are a higher risk of nerve trauma, with chronic groin pain described in up to 20% of patients.

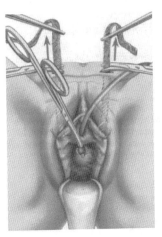

Fig. 22.5 Insertion of tension-free vaginal tape. The tape is placed in a U-shape under the urethra and the tension adjusted to prevent leakage as the woman coughs. Illustration reproduced by courtesy of ETHICON Women's Health and Urology.

Overactive bladder syndrome: overview

Definition
- OAB is a chronic condition, defined as urgency, with or without urge incontinence, usually with frequency or nocturia.
- It is used to imply probably underlying detrusor overactivity (DO), but this is a diagnosis made on urodynamic testing (Fig. 22.6).

Aetiology
- Idiopathic in most cases.
- Neurogenic DO is found in the presence of conditions such as multiple sclerosis, spina bifida, and upper motor neuron lesions.
- 2° to pelvic or incontinence surgery.
- OAB due to outflow obstruction is uncommon in women.

Clinical features of OAB
- Symptoms of OAB include urinary frequency, urgency, urge incontinence, and nocturia.
- Provocative factors often trigger it, such as cold weather, opening the front door, or hearing running water.
- Bladder contractions may also be provoked by ↑ intra-abdominal pressure (coughing or sneezing), leading to complaint of stress incontinence, which may be misleading.
- Quality of life can be significantly impaired by the unpredictability and large volume of leakage.

Investigations
Urine culture
Exclusion of infection is mandatory, as symptoms overlap those of UTI.

Frequency/volume chart
- Typical features are ↑ diurnal frequency associated with urgency and episodes of urge incontinence.
- Nocturia is a common feature of OAB.

Urodynamics
- Characterized by involuntary detrusor contractions during the filling phase of the micturition cycle, which may be spontaneous or provoked.
- Video-urodynamic testing is more appropriate in women with neurological diseases, to exclude vesicoureteric reflux or renal damage secondary to a persistent significant rise in intravesical pressure.

Diagnosis
- Urodynamic assessment is essential for the diagnosis of OAB in women with multiple and complex symptoms.
- Other factors, such as metabolic abnormalities (diabetes or hypercalcaemia), physical causes (prolapse or faecal impaction), or urinary pathology (UTI or interstitial cystitis), need to be excluded before the diagnosis of OAB is made.

Key points
- OAB is a common condition affecting around 1 in 6 women.
- The incidence of OAB increases with age.
- OAB is the second most common cause of urinary incontinence.
- OAB is the most common cause of incontinence in older women.
- Urodynamic assessment is required to make a diagnosis of DO.
- QoL is often severely affected by OAB symptoms.

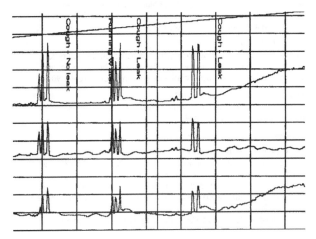

Fig. 22.6 Urodynamic trace showing detrusor overactivity. The upper trace of intravesical pressure (P_{ves}) vs. time shows a sharp increase of pressure within the bladder. The middle trace of pressure within the abdomen (P_{abd}) shows no similar increase. The lower trace, obtained by subtracting intra-abdominal pressure from intravesical pressure ($P_{det} = P_{ves} - P_{abd}$), shows significant detrusor overactivity.

Overactive bladder syndrome: management

Conservative management

It is wise to start with the simplest of conservative therapies and progress through to more radical treatments if necessary.

Behavioural therapy

- Advice to consume 1–1.5L of liquids per day.
- Avoid caffeine-based drinks (tea, coffee, cola) and alcohol.
- Various drugs, such as diuretics and antipsychotics, alter bladder function and should be reviewed.

Bladder retraining

- The principles of bladder retraining are based on the ability to suppress urinary urge and extend the intervals between voidings.
- Reported cure rates using bladder retraining alone are 44–90%.

Hypnotherapy and acupuncture

- These can be successful in some cases.
- The relapse rate is very high.

Pharmacological interventions

Anticholinergic (antimuscarinic) drugs

- These remain the mainstay of pharmacotherapy; they block the parasympathetic nerves, thereby relaxing the detrusor muscle.
- Patients should be advised about the side effects before starting treatment (some preparations may be better tolerated than others) (Table 22.2).
- The dosage may need to be titrated against efficacy and adverse effects.
- Adverse effects of anticholinergics may include:
  - dry mouth (up to 30%)
  - constipation, nausea, dyspepsia, and flatulence
  - blurred vision, dizziness, and insomnia
  - palpitation and arrhythmias.

Contraindications to anticholinergics

- Acute (narrow angle) glaucoma.
- Myasthenia gravis.
- Urinary retention or outflow obstruction.
- Severe ulcerative colitis.
- Gastrointestinal obstruction.

Oestrogens

- Intravaginal oestrogens may be tried in women with vaginal atrophy.
- Treatment with vaginal oestrogen often helps with symptoms of urgency, urge incontinence, frequency, and nocturia.

Use of botulinium toxin A for OAB

- Botulinium toxin A blocks neuromuscular transmission, causing temporary paralysis.
- Increasingly used as an intervention for refractory overactive bladder, with an efficacy of up to 90%.
- It is injected cystoscopically into the detrusor, usually under local anaesthetic.
- It can cause urinary retention in 5–10% of cases, in which case intermittent self-catheterization may be required.
- Repeat injections are required every 6–12mths.
- The long-term effects of repeat injections are unknown and are the subject of ongoing research.

Neuromodulation and sacral nerve stimulation

- Provides continuous stimulation of the S3 nerve root via an implanted electrical pulse generator and is thought to improve the ability to suppress detrusor contractions.
- It is being used increasingly in the treatment of refractory detrusor overactivity.
- Overall, neuromodulation has up to 50% clinical success rate.

Surgical management of OAB

- Surgery is reserved for those with debilitating symptoms and who have failed to benefit from medical, behavioural, and/or neuromodulation therapy.
- Procedures such as detrusor myomectomy and augmentation cystoplasty have limited efficacy and complication rates are high.
- Permanent urinary diversion is occasionally indicated in women with intractable incontinence.

Table 22.2 Anticholinergic drugs and their dosages

Drug	Delivery route	Adult dosage	Selectivity
Oxybutynin	(a) Oral	2.5–5mg, 1–4 times/day	Selective, predominantly M1 and M3
	(b) Transdermal patch	1 patch, twice weekly (3.9mg/24h)	
Propiverine	Oral only	15mg, 2–4 times/day	Non-selective
Solifenacin	Oral only	5–10mg daily	Selective, predominantly M3
Tolterodine	Oral only	(a) 2mg, bd (b) 4mg, od (sustained release)	Non-selective
Trospium	Oral only	20mg, bd	Non-selective
Fesoterodine	Oral only	4 or 8mg, od (sustained release)	Selective, predominantly M3

Anatomy of the pelvic floor

The pelvic floor consists of muscular and fascial structures that provide support to the pelvic viscera and the external openings of the vagina, urethra, and rectum (Fig. 22.7). The uterus and vagina are suspended from the pelvic side walls by endopelvic fascial attachments that support the vagina at three levels.

Three levels of vaginal support

- *Level 1:* the cervix and upper third of the vagina are supported by the cardinal (transverse cervical) and uterosacral ligaments. These are attached to the cervix and suspend the uterus from the pelvic sidewall and sacrum respectively.
- *Level 2:* the mid portion of the vagina is attached by endofascial condensation (endopelvic fascia) laterally to the pelvic side walls.
- *Level 3:* the lower third of the vagina is supported by the levator ani muscles and the perineal body. The levator ani, together with its associated fascia, is termed the pelvic diaphragm.

The axis of the vagina is also important. It normally lies in a horizontal plane, flat on the levator muscles. This protects it during coughing and other activities that increase intra-abdominal pressure (Fig. 22.7).

⚠ Damage occurring at the different levels of vaginal support causes different types of prolapse. It is therefore important to have an understanding of this anatomy.

Aetiology of prolapse

- *Pregnancy and vaginal delivery:* prolapse is uncommon in nulliparous women. Vaginal delivery may cause mechanical injuries and denervation of the pelvic floor. The risk is increased with large babies, prolonged second stage, and instrumental delivery (particularly forceps).
- *Congenital factors:* abnormal collagen metabolism, for example, in Ehlers–Danlos syndrome, can predispose to prolapse.
- *Menopause:* the incidence of prolapse increases with age. This may be due to the deterioration of collagenous connective tissue that occurs following oestrogen withdrawal.
- *Chronic predisposing factors:* prolapse is aggravated by any chronic increase in intra-abdominal pressure, resulting from factors such as obesity, chronic cough, constipation, heavy lifting, or pelvic mass.
- *Iatrogenic factors:* pelvic surgery may also influence the occurrence of prolapse:
  - hysterectomy is associated with subsequent vaginal vault prolapse (particularly when the indication was prolapse)
  - continence procedures, although elevating the bladder neck, may lead to defects in other pelvic compartments (Burch colposuspension may predispose to rectocele and enterocele formation).

(a)

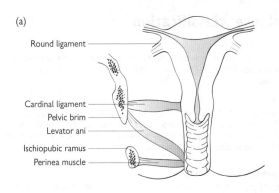

Round ligament

Cardinal ligament
Pelvic brim
Levator ani
Ischiopubic ramus
Perinea muscle

(b)

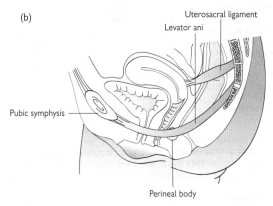

Uterosacral ligament
Levator ani

Pubic symphysis

Perineal body

Fig. 22.7 (a) Coronal view of the pelvis, showing cardinal ligaments and levator ani. (b) Lateral view of the pelvis, showing the uterosacral ligaments and levator ani. Reproduced with permission from Impey L. (1999). *Obstetrics and Gynaecology*. Oxford: Wiley-Blackwell Publishing.

Prolapse: classification

Definition

Prolapse is defined as protrusion of the uterus and/or vagina beyond normal anatomical confines. The bladder, urethra, rectum, and bowel are also often involved.

Incidence

The incidence of prolapse is difficult to define, as many women do not seek help and clinical examination does not necessarily correlate with symptoms. It is probably extremely common and is present in varying degrees in most older parous women.

Classification of prolapse

Types of uterovaginal prolapse are classified anatomically, according to the site of the defect and the pelvic viscera that are involved (Fig. 22.8).
- Cystocele is prolapse of the anterior vaginal wall, involving the bladder. Often there is an associated prolapse of the urethra, in which case the term cysto-urethrocele is used.
- Uterine (apical) prolapse is the term used to describe prolapse of the uterus, cervix, and upper vagina. If the uterus has been removed, the vault or top of the vagina, where the uterus used to be, can itself prolapse.
- Enterocele is prolapse of the upper posterior wall of the vagina. The resulting pouch usually contains loops of small bowel.
- Rectocele is prolapse of the lower posterior wall of the vagina, involving the anterior wall of the rectum.

Grading of prolapse

There are many grading systems. None is perfect, and some are complex and impractical. In 1996 the International Continence Society (ICS) Committee for Standardization published its POP quantitative scoring system.

For all measurements, the condition of the examination must be specified, i.e. position of the patient, at rest or straining, and whether traction is employed.

Grading of urogenital prolapse (Baden–Walker classification)

- *First degree*: the lowest part of the prolapse descends halfway down the vaginal axis to the introitus.
- *Second degree*: the lowest part of the prolapse extends to the level of the introitus and through the introitus on straining.
- *Third degree*: the lowest part of the prolapse extends through the introitus and lies outside the vagina.

▶ Procidentia describes a third-degree uterine prolapse.

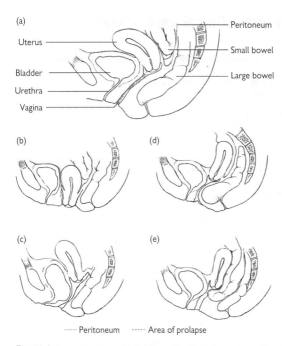

Fig. 22.8 Types of prolapse. (a) Normal pelvis, (b) uterine prolapse, (c) cystocele, (d) rectocele, (e) enterocele. Reproduced with permission from Impey L. (1999) *Obstetrics and Gynaecology*. Oxford: Wiley-Blackwell Publishing.

Prolapse: clinical assessment

Symptoms

Symptoms are often absent, but the most commonly reported are:
- *General:*
  - dragging sensation, discomfort, and heaviness within the pelvis
  - feeling of 'a lump coming down'
  - dyspareunia or difficulty in inserting tampons
  - discomfort and backache.
- *Cysto-urethrocele:*
  - urinary urgency and frequency
  - incomplete bladder emptying
  - urinary retention or reduced flow where the urethra is kinked by descent of the anterior vaginal wall.
- *Rectocele:*
  - constipation
  - difficulty with defecation (may digitally reduce it to defecate).

Symptoms tend to become worse with prolonged standing and towards the end of the day. In case of grade 3 or 4 prolapse, there may be mucosal ulceration and lichenification, resulting in vaginal bleeding and discharge.

Examination

- Exclude pelvic masses with a bimanual examination.
- Vaginal examination is best carried out with the woman in the left lateral position, using a Sims speculum.
- The walls should be checked in turn for descent and atrophy.
- If absolutely necessary, a volsellum may be applied to the cervix so that traction will demonstrate the severity of uterine prolapse (this can cause marked discomfort and should be performed very gently).
- Sometimes, prolapse may only be demonstrated with the woman standing or straining.
- An assessment of pelvic floor muscle strength should be carried out (see Box 22.1).

Quality of life assessment

- Symptoms can affect quality of life, causing social, psychological, occupational, or sexual limitations to a woman's lifestyle.
- Self-completion questionnaires allow a comprehensive assessment of prolapse symptoms and their impact, such as the Vaginal Symptoms module of the International Consultation on Incontinence Questionnaire (ICIQ-VS) (⌘ www.iciq.net).

Investigations

- USS to exclude pelvic or abdominal masses (if suspected clinically).
- Urodynamics are required if urinary incontinence is present.
- ECG, CXR, FBC, and U&E (if appropriate), to assess fitness for surgery.

Box 22.1 Modified Oxford system for grading pelvic floor muscle strength

A system of grading using vaginal palpation of the pelvic floor muscles.
- 0: No contraction.
- 1: Flicker.
- 2: Weak.
- 3: Moderate.
- 4: Good (with lift).
- 5: Strong.

Prolapse: conservative management

Prevention of pelvic organ prolapse
- Reduction of prolonged labour.
- Reduction of trauma caused by instrumental delivery.
- Encouraging persistence with postnatal pelvic floor exercises.
- Weight reduction.
- Treatment of chronic constipation.
- Treatment of chronic cough (including smoking cessation).

Physiotherapy
Physiotherapy has a role in the management of mild prolapse in younger women, who find intravaginal devices unacceptable and are not yet willing to consider definitive surgical treatment.
- *Pelvic floor muscle exercises (PFME):* are most effective when taught under the direct supervision of a physiotherapist; these will improve the tone in young parous women, but are unlikely to benefit older women with significant uterovaginal prolapse.
- Biofeedback and vaginal cones (see 📖 Stress urinary incontinence: conservative management, p. 664).

Intravaginal devices (pessaries)
Vaginal pessaries (Fig. 22.9) offer a further conservative line of therapy for women who decline surgery, who are unfit for surgery, or for whom surgery is contraindicated. They should be changed 6 monthly and topical oestrogen may be given to reduce the risk of vaginal erosion.
- *Ring pessary:* is most commonly used and is available in a number of different sizes (52–129mm); the ring is placed between the posterior aspect of the symphysis pubis and the posterior fornix of the vagina.
- *Shelf pessary:* can be used when a correctly sized ring pessary will not sit in the vagina and/or where the perineum is deficient (it may be difficult to insert and remove, so its use is becoming less common).
- *Hodge pessary:* can be used to correct uterine retroversion. It is of classical interest, but in practice is virtually never used now.
- *Cube and doughnut pessaries:* are, very rarely, used for significant prolapse, when others are not retained.

Factors influencing management of prolapse
- Severity of symptoms.
- Extension of the signs (asymptomatic grade 1 prolapse does not require treatment).
- Age, parity, and wish for further pregnancies.
- Patient's sexual activity.
- Presence of aggravating features such as smoking and obesity.
- Urinary symptoms.
- Other gynaecological problems such as menorrhagia.

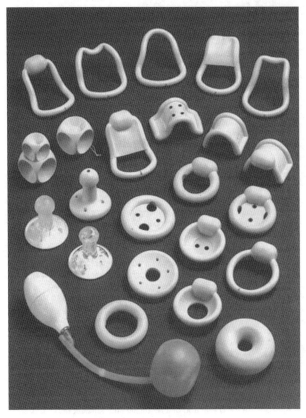

Fig. 22.9 Types of pessary for uterine prolapse include rings, cubes, shelf, and doughnuts. Reproduced by courtesy of Milex Products Inc., Chicago © 2002

Prolapse: surgical management, anterior and posterior compartments

Surgery offers definitive treatment of prolapse. Choice of procedure depends on patient and type of prolapse that exists.

Anterior compartment defect
Anterior colporrhaphy (anterior repair)
- Appropriate for the repair of a cysto-urethrocele.
- A longitudinal incision is made on the anterior vaginal wall and the vaginal skin separated by dissection from the pubocervical fascia.
- Buttressing sutures are placed on the fascia.
- The surplus vaginal skin is excised and the skin is closed.
- The repair is traditionally performed under regional or general anaesthesia; however, it can also be performed under local anaesthesia, allowing early mobilization and discharge home.
- Whilst morbidity is low, the long-term success rate of conventional anterior colporrhaphy is disappointing; recurrence rates of up to 30% have been reported. This may in part be due to failure to identify a co-existing apical defect.

Paravaginal repair
- Abdominal approach to correct an anterior defect.
- The retropubic space is opened through a Pfannenstiel incision and the bladder is swept medially, exposing the pelvic sidewall.
- The lateral sulcus of the vagina is elevated and reattached to the pelvic sidewall using interrupted sutures.
- A cure rate of 70–90% has been reported (may also be done laparoscopically).
- It isn't a commonly performed procedure, it is very invasive if performed via laparotomy, and the authors personal experience suggests higher recurrence rates than published data suggest.

Posterior compartment defect
Posterior colpoperineorrhaphy (posterior repair)
- Appropriate for correction of a rectocele and deficient perineum.
- It involves the repair of a rectovaginal fascial defect and removal of excess vaginal skin.

▶ Care must be taken when removing redundant vaginal skin, as vaginal narrowing can result in dyspareunia.

Perineoplasty is performed by placing deeper sutures into the perineal muscles, building up the perineal body to provide additional support.

Prolapse: surgical management, uterovaginal and vault

Uterovaginal (apical) prolapse

Vaginal hysterectomy

May be combined with the above procedures, in cases of significant uterine descent or menstrual problems (Table 22.3).

Manchester repair (or Fothergill repair)

- Now rarely performed.
- Cervical amputation is followed by approximation and shortening of the cardinal ligaments anterior to the cervical stump.
- This is combined with an anterior and posterior colporrhaphy.

Hysteropexy

- Can be performed if patient wishes to preserve uterus as an open or laparoscopic procedure (Fig. 22.10).
- Uterus and cervix are attached to sacrum using bifurcated non-absorbable mesh.
- Theoretical advantage of hysteropexy is stronger apical support when compared with vaginal hysterectomy.

Vaginal vault prolapse

Sacrospinous ligament fixation

- Involves suturing the vaginal vault to the sacrospinous ligaments, using a vaginal approach.
- Low immediate postoperative morbidity; success rate 70–85%.

⚠ As vaginal axis is changed by this procedure, there is risk of postoperative dyspareunia.

Sacrocolpoplexy

- The vault is attached to the sacrum using a non-absorbable mesh, and if can be performed either as an open procedure or laparoscopically.
- It has a higher success rate, of around 90%, and a better anatomical result than sacrospinous fixation.

⚠ Mesh erosion into the vagina, or rarely into the bladder or bowel, is a possible late complication.

Recurrent urogenital prolapse

- Approximately 1/3 of all prolapse surgery is for recurrent defects.
- Vaginal epithelium may be scarred and atrophic:
  - making surgical correction technically more difficult
  - increasing the risk of damage to the bladder and bowel.
- Use of synthetic meshes is becoming increasingly common for repair of recurrent prolapse, as they may offer more support where endopelvic fascia has proved to be deficient.

Table 22.3 Operations available for uterovaginal prolapse

Defect	Vaginal route	Abdominal route (open or laparoscoic)
Anterior	Anterior colporrhaphy	Paravaginal repair; sacrocolpopexy with placement of the mesh over anterior vaginal wall
	Transvaginal mesh repair	
Apical	Vaginal hysterectomy; sacrospinous fixation	Hysteropexy (laparoscopic or open); sacrocolpopexy
Posterior	Posterior repair; transvaginal mesh repair; perineal body reconstruction	Sacrocolpopexy to correct recto/enterocele

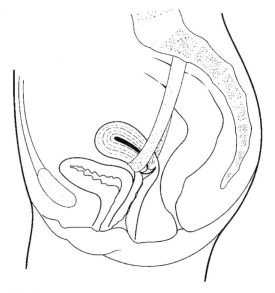

Fig. 22.10 Bifurcated mesh in position for sacrohysteropexy. Reproduced from Springer-Verlag London Ltd., Female Pelvic Reconstructive Surgery, 2002, p 187, Figure 13.10 Stanton and Zimmern. With kind permission of Springer Science and Business Media.

Benign and malignant gynaecological conditions

Benign neoplasms of the lower genital tract

Benign neoplasms are very common in the genital tract; most are innocent and easy to recognize.

Vulva

- *Bartholin's cyst:* arises from blocked Bartholin's duct in the lower third of the labia majora. It may present as a simple lump or an acute abscess after infection.
  - *Treatment*—incision and marsupialization; send pus to microbiology if infected (some are due to gonococcal infection and may need treatment and referral to GUM for contact tracing).
- *Sebaceous cysts, boils, and carbuncles:* very common and if symptomatic should be treated by incision and drainage. Tend to recur.
- *Cysts of the canal of Nuck* (embryological remnants): appear in the anterior part of the vulva.
- *Mucinous cysts:* may arise from the minor vestibular glands.
- *Mesonephric cysts:* generally seen on the labia majora.
- *Endometriotic lesions:* especially on an episiotomy wound.
- *Lipomas and fibromas:* also common.
- *Condylomata acuminata* (HPV 6/11): sessile polypoidal mass on the vulva.
  - *Treatment*—application of 80% trichloro-acetic acid. Laser or electro-diathermy under local anaesthesia reserved for larger lesions.

Urethra

- *Urethral caruncle:* most common in post-menopausal women and children. Appears as a bright red, tender swelling at the posterior margin of the urethral meatus. May present with dysuria, bleeding, and dyspareunia. The treatment is excision using diathermy.
- *Prolapse of the urethra:* presents as red lesion involving entire circumference of the urethral meatal margin. May be acute or chronic. Again, diathermy of the prolapsed mucosa is curative.

Vagina

- *Endometriotic deposits:* may present as small brown-black nodules.
- *Simple mesonephric (Gartner's) cysts and paramesonephric cysts:* usually appear in the fornices of the vagina. If symptomatic they should be marsupialized rather than excised.
- *Inclusion cysts:* can arise where vaginal epithelium is embedded under surface during perineal surgery. Treatment warranted only when patients are symptomatic.

Cervix

- *Cervical polyps (adenoma):* common; due to overgrowth of the endocervical mucosa. Sometimes arise in endometruim (pedunculated) and protrude from cervix. Very rarely malignant (1:6000), but they should be removed and hysteroscopy to rule out further polyps should be considered if symptoms warrant it.
- *Nabothian cysts:* mucous-retention cysts caused by blockage of endocervical mucous glands. Treatment is not required.

Benign neoplasms of the uterus

Uterine fibroids

These are the most common benign tumours arising from the myometrium of the uterus. Also called *leiomyomata*, these tumours are composed primarily of smooth muscles, but may contain fibrous tissue. Present in 20–40% of women in the reproductive age group, they have a higher incidence in Afro-Caribbean women and those with a family history of fibroids. Many women are asymptomatic, but may present with: dysmenorrhoea, menorrhagia, pressure symptoms (especially frequency), and pelvic pain. Infertility may be associated and, in <10% cases, caused solely by fibroids. In pregnancy can cause pain from degeneration, abnormal lie, and obstruction if cervical, and difficulty in CS. Association with miscarriage as yet unproven.

Types of uterine fibroids

- *Submucous*: >50% projection into the endometrial cavity.
- Intramural: located within the myometrium.
- *Subserous*: >50% of the fibroid mass extends outside the uterine contours.
- *Cervical*: relatively uncommon and can cause surgical difficulty due to the proximity to the bladder and the ureters.
- *Pedunculated*: mobile and prone to torsion.
- *Parasitic*: have become detached from the uterus and attached to other structures.
- *IV leiomyomatosis*: very rare, spread through the pelvic veins and vena cava to involve the heart.

Diagnosis

Clinical examination (hard, irregular uterine mass) may be sufficient. Transvaginal or abdominal ultrasound can differentiate the types and dimensions of the fibroids. Rarely MRI may be needed when the scan is inconclusive.

Endometrial polyps (adenoma)

These are focal overgrowth of the endometrium and are malignant in <1%. They are more common in women >40yrs, but may occur at any age. Treatment is usually resection during hysteroscopy and the polyp should be sent for histological assessment.

Treatment options for uterine fibroids

- No treatment may be necessary if minimal symptoms.
- GnRH analogues shrink fibroids, but should only be used for this purpose prior to surgery.
- *Myomectomy:* open, laparoscopic, or hysteroscopic depending upon location (especially when wish to preserve fertility and when the fibroids are distinctly isolated on scan—fibroids often recur).
- *Hysterectomy:* women who have either completed their family or are over 45yrs—guaranteed cure of fibroids.
- *Uterine artery embolization:* uterine artery is catheterized generally using the unilateral approach; polyvinyl alcohol powder or gelatin sponge is used as the embolic material (minimally invasive procedure with avoidance of a general anaesthetic).

Benign neoplasms of the fallopian tube

Hydrosalpinx, pyosalpinx, and tubo-ovarian masses following pelvic inflammatory disease or endometriotic adhesions may present as a benign mass in the pelvis. The diagnosis is essentially by ultrasound and laparoscopy. Most tumours of the fallopian tubes are malignant. Although they were thought to be rare, data from series of BRCA-positive women undergoing prophylactic bilateral oophrectomy and salpingectomy (BSO) suggest that 1° fallopian tumours may be more common than previously thought.

Benign ovarian tumours: diagnosis

Ovarian cysts are extremely common, and frequently physiological, due to follicular cyst (≤3cm) and corpus luteal cyst (≤5cm) formation during the menstrual cycle. In a woman who is having periods, a cyst of <5cm should not cause concern (or referral), unless there are other suspicious features or she is symptomatic (e.g. pain). A re-scan in 6wks is recommended (when she will be at another point in her cycle) to see if the cyst has resolved. Small cysts are also frequently seen in post-menopausal women (up to 14%) on TVS.

Ultrasound features and the tumour marker CA125 are used to determine the risk of malignancy index (RMI). This is useful for identifying patients with a high risk of cancer who should be referred to a cancer centre for treatment (sensitivity 87.4%, positive predictive value (PPV) 86.8% in recent series) (see Table 23.1).

Presentation
- Asymptomatic.
- *Chronic pain:*
  - dull ache
  - pressure on other organs (urinary frequency or bowel disturbance)
  - dyspareunia (endometrioma)
  - cyclical pain (endometrioma).
- *Acute pain:*
  - bleeding (into the cyst or intra-abdominal)
  - torsion
  - rupture.
- Abnormal uterine bleeding.
- Hormonal effects.

History and investigation

History
Menstrual history (LMP, cycle length, menorrhagia); pain (site, nature, radiation—typically down leg, duration, precipitating factors); bowel/bladder function; abdominal distension; medical and family history.

Examination
- *Systemic:* pulse; BP; anaemia; temperature.
- *Abdominal:* mass arising from pelvis; tenderness; signs of peritonism; upper abdominal masses or ascites suggest cyst less likely to be benign.
- *Pelvic:* PV discharge/bleeding; cervical excitation; adnexal mass or tenderness (mobile or fixed, smooth or nodular, size).

Haematological tests
- FBC.
- *Tumour markers:*
  - CA125
  - consider other tumour markers especially in a young woman (<40yrs) with solid mass: AFP, hCG, LDH, inhibin, and oestradiol.

Imaging
Abdominal/pelvic USS: presence and appearance of pelvic mass and ascites.

Modified risk of malignancy index

RMI = U x M x CA125
- U = ultrasound score (0, 1, or 3).
- M = menopausal status (1 = premenopausal, 3 = post-menopausal)
- CA125 = serum cancer antigen 125 level (U/L)

Ultrasound scoring system
- 1 point for each of the following features on USS:
  - multilocular cyst
  - evidence of solid areas
  - evidence of metastases
  - ascites
  - bilateral lesions.
- Final U score:
  - 0 if no features
  - 1 if 1 feature
  - 3 if 2 or more features.

📖 Tingulstad S, Hagen B, Skjeldestad FE, et al. (1996). Evaluation of a risk of malignancy index based on serum CA125, ultrasound findings and menopausal status in the pre-operative diagnosis of pelvic masses. *Br J Obstet Gynaecol* **103**(8): 826–31.

Table 23.1 RMI score and ovarian cancer risk

Risk	RMI score	Risk of cancer
Low	<25	<3%
Moderate	25–250	20%
High	>250	75%

Davies AP, Jacobs I, Woolas R, et al. (1993). The adnexal mass: benign or malignant? Evaluation of a risk of malignancy index. *Br J Obstet Gynaecol* **100**(10): 927–31.

Non-gynaecological causes of pelvic masses

Other benign masses due to non-gynaecological conditions in the pelvis should always be borne in mind as a differential diagnosis:
- Bladder tumours
- Intestinal tumours
- Diverticular disease
- IBD.

Benign ovarian tumours: histology

Histology

It is difficult to know the true incidences of benign ovarian tumours, as most will be functional cysts and are not removed; hence, ratios of functional/benign/malignant tumours are highly dependent on the age and selection of the population studied.

Non-neoplastic
- *Functional:*
  - follicular cysts (normally <3cm)
  - corpus luteal cysts (normally <5cm (may show signs of haemorrhage into cyst or cause haemoperitoneum)).
- *Pathological:*
  - *ovarian endometriotic cyst* (filled with old altered blood, 'chocolate cyst', see 📖 Endometriosis: overview, p. 582)
  - *polycystic ovarian syndrome* (generally bulky ovaries with multiple small follicles, fibrotic capsule, and smooth surface, 'ring of pearls' sign on TVUSS)
  - *theca leutin cysts* (multiple ovarian cysts, occur in conditions with ↑ hCG, e.g. hydatidiform molar pregnancy—resolve if ↑ hCG levels fall)
  - *ovarian oedema* (2° to ovarian torsion, the ovary is enlarged and boggy—exclude germ cell tumour in young woman).

Benign neoplastic
- *Epithelial tumours:*
  - *serous cystadenoma* (usually unilocular and 20–30% are bilateral, may have septations)
  - *mucinous cystadenoma* (often multiloculated, but usually unilateral (5% bilateral)—can get extremely large, >150 kg)
  - *Brenner tumours* (1–2% of ovarian tumours, unilateral, and have solid grey, white, or yellow appearance to cut surface, fibrous elements, and transitional epithelium).
- *Benign germ cell tumours:* mature teratoma or dermoid cyst (10% are bilateral, 90% occur in women of reproductive age, usually full of sebaceous material and hair, but may contain teeth, skin, cartilage, fat, or bone. Can cause chemical peritonitis if contents spill).
- *Sex-cord stromal tumours* (see 📖 Rare ovarian tumours: other, p. 728):
  - *fibroma* (commonest stromal tumour, up to 40% present with Meig's syndrome, ascites, and pleural effusion)
  - *Sertoli–Leydig cell tumour* (1% of ovarian tumours; produce androgens and present with virilization)
  - *thecoma* (produce oestrogens—present with abnormal vaginal bleeding)
  - *lipoma.*

Benign ovarian tumours: management

Most cysts presenting acutely will present with lower abdominal pain, but without signs of peritonism or systemic upset. Manage conservatively with analgesia; most will resolve spontaneously. However, if the woman presents with an acute abdomen and/or signs of systemic upset, due to ovarian torsion, rupture, or haemorrhage of a cyst, urgent diagnostic laparoscopy or laparotomy may be required. In these cases, blood should be sent for tumour markers at the time of surgery, as if cyst is not benign, this will aid follow-up.

Adolescent women Manage as for premenopausal women. Germ cell tumours are more common in this age group (up to 20% in some series), especially in those presenting with ovarian torsion. Aim for conservative surgery (cystectomy if possible) to diagnose, but preserve fertility.

Premenopausal women Malignant tumours rare in this age group (0.4–9:100 000). Aim to exclude malignancy and preserve fertility. Rescan in 6wks. If cyst is persistent then either monitor with USS and CA125 (e.g. 3 and 6mths (50% <5cm will resolve, less with larger cysts). Calculate RMI.

Management of low-risk cysts
- Transvaginal cyst aspiration under USS guidance has no advantage over expectant management.
- If cyst still persists or is >5cm then consider laparoscopic cystectomy.
  - *if cyst <5cm and simple*—cyst fenestration and wall biopsy for histology is acceptable.
  - *if cyst >5cm or is a dermoid*—aim to prevent spillage of contents, e.g. cystectomy and removal of cyst in an 'endobag'
  - *if suspicious findings at laparoscopy*—abandon procedure (take peritoneal biopsy for diagnosis). Refer to cancer centre for full staging laparotomy.

⚠ Do not use a morcellator and try not to spill cyst contents.

- If a dermoid cyst, this can cause a chemical peritonitis.
- If cyst ruptured and contents spill out, this can disseminate an otherwise early ovarian cancer (although rare in this age group).

Post-menopausal women
- *Low RMI (<25):* simple, <5cm cyst and normal CA125; follow up for 1yr with USS and CA125 every 4mths. If no change then discontinue monitoring. If change and RMI still low, or woman requests removal, laparoscopic oophorectomy (usually bilateral) is appropriate.
- *Moderate RMI (25–250):* oophorectomy (usually bilateral) in cancer centre recommended. May be acceptable to perform laparoscopically in some cases. If malignancy found then full staging laparotomy will be needed.
- *High RMI (>250):* refer to a cancer centre for a full staging laparotomy.

Further reading
RCOG. (2003). Ovarian cysts in post-menopausal women, RCOG guideline no. 34. ॐ http://www.rcog.org.uk/womens-health/clinical-guidance/ovarian-cysts-postmenopausal-women-green-top-34

Vulval dermatoses: lichen sclerosus

Skin conditions of the vulva can cause distressing symptoms, and be difficult to diagnose and manage. Irritation leads to scratching and excoriation, which may make the appearance clinically difficult to differentiate, especially when added to changes seen following secondary infection or use of topical creams.

Vulval dermatoses refers to a range of benign skin conditions, which generally cause white thickening of the vulval skin: lichen sclerosus; lichen planus; vulval dermatitis; vulval psoriasis.

Lichen sclerosus

- Chronic inflammatory condition (lymphocyte mediated).
- May be hereditary (association with HLA-DQ7).
- Usually confined to anogenital area.
- More common in women.
- Incidence estimated as 1:300–1:1000 women.
- Normally in peri-menopausal women, but can occur in young girls (2/3 improve at puberty—may be misdiagnosed as signs of abuse).
- Associated with other autoimmune diseases:
  - e.g. thyroid disease; diabetes; vitiligo; pernicious anaemia
  - 20–34% have association with autoimmune disease
  - up to 74% have autoantibodies.

See Colour plate 1.

> **Clinical presentation of lichen sclerosus**
> - Burning pain or itch, occasionally asymptomatic.
> - Figure of 8 appearance around vulva and anus.
> - White, shiny, wrinkly, atrophic appearance 'like tissue paper':
>   - may have white patches, purpura, or telangiectasia
>   - hyperkeratosis and lichenification if chronic scratching
>   - over time, can develop loss and fusion of labia minora, narrowing of introitus, resulting in problems with intercourse and micturation.

⚠ Long-term risk of vulval squamous cell carcinoma (~2%), so need long-term observation, follow-up, and biopsy of suspicious lesions. This can be in 1° care if symptoms well controlled.

Management of lichen sclerosus

- Biopsy for diagnosis, if not responding to treatment.
- Biopsy suspicious lesions (risk of vulval cancer) or if not responding to treatment made on clinical diagnosis.
- Check ferritin levels and treat if low.
- Screen for autoimmune conditions, if suggestive symptoms (FBC, TFTs, glucose, serum iron, autoimmune antibodies, intrinsic factor, and vitamin B_{12}).
- Potent corticosteroids: clobetasol propionate 0.05% bd initially once a night for 4wks, alternate nights for 4wks, once or twice weekly for 4wks, then use 'as required' for flares; the shiny appearance will remain.
- Follow-up at 3mths to check response.
- Annual review with GP and advise urgent contact if ulcers, bleeding, or suspicious lesions.
- Referral to specialist unit for tacrolimus if symptoms not responding.

Further reading

British Association of Dermatologists. ℘ www.bad.org.uk
℘ www.lichensclerosus.org
℘ http://www.macmillan.org.uk/Cancerinformation/Cancertypes/Vulva/Pre-cancerousconditions/Vulvallichensclerosuslichenplanus.aspx
RCOG. (2011). The management of vulval skin disorders, Green-top guideline 58. ℘ http://www.rcog.org.uk/files/rcog-corp/GTG58Vulval22022011.pdf

Other vulval dermatoses

Vulval dermatitis

- Dermatitis or eczema.
- If scratched so that thickening of skin → lichen simplex chronicus.
- Association with other atopic illnesses (asthma, hay fever, or eczema).
- *Common irritants:*
  - soaps, shower gels, condoms, deodorants, creams
  - if diagnosed as candidiasis, topical creams can be irritant.

> **Clinical presentation of vulval dermatitis**
> - Itch—burning and pain secondary to scratching.
> - Erythema ± scaling of skin.
> - No loss or fusion of labia.

Management
- Avoid irritant and apply general vulval skin care (see Box 23.1).
- Low vaginal swabs for secondary infection (e.g. *Candida*).
- Severe disease—treat with steroid cream—clobetasol propionate or betamethasone valerate, if less severe. Use bd initially; reduce to od, then twice weekly, as condition improves.
- Consider sedating antihistamine (e.g. chlorphenamine 4mg) at night to prevent scratching.
- Referral to dermatology for patch testing.

Lichen planus

Rare condition.

> **Clinical presentation of lichen planus**
> - Purplish papules and plaques; can have white streaks on top—'Wickham's striae'. May involve mouth too.
> - May cause painful, red, ulcerated areas around introitus. Occasionally can cause severe desquamative vaginitis.
> - Cause itch, pain, post-coital bleeding, or discharge.

Management
- As for lichen sclerosus, including follow up, as also have an increased risk of developing vulval cancer.
- Biopsy; potent steroids; good vulval skin care; local anaesthetic gel.

Vulval psoriasis

> **Clinical presentation of vulval psoriasis**
> Classically well-defined erythematous patches, may have scaling on pubic area, but not necessarily on vulval skin.

Management
- Good vulval skin care; bland emollients; mild topical steroids.
- Other psoriatic medications often too harsh for vulval skin.

Box 23.1 Vulval skin care

- Keep area clean but avoid soap:
  - *use soap substitutes*—soap-free shower gels; bath oil; just water
  - salt baths *may* help.
- Do not soak in hot bath.
- Allow air circulation to avoid sweating: loose underwear and bed clothes; avoid jeans, etc.
- Wear cotton next to skin: avoid synthetics (especially nylon) and wool (intrinsically itchy!).
- Avoid vaginal lubricants:
  - may be irritating;
  - can use saliva or oil (vegetable, olive, almond)—avoid perfumed oil.
  - oils weaken condoms!
- Refer for patch testing if vulval dermatitis.

Further reading

British Association of Dermatologists. ✆ www.bad.org.uk
http://www.macmillan.org.uk/Cancerinformation/Cancertypes/Vulva/Pre-cancerousconditions/
   Vulvallichensclerosuslichenplanus.aspx

Idiopathic vulval itch and pain

Pruritis vulvae
- Common (1 in 10 women).
- Persistent itch, often worse at night and may disturb sleep.

Management
- Identify cause and treat appropriately: may need swabs; skin scrapings; skin biopsy; U&E; LFTs.
- General vulval skin care and bland emollients.
- Short course of weak steroid cream (hydrocortisone 1–2wks).
- Sedating antihistamine at night (e.g. chlorphenamine 4mg) (break itch/scratch/itch cycle).

Vulvodynia/vestibulodynia
These are dysaesthesia, which involve pain in the vulva or around the introitus in the absence of a specific cause.
- Burning, stinging, or raw discomfort.
- Typically worse when sitting down.
- May occur as sequelae to inflammatory vulval condition, e.g. lichen sclerosus.
- Neuropathic pain.

Management
- Investigate and exclude other causes.
- General vulval skin care.
- Topical local anaesthetic gel.
- Amitriptyline; start on low dose (10mg) 3h before bed (to avoid morning 'hangover') and increase as tolerated/required by ~10mg/wk up to 80mg, reduce gradually after 3mths.
- Antiepileptics (used rarely and with specialist referral, e.g. chronic pain service): gabapentin and pregabalin.

Ulcers
- Aphthous ulcers.
- *Infectious:*
    - *herpes simplex virus*—multiple, extremely painful ulcers
    - *syphilis primary chancre*—painless unless infected
    - *tropical* (chancroid; granuloma inguinale; lymphogranuloma venerium).
- *Inflammatory/autoimmune:*
    - Crohn's disease
    - Behçet's disease (causes orogenital ulcers and ophthalmic inflammation; uncommon in women; HLA-B51 association).

Causes of pruritis vulvae

- *Infection:*
  - candidiasis
  - threadworms
  - *Phthirus pubis* (genital lice)
  - *Sarcoptes scabiei* (scabies, from Latin 'to itch').
- *Vulval dermatoses:*
  - lichen sclerosus
  - vulval dermatitis
  - lichen planus
  - vulval psoriasis.
- Vulval intraepithelial neoplasia or vulval carcinoma.
- Urinary incontinence.
- *Systemic conditions:*
  - liver failure
  - uraemia.
- Medication.
- Pregnancy/menopause.
- Idiopathic.

Further reading

http://www.patient.co.uk/health/pruritus-vulvae-vulval-itch
British Association of Dermatologists. Available at: www.bad.org.uk
Vulval Pain Society. Available at: www.vulvalpainsociety.org/

Cancer screening in gynaecology: overview

The intention of screening is early identification of a disease, prompt referral for diagnostic tests, and appropriate intervention and management. Screening test does not necessarily diagnose condition or disease, but may reduce associated incidence, mortality, and morbidity.

WHO principles of screening (1968)
- The condition should be an important public health problem.
- An effective intervention should be available.
- Clear, recognizable early stage and known natural history of condition.
- There should be a suitable screening test available.
- The test should be acceptable to the population.
- Benefits of the test should outweigh the risks.
- There should be an agreed policy on who to treat.
- The total cost of finding a case should be economically balanced.

Sensitivity, specificity, and positive and negative predictive values
- *Sensitivity:* the ability of the screening test to detect the disease— acceptable sensitivity detects most disease.
- *Specificity:* the ability of the screening test not to identify those who do not have the condition—acceptable specificity excludes most without the disease.
- *Positive predictive value (PPV):* the proportion with a positive test result who have the disease.
- *Negative predictive value (NPV):* the proportion with a negative test result who do not have the disease.

Ovarian and endometrial cancer screening

Ovarian carcinoma presents with advanced disease in nearly 75% of cases and, therefore, necessitates a reliable screening test. Cancers of the ovary are less well studied than other gynaecological malignancies and only a few aetiological factors have been identified.

The main predisposing factors to epithelial cancer of the ovary are:
- Nulliparity.
- Non-use of oral contraceptives (RR 0.40 if used for >36mths).
- Family history.

There is lack of robust evidence for other factors such as age at menarche, menopause, and first childbirth.

Genetic factors

If a first-degree relative develops ovarian cancer aged <50yrs, the risk increases 6–10-fold. If two or more close relatives are affected, the lifetime risk rises to 40%. Possibly 1% of families in the UK may belong to a very high risk group. This familial risk is associated with a mutation of the *BRCA1* gene on chromosome 17, but other loci may also be involved. *BRCA1* and *BRCA2* have been identified in almost all families with both breast and ovarian cancer and in 40% of families with breast cancer alone.

⚠ Genetic advice to women with one of these genes should be given by a clinical geneticist.

▶ Women with a family history of ovarian cancers in one first-degree relative should be reassured. Although their risk of ovarian cancer is increased the absolute risk remains small (lifetime risk of 2–5% vs. 1% in the general population).

▶ Salpingo-oophorectomy should not be used as a primary prophylactic procedure but may be considered in women who have a strong family history and have completed their family. The risk of other peritoneal cancers cannot be ruled out in these women.

Endometrial cancer screening

Ultrasound assessment of endometrial thickness and sampling of the endometrium have been described and clinical trials are on-going, but there is currently no evidence to use these as screening methods in the general population. Endometrial cancer tends to present early with aberrant bleeding and, as such, has a good prognosis, so screening is unlikely to be beneficial in the general population. Due to the increased risk of endometrial cancer in women with hereditary nonpolyposis colorectal cancer (HNPCC), guidelines from the American Cancer Society suggest annual screening from 35yrs of age with TVS/USS and endometrial sampling.

Ovarian cancer screening

The efficacy of screening for ovarian cancer is not proven. The results from a large UK Collaborative Trial of Ovarian Cancer Screening (UKCTOCS) are expected in 2015. Results of the Prostate, Lung, Colorectal, Ovarian (PLCO) cancer screening trial did not demonstrate reduced mortality from ovarian cancer using a cut-off level of CA125. Currently, any screening offered to women, should be as part of a clinical trial.

- Pelvic TVS can identify ovarian cysts. In a young woman most of these will be physiological, but features suggestive of malignancy are large size of cyst, internal septa, solid areas, and increased blood flow on Doppler examination. Operator expertise is extremely important in the screening process.
- CA125 is a glycoprotein shed by 85% of epithelial tumours. Normal levels are 30–65IU/L, but false +ves are commonly seen in other malignancies (liver, pancreas), endometriosis, PID, and early pregnancy. Sensitivity is improved using serial measurements and the trends. Up to 50% of stage 1 tumours will present with a CA125 level of <30IU/L.
- Both ultrasound examination and CA125 estimation can give rise to a false +ve result in nearly 2–3% of post-menopausal women. The use of the two tests together reduces the chance of false +ves.

UK Collaborative Trial of Ovarian Cancer Screening. ℛ www.ukctocs.org.uk/

Cervical cancer: pathology and screening

CIN is widely regarded as a necessary precursor lesion for carcinoma of the cervix. CIN is a histological diagnosis and needs persistent cervical infection with HPV to develop. There are about 15 high risk oncogenic subtypes of HPV, the most common being 16, 18, 31, and 33.

Risk factors for CIN
- Persistent high risk HPV infection.
- Multiple partners increases the risk of exposure to HPV infection.
- Smoking as a promoter.
- Immunocompromise, e.g. HIV, immunosuppressive agents.
- Use of the COCP has an association, probably due to non-barrier method and exposure to HPV.

Normal and abnormal physiology of transformation zone

The endocervix is composed of a thin secretory glandular epithelium; the ectocervix consists of a stronger stratified squamous epithelium. The two are in continuity and meet at the squamocolumar junction. Under the influence of oestrogen the glandular epithelium is pushed out onto the ectocervix and in response to low pH undergoes physiological squamous metaplasia—the *transformation zone* (TZ). The TZ is usually ectocervical in women of reproductive age, but tends to become endocervical in post-menopausal women.

As an area of high mitotic activity the TZ is vulnerable to HPV-driven neoplastic change, if persistent (i.e. not eradicated). Most work suggests an average of 8–10yrs from acquisition to development of cancer. Cervical cancer is therefore, in theory, a preventable disease.

Screening for cervical premalignancy

The NHS Cervical Screening Programme (NHSCSP) has been systematic since the 1980s and has since shown a 50% reduction in mortality from cervical cancer. Regular cervical screening reduces the risk of death from cervical carcinoma by 75% (but does not eliminate it).

Screening is based on the natural course of cervical cancer where CIN (dysplasia) precedes overt malignancy and is a progressive condition. However, in reality CIN may also revert back to normal. Routine screening carries a 50–70% sensitivity to detect CIN III.

HPV triage and test of cure was introduced in the UK in April 2012. Women with borderline nuclear changes or mild dyskaryosis have testing for high-risk HPV types. Women with high risk HPV are referred for colposcopy. Women without have smear follow-up at 3yrs. Similarly, following LLETZ for CIN, women without abnormal cytology or high risk HPV at the smear 6mths after treatment will return to 3-yearly smears. Women with high risk HPV or abnormal cytology will be referred back to colposcopy (see Table 23.2).

Current English criteria for cervical screening
- Sexually active women aged 25–64.
- Three-yearly for women aged 25–50, if normal, 5-yearly till 64.

▶Three-yearly screening identifies more than 95% of abnormalities tested by annual screening and is cost-effective.

▶ Screening in Scotland and Wales begins at 20.

Table 23.2 Management of abnormal smears

Papanicoulaou class	Histology	Management
Normal	0.1% CIN II–III	Repeat smear in 3yrs
Inflammatory	6% CIN II–III	Repeat in 6mths (colposcopy after 3 consecutive)
Borderline nuclear changes	20–30% CIN II–III	High risk HPV test—refer to colposcopy if +ve; repeat smear 3yrs if −ve
Mild dyskaryosis	30% CIN II–III	High risk HPV test—refer to colposcopy if +ve; repeat smear 3yrs if −ve
Moderate dyskaryosis	50–75% CIN II–III	Refer to colposcopy
Severe dyskaryosis	80–90% CINII–III	Refer to colposcopy
Invasion suspected	50% invasion	Refer to colposcopy
Abnormal glandular cells	Adenocarcinoma of the cervix	Refer to colposcopy

Further reading
NHSCSP. (2010). Colposcopy and programme management: guidelines for the NHS cervical screening programme. ℘ http://www.cancerscreening.nhs.uk/cervical/publications/nhscsp20.html

NHSCSP. (2011). HPV triage and test of cure protocol. ℘ http://www.cancerscreening.nhs.uk/cervical/hpv-triage-test-flowchart.pdf

Cervical cancer: cytology, colposcopy, and histology

Cervical cytology

The primary screening tool for cervical malignancy. NICE recommends liquid-based cytology for the cytological preparation of cervical cells—cleaner preparation, easier to read, inadequate cytology cut by 80%, and more cost-effective. High risk HPV testing can be performed on this sample, if indicated.

Dyskaryosis is a cytological term. False +ve and −ve rates are 10–15% and 5–15%, respectively. Due to these problems with sensitivity and specificity, abnormal cytology is further assessed by colposcopy.

Cytological markers seen with abnormal smears

- Increased nuclear/cytoplasmic ratio.
- Shape of the nucleus (poikilocytosis—abnormal shape).
- Density of the nucleus (koilocytosis—abnormal density).
- Inflammation, infection, and mitoses.

Colposcopy

Involves the magnified (6–40x) visualization of the transformation zone after application of 5% acetic acid (preferentially taken up by neoplastic cells) or Lugol's iodine (not taken up by glycogen-deficient neoplastic cells). Upon identification of colposcopic abnormalities either:
- Directed punch biopsy to gain histological confirmation; *or*
- Definitive treatment ('see and treat').

Adequate colposcopic assessment

- Visualization of the entire transformation zone.
- Any lesion identified must be completely seen (especially upper extent).
- *Problem areas:* post-menopausal, post-treatment, and post-partum.
See Colour plates 2–8.

Histology

CIN is a histological diagnosis and is characterized by loss of differentiation and maturation from the basal layer of the squamous epithelium upwards.
- Bottom 1/3 = CIN I.
- Bottom 2/3 = CIN II.
- Full thickness = CIN III.
- Mitotic figures are present throughout the epithelium in all grades.

Referral criteria for colposcopy
- Any smear showing borderline nuclear changes or mild dyskaryosis with high risk HPV.
- Any smear showing moderate or severe dyskaryosis.
- Any smear suggestive of malignancy.
- Any smear suggestive of glandular abnormality.
- Three consecutive inadequate smears.
- Keratinizing cells (?underlying CIN).
- Post-coital bleeding.
- Abnormal-looking cervix.

Colposcopic appearances of CIN
- Aceto-white epithelium (AWE).
- Vascular abnormalities, especially mosaic and punctuation.
- Bizarre or grossly abnormal vessels are suggestive of micro-invasive carcinoma.

Management of cervical intraepithelial neoplasia (CIN)

CIN can be managed conservatively, by excision, by destruction, or rarely by hysterectomy. Management depends upon the grade of CIN and patient preference, but excision is the preferred treatment modality. This is usually by LLETZ.

> **Benefits of LLETZ**
> - Easy and safe.
> - Usually possible with local anaesthetic.
> - Tissue available for histology and assessment of excision margins.

Low grade CIN (CIN I)

Will spontaneously regress in at least 50–60% of cases within 2yrs. Malignant potential is very low but still up to 10x greater than women with normal cytology. Management options are:
- Conservative monitoring with colposcopy and/or cytology every 6mths.
- LLETZ if persistent.

High grade CIN (>CIN I)

Will progress to cancer in up to 3–5% (CIN II) and 20–30% (CIN III) within 10yrs. Spontaneous regression occurs less often.
- LLETZ recommended.

Follow-up and management after LLETZ

- *Low grade:* follow-up cytology and HPV testing at 6mths. If –ve, smear in 3yrs.
- *High grade:* follow-up cytology and high risk HPV test-of-cure at 6mths. If –ve, smear in 3yrs.

> **Complications of LLETZ**
> *Short term*
> - Haemorrhage.
> - Infection.
> - Vaso-vagal reaction.
> - Anxiety (disproportionately high in colposcopy clinic attenders).
>
> *Long term*
> - Cervical stenosis (dysmenorrhoea and/or difficulty in follow-up).
> - Cervical incompetence and premature delivery (evidence suggests absolute risk of adverse effect on neonatal outcome is very low).

Further reading

NHSCSP. (2010). Colposcopy and programme management: guidelines for the NHS Cervical Screening Programme. ℘ www.bsccp.org.uk/docs/public/pdf/nhscsp20.pdf

NHSCSP. (2011). HPV triage and test of cure protocol. ℘ http://www.cancerscreening.nhs.uk/cervical/hpv-triage-test-flowchart.pdf

Management of cGIN and human papillomavirus

Dysplasia originating primarily in the glandular epithelium is known as cervical glandular intraepithelial neoplasia (cGIN). It is divided into low and high grade: the latter is a full-thickness abnormality. It can co-exist with CIN or stand alone and is associated with high risk HPV, especially HPV 18. It poses difficulties in management because:

- The endocervical epithelium extends beyond view (up to 10% of cGIN lesions will have higher 'skip' lesions).
- The natural history is less well understood than squamous CIN.
- No specific colposcopic appearances, unlike CIN.
- Follow-up is difficult and the only known guaranteed 'cure' is hysterectomy.
- The incidence of adenocarcinoma appears to be rising compared to squamous cell carcinoma.

Management of cGIN

All glandular cytological abnormalities should be referred for colposcopy. Colposcopy ± endometrial sampling may need to be performed. Endocervical curettage has a very low yield and is no longer recommended. In the presence of colposcopic abnormalities or high grade cytology a cylindrical shaped LLETZ or cone with deep 'top hat' or cold knife cone biopsy is recommended. Hysterectomy may be required after completion of family or if colposcopic assessment is incomplete with repeated cytological abnormality.

Prevention and the role of HPV vaccination

HPV is a necessity for the development of CIN and cancer. HPV vaccines have shown very promising results. They utilize the type-specific HPV-like particles (HPV-LPs). The two commercially available vaccines induce excellent antibody production against 4 and 6 HPV types, respectively, and in trials have been shown to reliably prevent CIN (types 16 +18 commonly) and anogenital warts (types 6 + 11).

HPV vaccines—what we know

- They reliably induce excellent type-specific antibody titres vs. HPV.
- There is good trial evidence for reliable prevention of CIN (and presumably therefore ultimately cancer) and anogenital warts.
- Due to type specificity they will not prevent all cancers—there are 15 high risk HPVs (current vaccines target 2h HPVs only).
- The long-term antibody response is not yet known, although current limited data suggest it is likely to be good.
- They need to be widely used in young girls before sexual debut to be most effective—recommended at 12yrs in the UK.
- They offer no protection once HPV-infected.

▶ Cost-effectiveness is still unknown and will take decades to determine, including whether they truly prevent cervical carcinoma.

CIN, VAIN, VIN + AIN

- The presence of any form of intraepithelial abnormality of the lower genital tract is a marker for a 'field change'.
- The vagina (VAIN), vulva (VIN), and peri-anal (AIN) area are all at risk in the presence of CIN and vice versa.
- When the cervical appearances are normal with abnormal cytology the abnormal cells may be derived from elsewhere—they should be examined at colposcopy.

Gynaecological cancer: a multidisciplinary approach

Optimal treatment of the gynaecological cancer patient is provided by coordination of care within a multidisciplinary team (MDT). This team is made up of doctors, nurses, and allied professionals with an interest in treating gynaecological cancer patients and should, at a minimum, consist of: gynaecological oncologist (surgeon); clinical oncologist; medical oncologist; radiologist; histopathologist; colposcopist; gynaecological cancer nurse specialist; and MDT coordinator. Ideally, because of the complex nature of gynaecological cancer patients, their treatments, and the complications they may encounter, teams should also include or have ready access to a:
• Palliative care team.
• Dietician; fertility specialist.
• Lymphoedema specialist.
• Lower gastrointestinal surgeon.
• Urological surgeon.
• Stoma therapy nurse.
• Psychologist.
• Psychosexual counsellor.

The role of the team is to provide the following areas of care:
• Diagnosis, staging, primary surgical, and adjuvant treatment, and coordination of follow-up care.
  • Psychological preparation for anticancer treatment and follow-up: psychosexual support is a vital aspect, since many of the treatments can have major impacts on sexual functioning, either physically or psychologically, and may deprive women of their sense of femininity.
• Information on diagnosis, treatment plans, likely side effects, and follow-up plans.
• Access to financial, social, and psychological support: often required as patients may be young and have either young or older dependants, for whom they may be either the financial provider or primary carer.
• Advice on future fertility and treatments available.
• Aiding rehabilitation and preventing complications, e.g. provision of dilators following pelvic radiotherapy.
• Support with issues of survivorship.
• Appropriate and timely transition from active care to palliative care.
• Recruitment to clinical trials.
• Training of junior doctors and nurses.
• Audit of practice.

The cancer nurse specialist is often the central point of contact for the patient and ideally is trained to fulfill a supportive, advisory, advocacy role, in addition to being experienced in caring for women with complex medical issues and treatments.

Provision of appropriate care within an MDT has been shown to not only improve outcomes in terms of life-expectancy and cure rates, but also benefit patients' functional, cosmetic, and psychological well-being.

Sources of information for patients

Excellent patient advice and information leaflets are available from:
- Macmillan Cancer Support. ✆ www.macmillan.org.uk
- Cancer Research UK. ✆ www.cancerresearchuk.org
- Ovacome, an ovarian cancer support network. ✆ www.ovacome. org.uk
- www.dipex.org (very useful website that uses patient experiences of disease to help patients and their carers)
- Jo's Cervical Cancer Trust. ✆ www.jostrust.org.uk/

Further reading

National Cancer Guidance Steering Group, Department of Health. (1999). *Improving outcomes in gynaecological cancers—guidance for commissioners: the manual.* London: NHS Executive. ✆ www.dh.gov.uk/en/publicationsandstatistics

Cervical cancer: aetiology and presentation

Cervical cancer is the second most common cancer in women world-wide (83% occur in developing countries), but mortality is declining in the UK due to the success of the cervical screening programme, introduced in the 1980s (decreased from 4000 to <1000 deaths/yr)—one of the few screening tests, that meets the WHO criteria for effectiveness (see 📖 Cancer screening in gynaecology: overview, p. 700). There are dual peaks in incidence (30–39yr age group and over 70s). The UK national screening programme is changing the spectrum of disease—↑ proportion of microscopic disease and adenocarcinomas.

Aetiology

The overwhelming majority of cervical cancer is associated with persistent infection with high risk HPV subtypes (mainly HPV 16 and 18). The natural history is well known; untreated high grade CIN leads to cervical cancer in 20–30% of women over 10yrs.

Risk factors for cervical cancer

- *Exposure to HPV:*
  - early first sexual experience
  - multiple partners
  - non-barrier contraceptive.
- COCP and high parity may have direct hormonal effect, but difficult to show independent role from indirect effect on sexual behaviour.
- *Smoking:* strong dose/response effect—reduces viral clearance.
- *Immunosuppression:* HIV and transplant patients especially.

Presentation

- Cervical smear demonstrating ?invasion (but not reliable, so if suspect cancer, clinically need biopsy).
- Incidental at treatment for pre-invasive disease (CIN).
- PCB.
- Post-menopausal bleeding (cervical cancer present in <1% of women with PMB).
- Rarer presentations (often suggestive of advanced disease):
  - heavy bleeding PV
  - ureteric obstruction
  - weight loss
  - bowel disturbance
  - fistula (vesicovaginal most common).

Histology of cervical cancers

- Squamous cell carcinoma (85–90%).
- Adenocarcinoma (10–15%).
- Neuroendocrine tumour (<1%):
  - originates from argyrophil cells in the cervix
  - may present with carcinoid syndrome (very rare)
  - median survival <2yrs.
- Clear cell carcinoma (<1%):
  - <25yrs 2° to DES exposure *in utero* (not now given)
  - >45yrs not associated with DES
  - treat as per adenocarcinoma, but prognosis worse.
- Glassy cell carcinoma (<<1%):
  - median age 35yrs
  - presents with bleeding—often normal smear history
  - similar prognosis to adenocarcinoma.
- Sarcoma botryoides of the cervix (<<1%):
  - type of embryonal rhabdomyosarcoma;
  - median age ~14yrs (range 5mths–45yrs);
  - local excision (conservative surgery if possible) ± chemotherapy.
- Lymphoma of cervix (0.06%):
  - no need for surgical excision
  - responds well to combination chemotherapy.

Cervical cancer: diagnosis

Investigation

History
- PCB.
- Abnormal menstruation.
- PMB.
- PV discharge.
- Risk factors.
- Parity.
- Fertility wishes.

Examination
- *Vaginal and bimanual examination:* roughened hard cervix, ± loss of fornices and fixed cervix, if there is extension of disease.
- *Colposcopy:* irregular cervical surface, abnormal vessels, dense aceto-white changes.

Histology
Take a punch biopsy or small diagnostic loop biopsy at colposcopy.

⚠ Do not try to treat with LLETZ if cancer is suspected clinically—it may bleed +++, or compromise further treatment.

Further investigations, if cancer confirmed on biopsy
- U&E, LFTs, FBC.
- CT abdomen and pelvis (staging and preoperative assessment).
- MRI pelvis (can be very accurate at staging and examining for suspicious lymph nodes, although staging still based on clinical examination *not* MRI or histology) (see Table 23.3).
- Examination under anaesthetic (EUA):
  - bimanual vaginal examination, cystoscopy, hysteroscopy, and PV/PR examination ± sigmoidoscopy
  - less often performed now as MRI is good and many tumours are microscopic, but it still has an important role in Ib1 tumours when considering surgery
  - can insert fiducial markers (small gold beads) at clinical extent of tumour in advanced disease to aid radiotherapy planning.

Table 23.3 FIGO staging of cervical cancer

Stage			Extent of disease	5-year survival
0			Cervical intraepithelial neoplasia (CIN)	
I			Limited to cervix	
	Ia		Microscopic disease	>95%
		Ia1	Microscopic disease: invasion ≤3 mm; width ≤7 mm	
		Ia2	Microscopic disease: invasion ≤5 mm; width ≤7 mm	
	Ib		Macroscopic disease or microscopic disease >5 mm depth and/or >7mm width	
		Ib1	<4cm in diameter	~90%
		Ib2	>4cm in diameter	~80–85%
II			Extended beyond uterus (parametria/vagina), but not out to pelvic side wall, or lower 1/3 vagina	~75–78%
	IIa		No obvious parametrial involvement	
	IIb		Obvious parametrial involvement	
III			Extension to pelvic sidewall and/or lower 1/3 vagina	~47–50%
	IIIa		Lower 1/3 vagina involved	
	IIIb		Extension to pelvic sidewall (includes all cases with hydronephrosis)	
IV			Extension beyond true pelvis or involvement of bladder/bowel mucosa	~20–30%
	IVa		Extension to adjacent organs	
	IVb		Distant metastases	

Cervical cancer: treatment

Management depends on stage and age. Age is not an independent adverse prognostic factor, but is associated with ↑ stage at presentation. RCTs show that for Ib disease Wertheim's hysterectomy and radiotherapy have equivalent survival. However, if +ve LN on histology, patient will need radiotherapy as well, which ↑ morbidity and mortality if both treatments required. If surgery appropriate, perform pelvic lymphadenectomy and check for LN involvement (either frozen section at time of hysterectomy or paraffin section in a two-stage procedure—?laparoscopic lymphadenectomy) and proceed with Wertheim's hysterectomy only if LN −ve.

Role of laparoscopic surgery

Increasingly laparoscopic surgery is used in cervical cancer treatment. Pelvic lymphadenectomy can be performed laparoscopically, and this may be done as a separate procedure to Wertheim's hysterectomy, to allow for formal paraffin-embedded histology of the LN, rather than frozen section. Wertheim's hysterectomy can also be performed laparoscopically.

Fertility-sparing surgery

In young women who are keen to preserve their fertility, fertility-sparing surgery (e.g. radical trachelectomy) is an option for early stage disease (stage 1a2 and early stage 1b1) if LNs are proven to be −ve following lymphadenectomy. This is a vaginal procedure and involves the removal of cervix and paracervical tissue, to the level of the internal os, with the introduction of a cerclage suture at the level of the internal os.

The procedure does not have long-term outcome data and may not be as safe as conventional treatment, but case series demonstrate good medium-term survival data and successful pregnancies can be achieved, although ↑ risk of late miscarriage, PPROM, and preterm delivery.

Treatment options for cervical cancer according to stage

- *Stage Ia1:* local excision or total abdominal hysterectomy (risk of +ve LN <1%).
- *Stage Ia2 and Ib1:* lymphadenectomy + Wertheim's hysterectomy if –ve LN (~5% +ve LN).
- *Stage Ib2 and early IIa:*
  - chemoradiotherapy
  - consider lymphadenectomy and Wertheim's hysterectomy in very selected LN –ve cases.
- *>Stage Ib2:* combination chemoradiotherapy.
- *Stage IVb:*
  - ?chemotherapy and pelvic radiotherapy, if response
  - ?best supportive care ± palliative radiotherapy to control symptoms.

Complications of treatment

- *Wertheim's hysterectomy and lymphadenectomy:*
  - bleeding
  - infection
  - DVT/PE
  - ureteric fistula
  - bladder dysfunction
  - lymphoedema
  - lymphocysts.
- *Radiotherapy:*
  - acute bowel and bladder dysfunction (tenesmus, mucositis, bleeding)
  - 5% late bowel and bladder dysfunction (ulceration, strictures, bleeding, fistula formation)
  - vaginal stenosis, shortening, and dryness.

Ovarian cancer: aetiology

Ovarian cancer is the leading cause of death from gynaecological malignancy in the UK, with around 6500 new cases per year. The ovary is a collection of several different cell types, each of which can have neoplastic development. However, 90% are epithelial ovarian cancers (EOCs) and are commonly referred to as ovarian cancer (and will be below unless otherwise stated). Peak incidence of ovarian cancer is in women aged 75–84yrs.

Aetiology

Believed to be due to irritation of ovarian surface epithelium by damage during ovulation.
- ↑ Risk if multiple ovulations and ↓ risk if ovulation suppressed:
  - nulliparity ↑ risk
  - early menarche and/or late menopause ↑ risk
  - COCP ↓ risk (RR 0.5)
  - pregnancy ↓ risk.

BRCA mutations
- BRCA1 and BRCA2 gene products involved in repair of damaged DNA.
- Mutations lead to ↑ risk of ovarian and breast cancer (see Table 23.4).

HNPCC (Lynch II syndrome)
Identified in families with strong history of colorectal, uterine, and ovarian cancer.
- Rarer than BRCA1 and BRCA2 mutations.
- Lifetime risk of ovarian cancer ~12%.
- If prophylactic surgery then consider hysterectomy in addition to BSO.

Screening of genetically high-risk individuals
- Need a blood sample from a consenting affected relative (often a problem as may have died). Mutations may occur anywhere within the BRCA1 and BRCA2 genes, so the entire sequence of the BRCA genes should be screened. However, a deletion may not be found, in which case patient is still at moderately high risk.

Table 23.4 Ovarian cancer risk in BRCA1 and BRCA2 positive women

Cumulative risk by age	BRCA1	BRCA2
30	0%	0%
40	3%	2%
50	21%	2%
60	40%	6%
70	46%	12%

Data from King MC, Marks JH, Mandell JB, et al. (2003). Breast and ovarian cancer risks due to inherited mutations in BRCA1 and BRCA2. Science **302**(5645): 643–6.

Clinical genetics counselling

Refer for if:

- Two primary cancers (breast and/or ovary) in one 1st or 2nd degree relative.
- Three 1st and 2nd degree relatives with any of the following cancers:
  - breast
  - ovary
  - colorectal
  - stomach
  - endometrial.
- Two 1st or 2nd degree relatives, one with ovarian cancer at any age, *and one* with breast cancer under 50.
- Two 1st or 2nd degree relatives with ovarian cancer at any age.

Management if *BRCA* mutation is identified

- Surveillance with repeated CA125/ TVS/USS—efficacy not proven (UKFOCCS trial results awaited).*
- *Prophylactic surgery:*
  - BSO
  - evidence that many tumours actually arise from the *fallopian tubes*, so remove as much tube as possible
  - counsel regarding risk of finding occult tumour at time of surgery
  - screen with CA125 and USS within 2mths prior to surgery (to ensure no evidence of cancer prior to prophylactic surgery, in which case a full staging laparotomy would be required rather than laparoscopic BSO)
  - can still develop primary peritoneal cancer post-surgery, so risk of cancer not reduced to zero
  - ↓ breast cancer risk following oophorectomy if premenopausal (even on combined HRT, but most will avoid).
- Theoretically ↓ risk of breast cancer further if only oestrogen HRT required (but would need hysterectomy).
- Hysterectomy only recommended if required for other reasons (fibroids, menorrhagia, etc.).

⅁ http://www.instituteforwomenshealth.ucl.ac.uk/academic_research/gynaecologicalcancer/gcrc/ukfocss/

Ovarian cancer: presentation and investigation

Presentation
Women present with a range of vague, common symptoms, which may be misinterpreted as other conditions, e.g. irritable bowel syndrome, diverticular disease, or 'middle-aged spread'. Approximately 50% of women will present to a specialty other than gynaecology. Combination of these symptoms should increase suspicion. 75% of women will present once disease has spread to the abdomen (FIGO stage III—see Table 23.5).

- **Common symptoms**: abdominal distension (often described as bloating, but persistent); increased girth; urinary symptoms; change in bowel habit; abnormal vaginal bleeding; detection of pelvic mass.

Investigation
History
Symptoms; risk factors; comorbidities; family history (if strong, consider referral for genetic screening).

Clinical examination
Pelvic/abdominal mass (fixed/mobile); ascites; omental mass (common site for metastasis, may involve whole omentum—'omental cake'); pleural effusion; supraclavicular lymph nodes.

Haematological tests
- FBC, U&E, LFTs—especially albumin.
- Tumour markers:
  - CA125: ↑ in 80% of epithelial cancers. RMI useful for identifying patients at high risk of cancer and who should be referred to a cancer centre for treatment (sensitivity 87.4%, PPV 86.8% in recent series) (see 📖 p. 691). NICE guidelines suggest performing CA125 in women with symptoms suggestive of ovarian cancer.
  - Carcinoembryonic antigen (CEA): raised in colorectal cancers, normal in ovarian cancer.
  - CA19.9: may be raised in mucinous tumours, which are more likely to have normal CA125 (also raised in pancreatic and breast cancer).
  - Tumour markers for rarer ovarian tumours if appropriate: AFP, hCG, LDH, inhibin, and oestradiol.

Imaging
- Abdominal/pelvic USS: presence of pelvic mass and ascites (recommended by NICE guidelines if CA125 raised).
- CXR: pleural effusion or lung metastases (for staging and preoperative-work up).
- CT abdomen/pelvis: omental caking, peritoneal implants, liver metastases, and para-aortic LN.

Management of ascites and pleural effusion

Diagnosis
- Ascitic or pleural fluid should be sampled and sent for:
  - cytology
  - microbiology
  - biochemistry (U&E).

▶ Send as much fluid as possible as it may be relatively acellular.

Symptom control
- Drainage of massive tense ascites or a pleural effusion preoperatively.
- For ascitic drainage use a pig-tail drain, aseptic technique, and instill LA into skin and through abdominal wall.

▶ USS guidance, especially if bowel metastases are suspected or previous abdominal surgery.

⚠ Albumin may ↓ precipitously following ascitic drainage. Suggest dietitian referral and use of high-protein supplements to avoid problems with hypoalbuminaemia and severe generalized oedema.

Table 23.5 FIGO staging of ovarian cancer

Stage		Extent of disease	5-yr survival
I		Limited to ovaries	75–90%
	Ia	One ovary	
	Ib	Both ovaries	
	Ic	Ruptured capsule, tumour on ovarian surface; or positive peritoneal washings/ascites	
II		Limited to pelvis	45–60%
	IIa	Uterus or tubes	
	IIb	Other pelvic structures	
	IIc	Positive peritoneal washings/ascites	
III		Limited to abdomen (including regional LN metastases)	30–40%
	IIIa	Microscopic metastases	
	IIIb	Macroscopic metastases <2cm	
	IIIc	Macroscopic metastases >2cm	
IV		Distant metastases outside abdominal cavity	<20%

Data from Shepherd JH. (1989). Revised FIGO staging for gynaecological cancer. *Br J Obstet Gynaecol* **96**(8): 889–92. Engel J, Eckel R, Schubert-Fritschle G, *et al.* (2002). Moderate progress for ovarian cancer in the last 20 years: prolongation of survival, but no improvement in the cure rate. *Eur J Cancer* **38**(18): 2435–45.

Ovarian cancer: treatment

Surgery

- Current standard care for patients with a high RMI is for a staging laparotomy to be performed through a midline incision.
- Ideally this should be performed at a cancer centre by a gynaecological oncologist, as studies have demonstrated that this ↑ prognosis.
- The laparotomy should aim to remove as much tumour as possible—ideally with no macroscopic tumour remaining.
- Achievement of optimal debulking is a positive prognostic factor.
- Full staging in stage Ia cancers is important as this affects whether adjuvant chemotherapy is required.

▶ Women with advanced ovarian cancer (bulky stage IIIc or IV) may benefit from neoadjuvant chemotherapy prior to interval debulking surgery after 3 cycles, followed by an additional 3 cycles postoperatively. Survival rates are similar, with reduced morbidity in the neoadjuvant group.

☞ There is no evidence to support routine 'second-look surgery' to see if there is still tumour present after chemotherapy.

☞ There is no consensus on the use of interval debulking surgery (IDS) (following 3 cycles of chemotherapy), if 1° surgery does not achieve optimal debulking.

☞ The role of supraradical surgery (diaphragmatic and extensive peritoneal stripping, liver resection, splenectomy, etc.) remains contentious.

Pseudomyxoma peritonei

Mucinous cystadenocarcinomas may present with a thick, jelly-like ascites with mucinous tumour deposits throughout the abdominal cavity. Frequently these may arise from a primary tumour of the appendix and an appendicetomy is recommended as part of the debulking surgery for diagnosis.

▶ Two specialist centres for pseudomyxoma peritoneii exist in the UK, at Manchester and Basingstoke. Optimal treatment requires extensive abdominal surgery (Sugarbaker technique) and intraperitoneal chemotherapy. Ideally, diagnosis should be made before surgery and patients referred for primary surgery at a specialist centre. If found intraoperatively, it is recommended that the main masses be removed (ovary and appendix) and the abdomen thoroughly washed out to remove as much jelly-like material as possible. More extensive primary surgery can limit ability of specialist centre to perform radical debulking and should be avoided, if possible.

This consists of a full surgical staging laparotomy

- Laparotomy.
- Hysterectomy.
- Bilateral salpingo-oophrectomy.
- Omentectomy.
- Lymph node sampling (pelvic and para-aortic).
- Peritoneal biopsies.
- Pelvic washings/ascitic sampling.

See Table 23.5.

Ovarian cancer: chemotherapy and follow-up

Adjuvant chemotherapy

Adjuvant chemotherapy (following surgery) is recommended for all patients other than those with low risk early stage disease (stage Ia–b low grade disease). For advanced disease (stage II and greater) RCTs have demonstrated that platinum agents are superior and that carboplatin = cisplatin in terms of prognosis, but has ↓ side effects.

▶ Normal regimen is 6 cycles of carboplatin ± paclitaxel every 3wks.

▶ Some patients with bulky stage IIIc/IV may benefit from neoadjuvant chemotherapy (3 cycles, IDS, 3 cycles).

▶ Systematic review evidence suggests that paclitaxel gives small additional survival benefit, although it increases side effects (uniformly causing alopecia as well as ↑ side effects caused by platinum agents). It has become the standard of care in women with an adequate performance status.

✎ RCTs have suggested that intraperitoneal (Ip) chemotherapy may improve survival (improved regional pharmacokinetics), although at the cost of increased side effects (many related to the Ip catheter or absolute dose of chemotherapy in Ip arm of trials) and should be used only as part of a clinical trial.

Investigations before starting chemotherapy

- Baseline CT scan (to assess response).
- Creatinine clearance, *or*
- ^{51}CrEDTA (to assess renal function).
- Histological diagnosis.

▶ Assessment of renal function is needed to determine platinum agent dosing.

Follow-up

Patients are monitored using clinical examination ± tumour markers, where previously raised (every 3mths for 1st year, every 4mths 2nd year, then, if no recurrence, every 6mths for up to 5yrs). Recent RCT demonstrated no benefit of monitoring CA125 in asymptomatic women during follow-up, since there is no improvement in overall survival if treated on CA125 rise only, in the absence of symptoms.

Various novel agents are being investigated in clinical trials for primary, relapsed disease and in a maintenance setting, including antibodies against VEGF (bevacizumab) and epidermal growth factor receptor (EGFR) (cetuximab), in addition to tyrosine kinase inhibitors (gefitinib).

Rare ovarian tumours: germ cell

Germ cell tumours account for <5% of ovarian tumours. Can arise anywhere down tract of embryological genital ridge, along which primordial germ cells migrate from yolk sac, although most occur in the ovaries. Degree of differentiation of primordial germ cell affects type of cancer produced: undifferentiated germ cells cause dysgerminomas; cells that have undergone initial differentiation can undergo embryonal or extra-embryonal differentiation, to produce choriocarcinoma/endodermal sinus tumours (yolk sac) or teratomas, respectively. Germ cell tumours most commonly occur in young women and account for 70% of ovarian tumours in the under 20s; when ~30% of these are malignant.

Dermoid cyst

Common benign ovarian tumour, often bilateral (10%), and commonly contain sebaceous material; sometimes hair and teeth.

Dysgerminoma

- Commonest malignant germ cell tumour.
- Female equivalent of a seminoma.
- 80% present at stage I and so treat with conservative surgery.
- Can be bilateral (10–20%) and require close follow-up of the conserved ovary.
- Common in XY karyotypically abnormal gonads, e.g. XO/XY Turner's syndrome mosaic, and prophylactic removal should be recommended.

▶ Dysgerminomas may require chemotherapy, if more advanced. Combination chemotherapy regimens include: bleomycin, etoposide, and cisplatin (BEP); vinblastin, bleomycin, and cisplatin (VBP); and cisplatin, vincristine, methotrexate, bleomycin, dactinomycin, cyclophosphamide, and etoposide (POMB/ACE).

⚠ Aim is to conserve fertility if appropriate in young women, but ↑ risk of secondary malignancies following chemotherapy.

Immature teratomas

- Present most commonly in girls 10–20yrs.
- Conservative surgery/chemotherapy unless stage Ia (BEP regimen).

Endodermal sinus tumours (previously yolk sac tumours)

- Median age 18yrs at presentation.
- Raised AFP levels.
- Conservative surgery and chemotherapy (BEP or POMB/ACE).
- 2yr median survival 60–70%.

Choriocarcinoma of ovary and embryonal carcinoma

- Presentation in women <20yrs.
- Raised hCG levels (choriocarcinoma) or hCG and AFP (embryonal carcinoma).
- Treat as other germ cell tumours.

Rare ovarian tumours: other

Sex-cord stromal tumours (~5%)

Granulosa cell tumour
- Solid ovarian tumours, which commonly produce oestrogens.
- Peak incidences in young girls and post-menopausal women.
- Present with PMB, menstrual problems, or precocious pseudo-puberty, depending on age.
- May be associated with concurrent endometrial cancer (2° to unopposed oestrogens).
- Often have raised inhibin (produced by granulosa cells to cause negative feedback on FSH levels from pituitary gland) and oestradiol levels—used as tumour markers for monitoring recurrence.
- Treat with surgery (conservative surgery in young woman, i.e. remove affected ovary, biopsy omentum and LN ± biopsy other ovary) as most (~80%) present at stage I and so fertility can be preserved.
- Often recur, which may be many years later and may require repeated surgical debulking.

Sertoli–Leydig cell tumour
- Produce androgens.
- Present with hirsuitism, amenorrhoea, and virilization (male pattern baldness, clitoromegaly, deepening voice, hairiness, oily skin, etc.).
- Normally benign tumours—treat surgically.

Fibroma
- Benign solid tumour.
- May present with ascites and pleural effusion (R > L)—Meig's syndrome.

Tubal carcinoma

- Present similarly to ovarian cancer (and may often be misdiagnosed as ovarian cancer and probably not as rare as previously thought).
- Normally serous cystadenocarcinoma.

See Table 23.6.

Table 23.6 Ovarian cancer: histological subtypes

Epithelial (85–90%)	Sex-cord stromal (5%)	Germ cell (5%)
Serous cystadenocarcinoma (75%)	Granulosa-stromal cell tumours	Dysgerminoma
Mucinous cystadenocarcinoma	Granulosa cell	Embryonal carcinoma
Endometrioid adenocarcinoma	Thecoma	Immature teratoma
Clear cell	Fibroma	Mature teratoma
Undifferentiated	Androblastomas	Stuma ovarii
	Sertoli cell	Carcinoid
	Sertoli–Leydig cell	Endodermal sinus tumour (yolk sac)
	Leydig cell	Choriocarcinoma

5% of ovarian tumours are 2° tumours: endometrium; cervix; fallopian tube; Krukenburg tumours (breast, stomach, colon); lymphoma; melanoma; carcinoid.

Borderline ovarian tumours

Borderline ovarian tumours arise from the ovarian surface epithelium. They are not benign tumours, and are staged as for ovarian cancer. They were previously known as 'tumours of low malignant potential' and account for ~15% of ovarian epithelial cancers, although they are more common in younger women.

Borderline tumours are:

• Often confined to ovary.
• Occur in premenopausal women: even in girls and teenagers.
• Can have metastatic implants: these may be non-invasive or invasive.
• Associated with a much better prognosis than epithelial ovarian cancer.
• Difficult to diagnose histologically.
• Of predominately serous histology.
• CA125 may be elevated and if so can be a useful tumour marker for recurrence.

Data suggest that women with borderline tumours without invasive implants do not benefit from chemotherapy. Surgery is the recommended treatment. In young women a conservative surgical approach is valid, with the aim of preserving fertility (i.e. unilateral oophorectomy with appropriate staging biopsies). In stage I disease an RCT found that conservative treatment was safe; relapse rate was 8% over 2–18yrs. They may relapse at a very late stage, after the traditional 5yr follow-up, and can occur anything up to 25yrs after initial presentation. Long-term follow-up study (Borderline Ovarian Tumour Study – BOTS) recently started to give more information about prognosis.

Further reading

Cancer Research UK. (2012). *A study to find out more about borderline ovarian tumours.* ℬ http://cancerhelp.cancerresearchuk.org/trials/a-study-find-out-more-about-borderline-ovarian-tumours

Endometrial hyperplasia

Endometrial hyperplasia is a premalignant condition, that can predispose to, or be associated with, endometrial carcinoma. It is characterized by the overgrowth of endometrial cells and is caused by excess unopposed oestrogens, either endogenous or exogenous, similar to endometrial cancer, with which it shares a common aetiology (see 📖 Endometrial cancer: aetiology and histology, p. 734).

Presentation

Endometrial hyperplasia was commonly diagnosed on endometrial biopsies of women investigated for infertility. However, these are not routinely performed, and it is now most commonly diagnosed in women over 40yrs old with irregular menstruation or in those with post-menopausal bleeding.

Histology

Endometrial sampling or formal endometrial curettage is necessary for diagnosis. Degree of hyperplasia (simple or complex) depends on the glandular:stromal ratio (much less stroma in complex hyperplasia). Atypia describes the appearance of the individual glandular cells (increased nuclear:cytoplasmic ratio—similar to CIN). Back-to-back atypical glandular cells (i.e. no stromal component) = endometrial carcinoma.

Management of endometrial hyperplasia (no atypia)

Depends on age of patient, histology, symptoms, and desire for retaining fertility.
- Exclude treatable causes of unopposed oestrogens:
  - oestrogen-only HRT
  - oestrogen-secreting tumour (e.g. granulosa cell tumour of ovary).
- Treat with progestagens, e.g.:
  - continuous oral progestagens daily for 3–6mths: 5mg norethisterone (premenopausal); 10mg medroxyprogesterone acetate (MPA) (perimenopausal); 20mg MPA (post-menopausal)
  - levonorgestrel intrauterine device if post-menopausal.
- Risk of progression to cancer:
  - simple hyperplasia ~1%
  - complex hyperplasia 3.5%.
- Rebiopsy only if abnormal bleeding continues.

Classification of endometrial hyperplasia
- Endometrial hyperplasia:
  - simple
  - complex (adenomatous).
- Atypical endometrial hyperplasia.

Atypical endometrial hyperplasia

◆ 46% of women with atypical hyperplasia will have a concurrent adenocarcinoma and, if not concurrent, there is a very high risk the woman will develop adenocarcinoma.

▶ Counsel about high risk of developing endometrial carcinoma.

▶ Unless fertility is desired or unacceptably high operative risk, recommend TAH (+ BSO if >45yrs).

▶▶ If conservative treatment, then treat with high-dose progestagens, e.g. MPA 100mg daily. Rebiopsy every 3–6mths until progression or regression, and continue with long-term surveillance. Mirena® coil often used for maintenance treatment (if not trying to conceive). Strongly consider hysterectomy once fertility not required.

Endometrial cancer: aetiology and histology

Endometrial cancer predominantly affects post-menopausal women (91% of cases in >50yr olds). Worldwide differences in prevalence reflect differences in risk factors (22:100 000 in North America compared with 3.5/100 000 in Africa), and incidence is rising with increasingly 'western' lifestyles.

Aetiology

Presence of unopposed oestrogen (i.e. no protective effect of progesterone), whether endogenous or exogenous.

- *Endogenous:*
  - peripheral conversion in adipose tissue of androstenedione to oestrone
  - oestrogen-producing tumour (granulosa cell tumour)
  - polycystic ovarian syndrome or anovulatory cycles at menarche or during climacteric period (lack of progesterone as no luteal phase).
- *Exogenous:*
  - oestrogen-only HRT
  - tamoxifen (oestrogen agonist in endometrial tissue).

Risk factors

- Obesity and conditions predisposing or associated with obesity (including type II diabetes mellitus, hypothyroidism, hypertension).
- *Reduced endogenous progesterone production:*
  - nulliparity (pregnancy associated with high progesterone levels)
  - PCOS (anovulatory cycles—no corpus luteum, no progesterone)
  - early menarche/late menopause (anovulatory cycles).
- *Genetic predisposition:* HNPCC (Lynch II syndrome) with high risk of colorectal, endometrial, and ovarian tumours (40–60% lifetime risk of endometrial cancer; inherited as autosomal dominant condition; inherited mutation in one copy of a mismatch repair gene)
- Breast cancer (shared lifestyle risk factors and tamoxifen usage).

Protective factors

- Parity (high progesterone dose in pregnancy).
- COCP (50% ↓ with up to 4yrs of use up to 72% with 12 or more years) (progesterone effect).

Histology

Endometrial cancer arises from the endometrial lining. The major prognostic indicators in endometrial cancer are their grade of differentiation and FIGO stage of disease. These factors guide use of adjuvant treatment.

⚠ Endometrial hyperplasia with atypia (but not without) is a premalignant condition and may have coincidental cancer in at least 50% of women.

Histological types of endometrial cancer

Adenocarcinoma
- Endometrial adenocarcinoma 87%.
- Adenosquamous carcinoma* 6%.
- Clear cell or papillary serous carcinoma* 6%.
- MMMT* 1%.

* High risk of advanced disease at presentation and recurrence—all G3. (See Grading below)

Grading
- Well differentiated (G1).
- Moderately differentiated (G2).
- Poorly differentiated or high risk cell type (G3).

Endometrial cancer: presentation and investigation

Presentation
Most commonly presents with PMB. Younger women present with menstrual disturbance (heavy or irregular periods). 1% are picked up on routine cervical smear tests.

⚠ 1 in 10 women with PMB will have endometrial cancer or atypical hyperplasia (Table 23.7).

▶▶ Endometrial sampling required for women >45yrs with abnormal menstrual symptoms.

⚠ PV discharge and pyometra may occur instead of bleeding—have a ↑ index of suspicion in post-menopausal women with ↑ PV discharge (50% of post-menopausal women with pyometra have underlying carcinoma).

Investigation
History
- Presenting symptoms.
- Menstrual history.
- Parity.
- Comorbidities.
- Drug history (COCP, HRT, tamoxifen, antihypertensives, oral hypoglycaemics).
- Family history.

Examination
- Rule out other causes of bleeding (vulval, vaginal, and cervical pathology) with vulval, vaginal, and speculum examination.
- *Bimanual examination:* uterine size, mobility, adnexal masses.

Haematological investigations
- FBC, U&E, LFTs.

Imaging investigations
- *TVUSS:* <4mm endometrial thickness/echo (ET) → very low risk of endometrial pathology in post-menopausal women (96% NPV)—no requirement for endometrial sampling.
- *CT chest/abdomen/pelvis:* G3 disease for preoperative staging as ↑ risk of disease outside of uterus.
- *MRI pelvis:* can be used to determine local extent of tumour and presence of grossly involved pelvic lymph nodes. Not routinely recommended as staging based on histology.
- CXR (staging).

Endometrial biopsy
Perform endometrial sampling if ET ≥4mm or persistent bleeding in woman with ET <4mm (in which case consider formal hysteroscopy).
- Blind outpatient sampling (e.g. pipelle, vabra).
- *Hysteroscopy:* under LA as outpatient or GA as inpatient.

Table 23.7 Histopathology findings in women with PMB

Histological diagnosis	%
Atrophy	49.9
Proliferatory/secretory	5.5
Benign polyps	9.2
Hyperplasia	
No atypia	27.8
Atypical hyperplasia	5.5
Adenocarcinoma	8.1
Not diagnostic	14.2
Other disorders	3.3

Data from Gredmark T, Kvint S, Havel G, et al. (1995). Histopathological findings in women with postmenopausal bleeding. *Br J Obstet Gynaecol* **102**(2): 133–6.

Endometrial cancer: treatment

Treatment

Surgery
TAH and BSO and pelvic washings: this can be performed via a transverse or midline incision. Increasingly, laparoscopic hysterectomy is gaining popularity and is approved by NICE, although longer-term survival data comparisons are lacking (no difference at 3yrs).

Pelvic lyphadenectomy
Role in low-grade early disease is controversial (and is debated fiercely across the Atlantic divide!). Two RCTs (and Cochrane systematic review) suggest no survival advantage in early disease (see Table 23.8).

Adjuvant radiotherapy
Adjuvant radiotherapy limited to vault brachytherapy, if intermediate risk (see below), EBRT ± vault brachytherapy boost for high risk (G3, stage Ib) or locally advanced disease.

Role of adjuvant chemotherapy in addition to ERBT in high risk disease being examined in clinical trial (PORTEC 3).

PORTEC and ASTEC trials
- These trials compared adjuvant radiotherapy vs. no adjuvant radiotherapy in women with intermediate risk early endometrial adenocarcinoma: G1 with deep myometrial invasion (>50%); G2 with any myometrial invasion (stage Ia or Ib); and G3 with superficial invasion (stage Ia).
- Radiotherapy reduced pelvic recurrences, but gave no survival advantage to women with stage Ib endometrial cancer and intermediate risk histology.
- This was because pelvic recurrences were amenable to radiotherapy in previously non-irradiated patients.
- Vault brachytherapy reduced risk of pelvic recurrence.

Hormonal
- High dose progesterone used for advanced and recurrent disease.
- Largely aiming for palliation of symptoms (bleeding)—no survival advantage demonstrated.

Palliative radiotherapy
- EBRT given at lower dose and in few fractions to control local symptoms (e.g. bleeding).

Further reading
NICE. (2010). *Treating endometrial cancer with keyhole hysterectomy.* ♪ http://www.nice.org.uk/nicemedia/live/12355/50833/50833.pdf

Table 23.8 FIGO staging of endometrial cancer

Stage	Extent of disease	5-year survival
I	Tumour limited to uterine body	85%
Ia	<1/2 myometrial depth invaded	
Ib	>1/2 myometrial depth invaded	
II	Tumour limited to uterine body and cervix*	75%
II	Invasion into cervical stroma	
III	Extension to uterine serosa, peritoneal cavity, and/or lymph nodes	45%
IIIa	Extension to uterine serosa, adnexae, or positive peritoneal fluid (ascites or washings)	
IIIb	Extension to vagina	
IIIc	Pelvic or para-aortic lymph nodes involved	
IV	Extension beyond true pelvis and/or involvement of bladder/bowel mucosa	25%
IVa	Extension to adjacent organs	
IVb	Distant metastases or positive inguinal lymph nodes	

*Endocervical involvement without stromal invasion now included in stage I.

Rare uterine malignancies

Uterine sarcomas

Uterine sarcomas are very rare, accounting for 3–5% of uterine cancers and have an incidence of 2:100 000 women. Abnormal bleeding is the most common presenting feature; other symptoms include pain and a pelvic mass. Polypoid masses may protrude through the cervical os.

⚠ Uterine corpus sarcomas account for 3–5% of all uterine cancers, but cause 26% of the mortality.

Types of uterine sarcomas
- Leiomyosarcoma (46%).
- Endometrial stromal sarcoma (12%).
- Carcinosarcoma (27%).
- Not specified/others (15%).

The peak incidence for leiomyosarcoma and endometrial stromal sarcoma is 50–64yrs of age. Peak incidence for carcinosarcoma is older, at 65–79yrs. Age, stage, and tumour type are important prognostic factors.
The 5-yr survival figures are:
- Leiomyosarcoma, stage I 65%, stage IV 0%.
- Carcinosarcoma, stage I 62%, stage IV 17%.
- Endometrial stromal sarcoma, stage I 85%, stage IV 37%.

Vulval intraepithelial neoplasia: overview

VIN can occur in any age group, but is more common in post-menopausal women. There has been an ↑ in incidence of VIN over 30yrs, especially in younger women, probably reflecting changes in sexual practice, as well as ↑ recognition. The natural history of VIN is not as well understood as CIN, but up to 9% of women with VIN may progress to vulval cancer over several years. VIN is difficult to treat and frustrating to patient and doctor.

Aetiology

VIN is a dysplastic lesion of the squamous epithelium. As with its cervical counterpart, CIN, it is associated with persistent infection with HPV in >90% of cases, especially HPV 16. HPV infection may cause multifocal disease, and patients with VIN should be carefully screened for CIN. Smoking is also associated with development of VIN.

Histology

The 2004 classification system now uses VIN to refer to previous VIN II–III, whereas VIN I is now thought to be non-specific inflammatory changes and is not premalignant.

Presentation and investigation

Symptoms are primarily those of itch, but include pain and ulceration; over 20% may be asymptomatic. Lesions may be raised and warty or flat and erythematous and are frequently found at multiple sites on the vulva (~50%). Diagnosis is made by punch or excision biopsy. Since HPV causes multifocal disease, patients require regular cervical smears.

Paget's disease of the vulva

- Non-mammary adenocarcinoma *in situ*: in breast, Paget's disease is normally associated with underlying malignancy, whereas only 10–12% with vulval Paget's disease have an invasive adenocarcinoma component, and another ~8% have an underlying adenocarcinoma (e.g. colorectal).
- Post-menopausal women.
- Presents with itching and vulval soreness.
- Eczematous or raised and velvety appearance—may weep serous fluid.
- Extent of disease spreads well beyond clinical lesion—difficult to excise completely.
- May be associated with rectal adenocarcinoma, especially if Paget's in perianal area.
- Treat with surgical excision and exclude underlying malignancy.
- Can recur and if does so is normally another adenocarcinoma *in situ*.

Vulval intraepithelial neoplasia: management

Although small, painful lesions can be excised, it must be remembered that there is normally a field change, and so it is difficult to completely excise the VIN, and recurrence rate is ↑ , even after radical vulvectomy. The aim of treatment is therefore to minimize symptoms and side effects of disease and to exclude development of vulval cancer.

Surveillance

Careful follow-up of patients with VIN is required and suspicious lesions should be biopsied.

Surgery

Excision of painful/irritating lesions can be performed, but skinning vulvectomy or laser ablation is rarely recommended, due to the high recurrence rate (40–70%) and poor functional outcome. Development of pain is associated with ↑ risk of vulval cancer.

Immunotherapy

Imiquimod, an immune modifier, has been shown to help clearance of genital warts. Stimulates monocytes and macrophages; these secrete cytokines which result in T-helper cell coordination of a cell-mediated immune response. Apply cream 2–3 times weekly for 12wks. ~30% response rate, most will relapse. Treatment can be limited by side effects—soreness and burning. Evidence suggests reduction in need for excision.[1]

Vaccination

HPV vaccination for prevention of CIN may help to reduce VIN, but no role in treatment of existing VIN.

Chemotherapy

✿ Topical 5-fluorouracil (5-FU). This is usually ineffective and badly tolerated and is no longer recommended.

1 Pepas L, Kaushik S, Bryant A, *et al.* (2011). Medical interventions for high grade vulval intraepithelial neoplasia. *Cochrane Database System Rev* Issue 4. Art. No.: CD007924. DOI: 10.1002/14651858. CD007924.pub2.

Vulval cancer: aetiology and investigation

Vulval carcinomas are uncommon, but approximately 90% are squamous cell carcinomas and ~5% are vulval melanomas, with basal cell, Bartholin's gland carcinoma, and rarely sarcomas, accounting for the rest. Most occur in older women (median age at presentation 74yrs), although younger women are at risk, especially those with multifocal VIN.

Aetiology

Vulval squamous carcinomas (vulval cancer) commonly arise on a background of lichen sclerosus or VIN.

Presentation

Vulval cancers commonly present with a lump, pain, irritation, or bleeding. There may be an obvious ulcer present. Older women in particular may delay presentation due to embarrassment. Referral to secondary care may also be delayed if there is not an adequately high index of suspicion.

Investigation

History

Vulval symptoms, treatments (prescribed or self), past medical history, and performance status (see Table 23.9).

Clinical examination

Palpable groin LN, size and location of lesion, general medical condition. May be too painful for examination unless under GA, so if obvious tumour, do this at time of biopsy.

Haematological investigations

FBC, U&E, LFTs.

Imaging investigations

• CXR (staging and preoperative).
• As yet, no role of imaging groins for LN (see p. 746).

Anaesthetic review

Patients with vulval cancer are often very old and may be quite frail. Involve an anaesthetist at an early stage in the preoperative work-up. Remember that regional anaesthetic may be a preferred option in some patients.

Histology

All suspicious vulval lesions should be biopsied. Small lesions can be excised and larger lesions should have a wedge biopsy taken, including the edge of the lesion if possible (in ulcerated lesions, it may be difficult to get a diagnosis from the sloughed tissue central to the lesion).

Table 23.9 ECOG performance status

Grade	Performance criteria
0	Fully active
1	Reduced physical activity, but ambulatory and able to perform light work, e.g. light housework, office work
2	Ambulatory and capable of all self-care, but unable to carry out work activities. Up and about more than 50% of waking hours
3	Limited self-care, confined to bed or chair more than 50% of waking hours
4	Totally confined to bed or chair, cannot carry out any self-care

Vulval cancer: treatment

Surgery

Surgery is the mainstay of treatment in vulval cancer, both for curative intent and also for palliation.

- Patients with disease >1mm invasion should have groin lymphadenectomy performed.
- Lateral disease can have an ipsilateral LN dissection: if +ve LN, bilateral groin LN dissection is required.
- Central disease requires bilateral groin LN dissections.

The importance of lymphadenectomy was recognized in the 1940s by Way and Taussig, who developed the 'butterfly' incision *en bloc* dissection, which removed the entire vulva and inguinal LNs with all connecting tissue. These wounds frequently broke down and took many months to heal by secondary intent. The triple incision vulvectomy, with separate groin incisions, was subsequently developed to reduce morbidity. Current treatment aims for wide local excision (ideally margins >1cm) of the vulval lesion and LN dissection through separate incisions along the inguinal ligament. Occasionally, plastic surgical reconstruction is required.

▶ Groin recurrence is very difficult to treat and carries a very ↑ rate of mortality.

Complications

- Wound breakdown and infection.
- Lymphocysts.
- Lymphoedema.
- DVT/PE.

Radiotherapy +/− chemotherapy

- Can be used before surgery to shrink primary to reduced morbidity of surgery (e.g. if urethra or anus involved).
- Is used after surgery if positive groin LNs, to prevent regional recurrence. External beam radiotherapy given to treat potentially +ve pelvic LN.
- Can combine with chemotherapy.

▶ Should not be used as an alternative to groin dissection (RCT halted early as 5/26 had groin recurrences, compared with none in surgical arm).

Sentinel lymph node biopsy

Morbidity ↑ from groin LN dissection. The theory is that there is a single LN, which primarily drains the tumour. If this is identified and is negative, patient can be spared full groin dissection. Identify sentinel LN with blue dye and radiolabelled tracer. Currently under RCT investigation for safety comparing sentinel LN dissection +/− radiotherapy with groin node dissection +/− radiotherapy. GROINS II Trial changed at interim analysis, as high recurrence in +ve sentinel node + radiotherapy arm, so now full groin node dissection required if +ve sentinel node (see Table 23.10).

Vulval/vaginal melanoma

- Staged, like other melanomas, rather than vulval cancer: Breslow depth and American Joint Committee on Cancer (AJCC) staging (2002).
- Most common site is the lower anterior vaginal wall (so easy to miss on speculum examination).
- Very poor prognosis—5-yr survival 13–19%.

Table 23.10 FIGO staging of vulval cancer

Stage	Extent of disease	5-yr survival
0	Intraepithelial neoplasia (VIN)	
I	Tumour limited to vulva or perineum <2cm diameter (–ve lymph nodes)	98%
Ia	<1mm depth of invasion	
Ib	>1mm depth of invasion or >2cm	
II	Tumour of any size with spread to adjacent perineal structures (lower 1/3 vagina, lower 1/3 urethra, anus) with negative lymph nodes	
III	Tumour of any size with or without extension to adjacent perineal structures	
IIIa	1 LN metastasis >5mm; 2–3 LN metastases <5mm	
IIIb	≥2 LN metastases (>5mm); ≥3 LN metastases (<5mm)	
IIIc	+ve LN with extracapsular spread	
IVa	Tumour spread to upper urethra, bladder, bowel, pelvic bones, and/or fixed/ulcerated inguinal lymph nodes	
IVb	Distant metastases and/or +ve pelvic lymph nodes	

Vaginal cancer

All primary vaginal carcinomas are rare and account for only 1% of gynae-cological malignancies. Most vaginal tumours are metastases from either above (cervical or uterine) or below (vulval). Of the remaining true vaginal tumours, most are squamous cell carcinomas and present in older women. Many will have a previous history of intraepithelial neoplasia or invasive carcinoma of the vulva, vagina, or cervix. Other predisposing factors include pelvic radiotherapy and long-term inflammation due to a vaginal pessary or procidentia. Squamous cell carcinoma, similar to cervical carcinoma, is commonly HPV-related.

Vaginal clear cell adenocarcinoma

Occur in younger women and are strongly associated with DES exposure *in utero*. DES was administered to several million pregnant women at risk of miscarriage or premature delivery between 1940 and 1971. The critical time for exposure was in the first 20wks of pregnancy.

Treatment of vaginal clear cell adenocarcinoma

Aim to preserve reproductive function in (often) young women. Stage I tumours treated with wide local excision. In more advanced stage disease, radiotherapy is indicated (see Table 23.11).

Embryonal rhabdomyosarcoma (sarcoma botryoides)

- Rare tumour with a multicystic grape-like form (sarcoma botryoides).
- Derived from rhabdomyoblasts.
- Presents in infancy (girls <3yrs).
- Cervical rhabdomyosarcoma can occur in teenagers, and uterine rhabdomyosarcoma has been described in post-menopausal women.
- Presents with a grape-like mass arising from the vagina; can present with vaginal bleeding or a single polyp.
- Treatment—preserve fertility and vaginal function:
  - smaller tumours excised followed by combination chemotherapy (vincristine, dactinomycin, and cyclophosphamide)
  - neoadjuvant chemotherapy given for larger tumours, to reduce their size prior to surgery.
- Survival rates of 90% can be achieved: refer to centres with expertise—may need reconstructive surgery.

Vaginal clear cell adenocarcinoma in DES-exposed women

- Probably only of historical significance.
- Appear after 14yrs of age; peak incidence of 19yrs.
- RR of developing clear cell adenocarcinoma is 40.7 (95% CI, 13.1–126.2).
- Cumulative incidence rate only 1.5:1000 DES-exposed women.

Vaginal clear cell adenocarcinoma in women not exposed to DES

- Peak incidence 50–60yrs.

⚠ The DES-exposed cohort is only just reaching this age, so the total effect of DES exposure is not yet known.

Table 23.11 FIGO staging of vaginal cancer

Stage	Extent of disease	5-yr survival*
0	Intraepithelial neoplasia (VAIN)	95%
I	Tumour limited to vaginal wall	~67%
II	Tumour limited to vagina and subvaginal tissue, but not extending to pelvic sidewall	<39%
III	Tumour spread to pelvic sidewall	~33%
IV	Tumour spread beyond true pelvis and/or into bladder/bowel mucosa	<19%
IVa	Tumour spread to bladder/bowel or directly invading beyond true pelvis	
IVb	Distant metastases	

* Beller U, Maisonneuve P, Benedet JL, et al. (2003). Carcinoma of the vagina. *Int J Gynaecol Obstet* **83**(Suppl 1):27–39.

Gestational trophoblastic disease: hydatidiform mole

Gestational trophoblastic disease (GTD) covers a spectrum of diseases caused by overgrowth of the placenta. This includes hyatidiform mole, choriocarcinoma, invasive mole, and placental site trophoblastic tumour.

- *Incidence:* 0.6–2.3:1000 pregnancies.
- *Background:* 50% of cases follow hyatidiform mole, 25% a normal pregnancy, and 25% a miscarriage or ectopic pregnancy.

Hyatidiform mole

Can be subdivided into complete and partial mole based on genetic and histological features.

Complete mole

- Consists of diffuse hydropic villi with trophoblastic hyperplasia.
- This is diploid, derived from sperm duplicating its own chromosome following fertilization of an 'empty' ovum. This is mostly 46XX with no evidence of fetal tissue.

Partial mole

- Consists of hydropic and normal villi.
- This is triploid (69XXX, XXY, YYY) with one maternal and two paternal haploid sets. Most cases occur following two sperms fertilizing an ovum, and a fetus may be present.

Diagnosis

Symptoms and signs (with approximate frequency)

- Irregular first-trimester vaginal bleeding (>90%).
- Uterus large for dates (25%).
- Pain from large theca lutein cysts (20%) resulting from ovarian hyperstimulation by high hCG levels.
- Vaginal passage of vesicles containing products of conception (10%).
- Exaggerated pregnancy symptoms:
  - hyperemesis (10%)
  - hyperthyroidism (5%)
  - early pre-eclampsia (5%).

▶ Serum hCG is excessively high with complete moles, but levels may be within the normal range for partial moles.

Risk factors for hyatidiform mole

- *Age:* extremes of reproductive life (>40yrs and <15yrs of age) in complete moles, not partial moles.
- *Ethnicity:* x2 higher in east Asia, particularly Korea and Japan.
- *Previous molar pregnancy:* x10 higher risk of developing future molar pregnancy.

USS findings (see Fig. 23.1)

Complete mole
- 'Snowstorm' appearance of mixed echogenecity, representing hydropic villi and intrauterine haemorrhage.
- Large theca lutein cysts.

Partial mole
Fetus may be viable, with signs of early growth restriction or structural abnormalities.

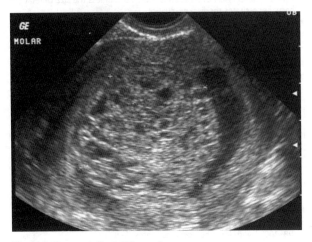

Fig. 23.1 Ultrasound of hydatidiform mole.

Hydatidiform mole: management

Management

- *Complete mole:* surgical evacuation is advisable and should be performed by an experienced surgeon as risks of uterine perforation and haemorrhage are significant. Oxytocin may be required to reduce the risk of haemorrhage, but its use is associated with a theoretical risk of tissue dissemination leading to metastatic disease to the lungs or brain and should be avoided until the uterus is evacuated if possible.
- *Partial mole:* surgical evacuation is preferable, unless the size of fetal parts necessitates medical evacuation.
- Histological examination of products of conception is essential to confirm diagnosis.

Treatment of persistent gestational trophoblastic disease

Risk of requiring chemotherapy is 15% after a complete mole and 0.5% after a partial mole.

> **Indications for chemotherapy**
> - Serum hCG levels >20 000IU/L at 4wks after uterine evacuation.
> - Static or rising hCG after uterine evacuation in absence of new pregnancy.
> - Persistent symptoms, e.g. uterine bleeding and/or abdominal pain.
> - Evidence of metastases.
> - Histological diagnosis of choriocarcinoma.

Prognosis

- With effective registration and treatment programme, cure rate is high (98–100%) with low chemotherapy rates (5–8%).
- Recurrence rate is low (1/55).
- Women should be advised not to conceive until hCG level has been normal for 6mths.
- hCG levels should be checked 6 and 10wks after each subsequent pregnancy.

Contraception and hormone replacement therapy

- Barrier contraception should be used until serum hCG is normal.
- The COCP and HRT are safe to use after hCG levels have returned to normal.

Specialist follow-up for molar pregnancy

In the UK, all women with any molar pregnancy should be registered at one of the three specialist centres (Sheffield, Dundee, London). The protocol for follow-up varies amongst the specialist centres. At Charing Cross Hospital (London), follow-up with hCG ranges from 6mths to 2yrs after uterine evacuation.

- Serum hCG should be checked fortnightly until levels are normal (<4IU/L).
- Following this, urine hCG is requested at 4-weekly intervals until 1yr post-evacuation, then every 3mths in the 2nd year of follow-up.
- If hCG normalizes within 8wks, follow-up will be limited to 6mths.
- Patients who do not have normal hCG values within 8wks of evacuation should have the 2-yr follow-up.

Further reading

Hydatidiform Mole and Choriocarcinoma UK Information and Support Service. ℘ www.hmole-chorio.org.uk

RCOG. (2010). *The management of gestational trophoblastic neoplasia*, RCOG Guideline No. 38. ℘ http://www.rcog.org.uk/files/rcog-corp/GT38ManagementGestational0210.pdf.

Sheffield Trophoblastic Tumour Screening and Treatment Centre. ℘ http://www.chorio.group.shef.ac.uk/clin.html

Gestational trophoblastic disease: choriocarcinoma

This is a highly malignant tumour consisting of syncytio- and cytotrophoblast with myometrial invasion. Local spread and vascular metastases to the lung are common. 50% of cases are preceded by hyatidiform mole, 40% by normal pregnancy, 5% by miscarriage or ectopic pregnancy, and 5% are non-gestational in origin.

Incidence
1:30 000 pregnancies in western countries and 1:11 000 in east Asia.

Diagnosis
Signs and symptoms
- Vaginal bleeding.
- Abdominal or vaginal swelling.
- Amenorrhoea.
- Dypnoea and haemotypsis (2° to lung metastases).
- Intra-abdominal haemorrhage (due to uterine perforation by tumour tissue).
- Less common sites for metastases include brain, kidney, liver, or spleen; these present with symptoms related to their site.

Investigations
- USS.
- Serum hCG.
- CXR ('cannonball' or 'snowstorm' appearance).
- CT of chest and abdomen.

Treatment
The chemotherapy regime used is determined by a FIGO prognostic scoring system which is based on:
- Age of patient and type of antecedent pregnancy.
- Extent of tumour burden (hCG level, number, site, and size of tumour, site of metastases).
- Interval from antecedent pregnancy.
- Response to previous chemotherapy.

Prognosis
- Overall survival rate is >90%.
- Poorer prognosis is associated with patient aged >40yrs, antecedent pregnancy being term pregnancy, time interval from antecedent pregnancy to chemotherapy >4mths, large tumour burden, and poor response to previous chemotherapy.

Chemotherapy for GTD

- Chemotherapy continued until hCG normal for 6wks.
- More likely to have earlier menopause.
- *Low risk patients (≤6):*
  - methotrexate and folinic acid (well tolerated with main side effects of mucositis and pleuritic chest pain)
  - cure rate almost 100%.
- *High risk patients (≥7):*
  - intensive weekly schedule of EMA (etoposide, methotrexate, and dactinomycin) alternating with CV (cyclophosphamide and vincristine)
  - salvage surgery may be required (craniotomy, pleurotomy, hysterectomy)
  - cure rate 95%
  - increased risk of 2° cancers
  - small increased risk of miscarriage and stillbirth, but no increase in fetal abnormalities in subsequent pregnancy.

Principles of chemotherapy

Chemotherapy, together with radiotherapy and surgery, is used in the treatment of gynaecological cancers for control (and in some cases cure) of these diseases or palliation of their symptoms.

The cell cycle

- Chemotherapeutic agents interfere with cell division by acting on a specific phase of the cell cycle (see 📖 Principles of chemotherapy, phases of the cell cycle, p. 757) (e.g. taxanes active against cells in G2/M) or non-specifically (e.g. alkylating agents exert their effects throughout the cell cycle).
- One of the characteristics of cancer cells is uncontrolled proliferation. As chemotherapy has a propensity for actively proliferating cells, they are more vulnerable than normal cells. However, they do act on normal cells so side effects are not unusual (see 📖 Side effects of chemotherapy: haematological and gastrointestinal, p. 758).

Practical aspects

Before embarking on chemotherapy, and indeed any other form of therapy, the intent of treatment (i.e. curative or palliative) for each patient should be discussed within the MDT and clearly explained to the patient.

It is important to weigh up the potential risks and anticipated benefits so that optimal survival and quality of life may be achieved. Factors to consider are:
- *Disease-related:*
  - type and stage of cancer
  - response to previous treatment.
- *Patient-related:*
  - performance status (PS; the general condition of the patient); in general, chemotherapy is not indicated if PS >2
  - concurrent medical problems
  - nutritional status
  - patient's wishes.
- *Chemotherapy is generally delivered on an outpatient basis:*
  - for most ovarian chemotherapy, each course of systemic treatment is composed of 6 cycles, depending on response assessed after the 3rd one
  - each cycle lasts 21–28 days
  - the gap between consecutive cycles enables damaged 'normal' cells to repair and regenerate.
- *Response to treatment is assessed by:*
  - changes in evaluable disease on CT/MRI scans (RECIST (response evaluation criteria in solid tumours) criteria)
  - trends in tumour markers (e.g. CA125 levels for ovarian cancer)
  - symptoms
  - signs.

Phases of the cell cycle

- *G0:* resting phase.
- *G1:* RNA and protein synthesis.
- *S:* DNA synthesis.
- *G2:* protein synthesis, mitotic spindle formation.
- *M:* mitosis.

ECOG performance status

- *Grade 0:* asymptomatic, fully active.
- *Grade 1:* restricted in strenuous activity by symptoms but fully ambulatory.
- *Grade 2:* symptomatic, able to self-care, but not work, in bed <50% of the day.
- *Grade 3:* symptomatic, in bed >50% of the day.
- *Grade 4:* confined to bed or chair, unable to self-care.
- *Grade 5:* dead.

RECIST criteria

- *Complete:* disappearance of all lesions with no evidence of new lesions on two occasions of at least 4wks apart.
- *Partial:* ≥30% decrease in sum of longest diameters of lesions.
- Stable disease.
- *Progression:* ≥20% increase in the sum of longest diameters of lesions or presence of new lesions.

Some classes of cytotoxic agents

- *Antimetabolites:* interfere with DNA and RNA synthesis, e.g. 5-FU, gemcitabine, methotrexate.
- *Alkylating agents:* form covalent bonds with DNA bases, e.g. cyclophosphamide, ifosfamide.
- *Intercalating agents:* bind to DNA, thus inhibiting its replication, e.g. cisplatin, carboplatin (most widely used in gynaecological cancer).
- *Antitumour antibiotics:* complex mechanism of action leading to inhibition of DNA synthesis, e.g. bleomycin, doxorubicin, etoposide.
- *Drugs against spindle microtubules:* prevent mitosis, e.g. paclitaxel, vincristine.

Side effects of chemotherapy: haematological and gastrointestinal

Chemotherapy is associated with a range of side effects due to its action on normal cells, as well as cancer cells. Pattern of toxicity varies between drugs, as well as between individuals. Most side effects are self-limiting. It is important to recognize and seek ways to prevent and manage them, whenever possible, to maintain good quality of life.

Haematological

Bone marrow suppression leads to a gradual fall in blood count, which eventually recovers. The *nadir* (period of lowest count) occurs around 7–14 days after chemotherapy.

- *Neutropenic sepsis:* potentially fatal, urgent action required
  - neutropenia = neutrophil count ≤1.0 × 10^9/L
  - must have a high level of suspicion in any patient having chemotherapy presenting with a temperature of ≥38°C and feeling unwell
  - take FBC, cultures—blood, urine, etc., start IV broad-spectrum antibiotics as per hospital protocol (e.g. pipercillin and tazobactum, and gentamicin), and inform an oncologist
  - prophylaxis with granulocyte colony-stimulating factor (GCSF) and oral antibiotics, such as ciprofloxacin, may be appropriate if there have been previous episodes of neutropenic sepsis.
- *Anaemia* (Hb ≤11g/dL):
  - may be seen after several cycles of chemotherapy
  - treatment depends on severity and includes blood transfusion, iron tablets, erythropoietin.
- *Thrombocytopaenia* (platelet count ≤100):
  - rarely problematic with chemotherapy used for gynaecological cancers
  - avoid invasive procedures.

Gastrointestinal

Gastrointestinal side effects are due to loss of epithelial cells.

- *Nausea and vomiting:* can be prevented in most cases with effective antiemetics (e.g. steroids, domperidone, metoclopramide, and/or 5-HT3 antagonists).
- *Mucositis:*
  - resolves spontaneously with epithelial healing
  - helpful measures are good mouth care, use of local anaesthetic agents, treatment of oral candidiasis
  - commonly occurs with methotrexate and 5-FU.
- *Constipation:* pay attention to diet and fluid intake; short-term use of laxatives.
- *Diarrhoea:*
  - exclude infection/constipation
  - control with codeine phosphate, loperamide, and rehydration.

Side effects of chemotherapy: other

Alopecia
- Taxanes (e.g. paclitaxel), doxorubicin, and etoposide commonly cause temporary hair loss.
- Carboplatin and cisplatin are not usually associated with this side effect.
- Has a psychological impact on some women. Individual preference for wigs, scarves, or hats.

Neurological
These are dose-related side effects that slowly subside on dose reduction or on stopping the offending drug.
- *Peripheral neuropathy:*
  - usually sensory changes such as numbness and tingling
  - commonly seen with paclitaxel and cisplatin.
- *Tinnitus:* associated with cisplatin and taxanes.

Constitutional
These symptoms tend to have cumulative effects as treatment progresses, but resolve on its cessation.
- Lethargy.
- Anorexia.

Reproductive function
- *Fetal abnormality:*
  - most chemotherapeutic agents are teratogenic and should be avoided during the 1st trimester. Some agents may be used after 12wks if necessary—data are generally reassuring but limited
  - contraception is necessary until a period of time has elapsed following completion of treatment.
- *Ovarian failure:*
  - more likely to be caused by alkylating agents than other chemotherapy
  - permanent ovarian failure in premenopausal patients results in early menopause and infertility
  - young women with premature menopause are predisposed to osteoporosis, cardiovascular disease, and post-menopausal symptoms; hormone replacement therapy can be used without evidence of increase risk of cancer recurrence in most cancers.
  - cryopreservation of embryos and ovarian tissue is possible for women who wish to preserve their fertility options prior to chemotherapy.

Chemotherapy for gynaecological cancer

General points
- Chemotherapy has a narrow therapeutic index; close monitoring whilst on treatment is essential.
- Before the start of each cycle of treatment, blood tests (FBC, U&E, LFT) are taken, and patient's performance status and side effects are assessed.
- Chemotherapy when used alone normally has a palliative rather than curative role, except for choriocarcinoma, which is highly chemosensitive.
- Response rate is better when chemotherapy is used in combination with surgery or radiotherapy—this may be given:
  - *neoadjuvantly*—before definitive treatment (i.e. surgery or radiotherapy) to reduce tumour bulk
  - *adjuvantly*—after definitive treatment to reduce the risk of recurrence.

The future
Standard chemotherapy agents do not differentiate between cancer cells and normal cells. Side effects are common because these agents damage DNA of potentially all cells. It is known that cancer cells have certain characteristics that enable them to continue to proliferate. Much attention has been focused on exploiting the differences between normal and cancer cells in order to develop targeted therapy.
- Targeted therapy is defined as a drug that acts on a defined target or biological pathway that is present on the cancer cells only; because normal cells are relatively unaffected, side effects are likely to be less problematic.
- Targeted agents that have shown some response in ovarian cancer are:
  - *bevacizumab*—a VEGF inhibitor. VEGF is needed for blood vessel formation (angiogenesis); successful angiogenesis will enable the tumour to be supplied with oxygen and nutrients for its continued growth
  - *cediranib*—tyrosine kinase inhibitor of VEGF receptor; ICON6 RCT investigation in relapsed ovarian cancer—results awaited.

Common chemotherapy regimens for gynaecological cancers

- *Ovarian cancer:*
  - sensitive to platinum-based regimens, response rate ~70%
  - carboplatin +/− paclitaxel (may be used neoadjuvantly, adjuvantly, or palliatively)
  - >50% of patients will relapse and require further treatment; if >6mths have elapsed since initial chemotherapy, tumour more likely to be sensitive to carboplatin and therefore it is often given again
  - Ip chemotherapy (instillation of agents such as cisplatin directly into the peritoneal cavity) has shown clinical benefit, but with increased toxicity; recommended to be used as part of clinical trial only).
- *Endometrial cancer:*
  - chemotherapy has a limited role, reserved for recurrent or metastatic disease
  - carboplatin +/− paclitaxel
  - doxorubicin and cisplatin.
- *Cervical cancer:*
  - cisplatin combined with radiotherapy has been shown to reduce risk of relapse for those undergoing radiotherapy after surgery
  - cisplatin may be used for metastatic disease but the response rate is low.
- *Vulval cancer:*
  - cisplatin can be used in combination with radiotherapy for patients unfit for surgery
  - cisplatin may be used as sole therapy for symptom control in metastatic disease.
- *Trophoblastic tumour:*
  - chemotherapy alone may be curative
  - treatment given at specialist centres
  - see p. 750.

Radiotherapy: principles

Radiotherapy, unlike chemotherapy, is local and not systemic treatment. It may be used with curative and palliative intent in some gynaecological cancers.

Radiobiology

- Radiotherapy kills cells by the use of ionizing radiation:
  - X-rays
  - gamma-rays
  - β-particles.
- Radiation can lead to breakage of DNA directly or indirectly via production of free radicals.
- Sensitivity of any cell to radiation depends on:
  - cell type (for example, cells of the small bowel have low tolerance to radiation)
  - cell cycle (cells in G0, resting, phase are relatively resistant, whereas cells in G1 and G2 phases are sensitive)
  - micro-environment (cells in areas of low oxygen are radioresistant).
- Many cells are able to repair a certain amount of DNA damage but cancer cells do this less effectively; thus a significantly higher proportion will be destroyed.
- The total dose of radiotherapy that can be given to one area is limited by the tolerance of the surrounding normal tissue of that area.

Delivery of radiotherapy

Radiation may be given by external beam therapy and/or brachytherapy.
- *External beam therapy:*
  - radiation is distant from the patient
  - delivered from a linear accelerator
  - use of conformal radiotherapy (i.e. shaping the radiation beam to shape of tumour) encompasses less normal tissue within the field and therefore reduces side effects.
- *Brachytherapy:*
  - placement of radioactive source directly within or around the tumour site (e.g. intravaginal/intrauterine brachytherapy for cervical cancer)
  - *advantage*—higher radiation dose to the tumour, lower exposure to normal tissue.
- Side effects may be reduced by giving radiotherapy in divided doses so that normal tissues can recover.

Radiotherapy: side effects

The side effects of radiotherapy depend on the site being irradiated. In gynaecological cancers this is the pelvis, and therefore tissues in this area are prone to damage. Problems may become apparent during and immediately after treatment (early effects) or occur months or years later (late effects).

Early side effects

- Due to damage of rapidly dividing cells such as the mucosa. Usually self-limiting.
- *Skin:*
  - erythema
  - moist desquamation
  - *management*—aqueous cream, hydrocortisone cream.
- *Mouth/bowel:*
  - *mucositis*—treat with mouthwash, analgesia, nystatin if thrush present
  - *nausea* (less so vomiting)—antiemetics for prophylaxis or treatment
  - *diarrhoea*—exclude infection, treat with loperamide or codeine phosphate.
- *Bladder:*
  - cystitis causing frequency and dysuria
  - *management*—exclude infection, ensure adequate fluid intake, oxybutynin may help.
- *Tiredness:*
  - treat anaemia if present
  - rest.
- Bone marrow suppression.

Radiotherapy: gynaecological cancers

Management of gynaecological cancers is multimodal in nature, combining surgery, chemotherapy, and radiotherapy. Surgery is the mainstay of treatment whenever possible. The choice of treatment depends on the type of cancer, the extent of disease, and the patient's fitness and wishes.

Cervical cancer

- *Early disease (stage Ib):*
  - radiotherapy is as effective as radical hysterectomy (cure rate ~80%)
  - for those who have had surgery, radiotherapy may be given afterwards (adjuvant treatment) to reduce the risk of pelvic recurrence.
- *Locally advanced disease (stage II–IVa):* adjuvant use of external beam radiotherapy and brachytherapy ± chemotherapy.
- *Recurrent disease:* localized recurrence may be treated by surgical resection or radiotherapy.
- *Distant metastatic disease (stage IVb):* best supportive care, palliative radiotherapy; or palliative chemotherapy.

Endometrial cancer

- *Early disease (stage I):*
  - if patient unfit for surgery, radiotherapy used as primary treatment
  - if fit for surgery, brachytherapy +/– external beam therapy to the pelvis adjuvantly, especially if high risk features present (e.g. poorly differentiated tumour, deep myometrial involvement).
- *Locally advanced disease (stage II–IIIc):* postoperative (adjuvant) radiotherapy.
- *Recurrent disease:* as for cervical cancer.

Vulval cancer

- *Early disease:* primary radiotherapy if unfit for surgery.
- *Locally advanced disease:*
  - radiotherapy to the pelvis after surgery if lymph nodes found to be involved
  - radiotherapy in combination with chemotherapy being evaluated to shrink extensive disease before surgery.
- *Recurrent disease:* may be possible if the maximum dose has not been exceeded.

Ovarian cancer

- No evidence to support the use of radiotherapy in the primary or adjuvant setting.
- Radiotherapy may have a role in the palliation of localized symptoms.

Radiotherapy for symptom palliation

Radiotherapy is used to control some symptoms caused by metastatic disease. Examples are:
- Pain from bone/brain metastases.
- Bleeding from fungating tumour.

Pain and its management

Most patients with advanced cancer experience moderate to severe pain that can be attributed directly to the cancer.

Type of pain
- Somatic (e.g. bone pain).
- Visceral (e.g. liver capsular pain).
- Neuropathic (e.g. lumbosacral plexus involvement, often described as burning, sharp).

Assessment
- Ask questions about pain (SOCRATES) to assess its nature and distinguish whether acute or chronic.
- Measurement of pain may be done using scales; for example, by asking the patient to score her pain out of 10.
- Consider psychological factors that might contribute to or exacerbate pain, such as anxiety and depression.

'SOCRATES'
- Site.
- Onset.
- Character.
- Radiation.
- Associations.
- Timing.
- Exacerbating/relieving factors.
- Severity.

Methods for the management of pain
- *Non-pharmacological:*
  - relaxation/massage
  - acupuncture
  - TENS
  - radiotherapy
  - nerve block.
- *Pharmacological:*
  - use analgesia according to WHO ladder
  - increase dose of analgesia at each step to its maximum; if pain is still not controlled, move up the ladder
  - give regularly
  - anticonvulsants (gabapentin, pregabalin) ± antidepressants (amitriptyline) for neuropathic pain
  - corticosteroids for pressure due to metastases
  - bisphosphonates for bone pain due to metastases.

▶ Remember to *assess and reassess* frequently to maintain good pain control.

WHO analgesic ladder
- *Step 1:* non-opioid (e.g. paracetamol, NSAIDs).
- *Step 2:* weak opioid (e.g. codeine) + non-opioid.
- *Step 3:* strong opioid (e.g. morphine) + non-opioid.

Side effects of opioids
- Commonly:
  - nausea
  - constipation
  - sedation (advise amitriptyline should be taken 3 h before bed to avoid morning 'hangover').
- Inform patient of potential problems.
- Give antiemetics and laxatives.

⚠ Do not allow concerns about potential dependence prevent you from prescribing adequate amounts of opiates.

Symptoms of advanced gynaecological cancer

Gastrointestinal symptoms

Nausea and vomiting

- *Causes:*
  - ascites
  - constipation
  - metabolic (e.g. Ca^{2+})
  - bowel obstruction
  - brain metastases
  - medication.

- *Treat cause, if possible:*
  - radiotherapy and corticosteroids for brain metastases
  - paracentesis for ascites
  - hydration and bisphosphonates for hypercalcaemia.
- Antiemetics.

Constipation

- *Causes:*
  - ↓ fluid intake
  - immobility
  - lethargy
  - bowel obstruction
  - metabolic (e.g. Ca^{2+})
  - medication (especially opioids).

- Treat cause, if possible.
- Laxatives.

(Subacute) bowel obstruction

- Caused by tumour seedling within the peritoneum.
- Exclude constipation with AXR.
- Best to manage conservatively; however, if patient is reasonably fit and there is only one area of obstruction, surgery may be an option.

Other symptoms

- *Vaginal discharge and bleeding:*
  - may be infective, therefore give metronidazole
  - tranexamic acid +/– embolization for bleeding.
- *Fistulae:* difficult to manage, limited role for surgery.
- *Fatigue:* dexamethasone may give a sense of well-being.
- *Anorexia and cachexia:*
  - caused by the secretion of pro-inflammatory cytokines
  - dexamethasone or megestrol/medroxyprogesterone may improve appetite
  - total parenteral nutrition is rarely indicated.
- *Dyspnoea:*
  - causes—pleural effusion, cachexia, lymphangitis, anaemia, lung metastases, pulmonary embolism
  - suspect pulmonary embolism if acute onset of shortness of breath.

Principles of palliative care

The WHO defines palliative care as the 'active, holistic care of patients with advanced, progressive illness'.

Good communication and rapport with the patient (and her family) are essential to facilitate frank discussion of prognosis and formulate a plan of care that is most suited to her.

Goals of palliative care

- To achieve optimal symptom relief.
- To promote the best quality of life.

In order to palliate effectively, it is necessary to individualize each patient's care and take her wishes into account. Aspects to explore include:

- Physical symptoms.
- Psychological symptoms.
- Social issues.
- Spiritual issues.

Multidisciplinary approach

- Symptoms may be controlled by pharmacological or non-pharmacological means.
- The expertise of different specialties may be needed depending on the nature of the patient's problems, e.g. advice from dietitians about nutrition, from clinical oncologists about radiotherapy for bone pain, from surgeons about feasibility of resection for bowel obstruction.
- Palliative care is delivered at home, in a hospice, or in hospital.

Terminal care

- Institute Liverpool Care Pathway.
- Aim for a peaceful and dignified death.
- Maintain comfort and offer psychosocial-spiritual support.
- Avoid unnecessary/uncomfortable procedures.
- Review medication. Most can be stopped, but continue the following:
  - analgesics
  - antiemetics
  - anxiolytics
  - anticonvulsants.

Miscellaneous gynaecology

Injuries in obstetric and gynaecological practice: overview

Because of their close anatomical relationship, operating on the genital tract may also incur injury to the urinary tract. Complicated gynaecological procedures increase the risk of urinary tract injury. If an injury occurs, prompt recognition and appropriate management are important both to prevent long-term sequelae (urinary incontinence, fistulae, and, rarely, renal failure) and to reduce litigation related to the injury.

Medico-legal implications

Up to 6% of all medical malpractice claims in gynaecological practice are related to urinary tract injuries. The quantum of claims is probably related to the degree of suffering or perceived suffering by the patient. Thus, urinary tract injuries that lead to litigation are likely to be associated with significant physical and psychological morbidity or loss of income.

Claims have increased over time and every attempt should be made to reduce the risk—despite every effort, occasional injury is inevitable, particularly with highly challenging surgery.

In the event of an adverse event

Remember the GMC guidance on being open and honest with patients:
- If a patient under your care has suffered harm or distress, you must act immediately to put matters right, if that is possible. You should offer an apology and explain fully and promptly to the patient what has happened, and the likely short-term and long-term effects.
- Patients who complain about the care or treatment they have received have a right to expect a prompt, open, constructive, and honest response including an explanation and, if appropriate, an apology. You must not allow a patient's complaint to affect adversely the care or treatment you provide or arrange.

Remember, doctors who are open, honest, and non-defensive are less likely to be sued for negligence and less likely to have formal complaints made about them, regardless of what has gone wrong.

Ureteric injury

Incidence
0.5–2.5% of iatrogenic ureteric injuries occur during routine pelvic surgery, mainly gynaecological. Ureteric injury occurs in 0.03% of CS deliveries compared with 0.001% of vaginal births.

Mechanism of injury
- *Avulsion:* liable to occur when tissues are fragile.
- *Transection commonly at:*
  - the pelvic brim (vascular ovarian pedicle is close to the ureter)
  - the base of the broad ligament where the uterine arteries cross (commonly during hysterectomy as the ureters enter the bladder above the lateral vaginal fornix just 2cm lateral to the cervix)
  - the ureterovesical junction.
- *Ligation:* especially during vaginal hysterectomy and repair of procidentia when the ureters also prolapse.
- *Crush:* by clamps causing necrosis or stricture.
- *Devascularization:* causing ischaemia and necrosis.

Presentation
Only 15–20% of iatrogenic injury presents at the time of surgery.

Diagnosis
- IVU.
- Cystoscopy and bilateral retrograde pyelography to identify site of injury, extravasation, or ureteric dilatation.
- CT for suspected urinoma.
- USS may also diagnose hydronephrosis or urinoma.

Treatment
⚠ Intraoperative repair has a better long-term prognosis than postoperative interval repair. Assistance from the urological team should be requested as soon as injury is suspected.

Injuries at or below the pelvic brim
- *Psoas hitch:* shortens the ureterovesical gap and reduces tension.
- *Boari flap:* creation of a tension-free anastomosis.

Higher-level injuries
- May require nephrostomy or downward displacement of the kidney with end-to-end ureteric anastomosis with the ipsilateral ureter.
- Ureteroileal anastomosis may be necessary in extensive upper ureteral injury (very rare).
- May need cutaneous ureterostomy or transuretero-ureterostomy.

Presentation

Postoperatively, uretric injury presents with:
- Fever (sepsis).
- Flank pain from hydronephrosis.
- Vaginal fistulae.
- Non-specific symptoms of malaise, ileus, or the presence of a pelvic mass ('urinoma').
- Bilateral ureteric injury is very rare, so renal function is usually normal.

Risk factors for ureteric injury

- Previous surgery.
- Bulky tumours distorting anatomy and/or displacing ureters.
- Endometriosis with peritoneal scarring or frozen pelvis.
- PID and tubo-ovarian abscesses.
- Carcinoma of the cervix with parametrial involvement.
- Situations that require haste (e.g. CS).
- Angular or broad ligament tears during CS.

Prevention is better than cure!

Identification of the ureters prior to ligation of the uterine and ovarian arteries during hysterectomy should be routine practice. If difficult surgery is anticipated or encountered identification aids include:
- Preoperative ureteric stents (can be 'lighted').
- IV administration 10mL indigo carmine or methylene blue with 20mg of furosemide. Leakage of dye or contrast is demonstrated with ureteric injury.
- Retrograde pyelography under fluoroscopic guidance (identifies ureteric strictures).

Bladder and urethral injury

Incidence

Approximately 50% of all bladder injuries are the result of surgical procedures (may occur during hysterectomy and usually involves the anterior bladder wall). Obstetric bladder injury occurs in 1.4% of CS compared with 0.01% of vaginal deliveries.

Mechanisms of injury

- Mobilization of the bladder to expose the cervix or the lower uterine segment during a hysterectomy. Previous scarring (CS, myomectomy, PID, or endometriosis) contributes to ↑ risk.
- Perforation of the bladder may occur during laparoscopy, hysteroscopy, and sling procedures (TVT).
- Ischaemic injury may occur as a result of an inadvertent suture in the bladder.
- Prolonged and obstructed labour may compress the bladder leading to avascular necrosis and vesicovaginal fistula.
- High forceps deliveries (especially if the bladder is not emptied beforehand).

Presentation

Bladder injuries commonly present with haematuria and abdominal pain, but can present with abdominal distension, suprapubic tenderness, and an inability to void.

Diagnosis

- Bladder injury may be obvious at the time of surgery as the catheter balloon may become visible.
- Instillation of methylene blue dye into the bladder through a Foley's catheter may demonstrate leakage into the peritoneal cavity under direct visualization at surgery.
- Cystoscopy is commonly used when bladder injury is suspected postoperatively.
- A cystogram will also demonstrate urinary leakage.
- Instillation of methylene blue dye into the bladder through a Foley's catheter with swabs inserted into the vagina may help identify a vesicovaginal fistula ('three-swab test').

Treatment

- Iatrogenic injuries may be repaired surgically or managed with catheter drainage depending on size and location of injury.
- Bladder perforation is repaired in two layers using absorbable sutures.
- Foley catheter is recommended for 7–10 days with antibiotic cover.
- Thorough assessment of whether the ureteric orifices have been involved needs to be made at time of repair particularly if injury is large, posterior, or basal.

It is good practice and medico-legally prudent to involve specialist urological advice and help when there has been an inadvertent urinary tract injury.

Urethral injury at a glance

Female urethral injuries are rare, and they occur commonly with urethral instrumentation, vaginal surgery, and obstetric complications. Most commonly the result of difficult catheterization where it is forced and there is rupture or subsequent scarring of the urethra.

Presentation
- Diagnosis can be difficult, but they can present with urethral bleeding or an inability to void (retention or poor stream and dribbling).
- Fistulae will present with labial swelling or with leaking of urine through the vagina.

Diagnosis
- IVU.
- Voiding cystourethrography.
- MRI.
- Cystoscopy.

Treatment
- For most cases urethral catheterization is sufficient if this is possible.
- Suprapubic catheterization may be necessary prior to formal repair.
- Larger tears are surgically repaired using layered closure.
- Proximal damage to the urethra requires reconstruction surgery including bladder flap–urethral tube reconstruction and vaginal flap urethroplasty.
- Long-term suprapubic catheterization may be necessary in the small group of women for whom urethral repair is unsuccessful.

Urethral surgery is very difficult and requires expert urological input.

Risk factors during Caesarean section
- Emergency CS, particularly category 1.
- Low station of the presenting part (especially at full dilatation as the bladder is stretched up the lower segment and is 'higher than expected').
- Prolonged labour prior to section.
- Preterm delivery (<32wks gestation).
- Previous CS (risk increases with increasing number of CS).
- Previous extensive abdominal and pelvic surgery, especially previous myomectomy.
- The presence of lower uterine and cervical fibroids.
- Operator skill.

Communication and record keeping

Good communication, in particular, is as highly valued by patients as any knowledge or technical ability. Repeatedly, the biggest cause of complaints is poor communication (patients will rarely complain about a doctor they like!). Just about every patient complaint, regardless of the underlying issue, is compounded by perceived gaps in communication. The biggest cause of lost medico-legal cases is poor documentation.

Good communication

- Treat your patients as you would like to be treated yourself.
- Always introduce yourself and explain the purpose of any consultation.
- Generally ask 'open' questions ('could you describe the pain you have?') and signpost changes of enquiry ('can I now ask you about any medication you are taking?').
- Give the patient time to talk (it is her story, not yours, and remember, the patient knows her symptoms better than you do!).
- Listen to the answers (if you don't listen, why ask the question?)— patient complaints frequently cite that 'the doctor just wasn't listening' or 'nobody was listening to me'.
- Summarize your history and invite questions from the patient.
- Always close the consultation with a clear plan of action.
- Acknowledge fear, upset, or if someone looks worried—do not avoid it; the patient nearly always feels better for discussing it.
- Do not be dismissive or appear rushed.
- Doctors who come across as arrogant or patronizing induce anger and resentment in their patients—be wary of this—you will also be complained about or sued if you make a mistake!
- Don't take anger or criticism personally (part of a doctor's job is listening, even when we don't want to hear it).
- Be honest at all times, including when things go wrong or if you are unsure about a particular problem or management plan— patients understand that things sometimes go wrong and that doctors don't know everything.
- Apologize when appropriate. Often this is all a patient wants—things do go wrong, and apologizing is not an admission of guilt or culpability.

Good documentation

- Always record correct date and time of every patient encounter.
- Ensure name, date of birth, and identifying number are on every sheet of paper.
- Always write legibly in black ink.
- If entries need to be changed/altered then cross out old entry, but leave it visible and legible and sign and date new changes.
- Never alter or remove pages from notes when things may have gone wrong—they have usually been photocopied already!
- Always identify yourself by signature, printed name, and position.
- Identify all people present for any discussions (especially interpreters).
- Keep notes contemporaneously wherever possible (you never remember things quite as they were if there is a time delay).
- If you need to back-date an entry (e.g. if you are called to deal with an emergency) then indicate that this is back-dated and what time the actual event refers to.
- Document discussions fully, particularly possible complications; 'complications of laparoscopy explained' will not stand up to scrutiny or challenge after a bowel injury!—see 📖 Consent to treatment, p. 782.
- For operative procedures or diagnostic imaging, take hard-copy prints or preferably archive images wherever possible—a diagram may also be useful.
- If you need to deviate from a guideline then fully document your reasons for doing so in the given clinical situation including when discussed with a colleague.
- Avoid abbreviations and acronyms wherever possible, or explain them (IUD = intrauterine device or intrauterine death!?).
- Never make jokes or flippant comments: they are distasteful, notes are a legal document, and patients can access their files—how would you feel if your notes said 'needs a checkup from the neck up'?
- For operative procedures or diagnostic imaging, take hard-copy prints or preferably archive images wherever possible—a diagram may also be useful.

Medico-legal aspects of obstetrics and gynaecology: overview

It is good medical practice for all doctors to have a basic understanding of the law and its relationship with medicine. For the obstetrician and gynaecologist it is essential, because of the many complex medico-legal issues dealt with on a daily basis. The two largest areas for medico-legal claims are A&E and obstetrics.

UK law and the court system

The legal system in England and Wales is quite different from that in Scotland, although many of the principles are the same. What is described here is the English system. Medico-legal cases may be heard in different types of court. The court system is hierarchical. The Supreme Court is the most senior court in the land followed by the Court of Appeal and the High Court. Laws are made in a variety of different ways.

Common law

This is law that is developed over time through decisions made by judges. These decisions establish legal principles or 'precedent' which can be applied to future cases. Precedent set by a higher court such as the Supreme Court overrules that of a lower court. Medical law regarding clinical negligence is largely derived from common law.

Statute law

These are laws made by parliament. Statute law overrides common law developed by the courts. Many medico-legal issues in obstetrics and gynaecology are governed by statutes, such as the Abortion Act 1967.

Medical negligence

In order to establish that negligence has occurred, it must be shown that on the balance of probabilities:

- The doctor or hospital had a duty of care.
- There was a breach of that duty.
- The breach of duty caused harm to the patient.

What is medical negligence?

- Claims for medical negligence are both more common and more costly in obstetrics and gynaecology than in any other specialty.
- The National Health Service Litigation Authority (NHSLA) has dealt with nearly £2 billion of claims by patients since 1995.
- Claims are usually made against doctors (in practice a claim is made against a hospital trust) in civil law rather than criminal charges.
- Medical negligence is the legal term used when harm arises because of a breach of duty by an individual clinician or a hospital:
  - an inappropriate treatment or failure to make a correct diagnosis may be found negligent if the patient suffers harm as a result
  - it may be judged negligent to fail to warn a patient about a risk inherent in an operation, e.g. ureteric injury during hysterectomy.
- The standard used to decide if a doctor breached his or her duty of care is whether a responsible body of medical opinion, acting in a logical manner, would have acted differently in the same circumstances.
- It also has to be proved that, on the balance of probabilities, it was the breach of duty that caused the harm. Thus, where an abnormal CTG was not acted upon and a baby develops CP, negligence will only be established if the CP is shown to be caused by hypoxia during labour and not another cause.

Consent to treatment

⚠ Treating an adult without her consent may lead to claims of negligence or, more rarely, a claim of battery.

> **Consent**
> In order for consent to be valid the patient must:
> - Have the capacity to give consent.
> - Give consent voluntarily.
> - Be given appropriate information regarding the procedure.

Capacity

- The Mental Capacity Act 2005 has defined capacity in law.
- The pain and distress caused by labour is not enough to determine that a woman lacks capacity to consent.

> **Assessment of capacity**
> The person will lack capacity if there is a disturbance in the functioning of the mind or brain so she cannot:
> - Understand the information relevant to the decision.
> - Retain the information.
> - Use or weigh the information.
> - Communicate the decision.

Voluntary consent

Consent must be given freely, without undue influence or pressure from others.

Information

To avoid a claim of battery, a patient must be aware of the nature and purpose of any procedure to which she consents. For example, when a medical student is to perform a vaginal examination, it must be clear to the patient that the purpose is to enhance the student's training and not for the benefit of the woman. More commonly, lack of information during the consent procedure may give rise to a claim of negligence.

Consent for operations

The law does not specify who can take the consent for an operation, but the person obtaining consent should, at the very least, be familiar with the procedure and be able to explain it in detail. Thus in complex cancer or laparoscopic surgery it may be wise for the operating surgeon to obtain the patient's written consent.

The Department of Health has published guidance on what information should be given to patients before an operation. This includes:
- Details of the proposed procedure.
- The nature of the condition being treated.
- The benefits of treatment.
- Alternative treatments.
- Serious and frequently occurring risks.
- Additional procedures that may be necessary, e.g. blood transfusion.

Consent: other issues

Refusal of treatment

The law allows a competent adult to refuse medical treatment without reason or justification.

Blood products

Religious groups such as Jehovah's Witnesses may refuse all blood products and it is essential that such wishes are very carefully documented. In cases where advanced refusal of blood products is known and the potential for bleeding anticipated (e.g. laparoscopy for ectopic pregnancy) the most senior person available should perform the procedure.

Caesarean section

Several cases have been brought to court challenging a woman's right to refuse a CS thought by doctors to be in the best interests of her or her fetus.

The law is clear that the fetus *in utero* has no legal rights up until the moment of birth. Therefore, a woman may refuse to consent to CS even if the consequences for herself or the fetus are death or severe injury.

Subfertility

The Human Fertilization and Embryology Authority (HFEA) Act 1990 regulates the area of reproductive medicine covering:
- Infertility treatments using donated genetic material.
- Infertility treatments involving stored genetic material.
- The creation of embryos outside the body.
- Embryo research.

The Act established the HFEA. This body licenses, monitors, and reports on establishments that provide fertility treatments. Individuals undergoing fertility treatments covered by the Act must give written consent to treatment as well as to storage of gametes and embryos. When couples have fertility treatment together, both must consent to the treatment and either may withdraw their consent at any time.

Consent in children

It is not uncommon for child <16yrs to request contraception or a TOP without parental knowledge. In the case of Gillick vs. West Norfolk and Wisbech AHA (1985), the courts ruled that doctors may treat children without parental consent if certain conditions are fulfilled:
- The child understands the advice or treatment being given.
- Attempt has been made to persuade the child to inform the parents.
- In case of seeking contraception, the child is likely to have unprotected intercourse whether or not contraception is prescribed.
- The physical or mental health of the child is likely to suffer if the treatment is not provided.

Consent for common gynaecological procedures: overview

The principles of consent are universal for all procedures and outlined in the 2008 GMC document:

Consent

Patients and doctors must make decisions together:

- You must work in partnership with your patients.
- You should discuss their condition and treatment options in a way they can understand.
- You should respect their right to make decisions about their care.
- Gaining their consent is an important part of the process of discussion and decision-making, not something that happens in isolation.
- The information you share should be in proportion to the nature of their condition, the complexity of the proposed investigation or treatment, and the seriousness of any potential side effects, complications, or other risks.
- *Risks of procedures will usually include:* side effects, complications, and failure of an intervention to achieve the desired aim.
- In the event an adult patient cannot consent, e.g. unconscious, remember the laws on capacity and that nobody can consent on behalf of another adult without power of attorney.
- All necessary information on consent in difficult circumstances, e.g. in children <16yrs, those without capacity, guidance can be found at ℘ http://www.gmc-uk.org/guidance/index.asp

Some practical tips on consent

- If you are the surgeon, consent the patient personally, do not delegate the responsibility unless unavoidable.
- If consent has already occurred, but there is a significant time gap (more than 1mth) then check it is still clinically appropriate and consider reconsent for the procedure.
- If you do not document what you have discussed it didn't occur!
- 'Risks of procedure fully discussed' is not adequate—you need to be procedure specific including realistic possible outcomes.
- Even if a patient's decisions about her procedure seem inappropriate they are her right to make—if you feel uncomfortable about a patient's decision or are feeling manipulated into performing something you do not feel is appropriate then do not do the procedure!—get a second opinion.
- Always record their LMP and current method of contraception in the reproductive age group.
- If there is even a remote chance the patient may be pregnant (especially in the luteal phase) then it is better to postpone the procedure—the commonest reason for a pregnancy post-sterilization is that the patient was pregnant at the time of the procedure!

If you are in any doubt about the appropriateness of surgery, the patient's decision, or unexpected anaesthetic issues on the day (e.g. temperature or unexpected low Hb) at the time of consent, then it is generally better to postpone the operation—if something adverse occurs, the first question will always be 'did she need an operation at all or on that day?'

Further reading

RCOG. (2008). *Obtaining valid consent*. Clinical Governance Advice 6. ℘ http://www.rcog.org.uk/womens-health/clinical-guidance/obtaining-valid-consent

Consent for surgery that breaches the peritoneum

Laparoscopic, open abdominal procedures and vaginal procedures that breach the peritoneum (e.g. vaginal hysterectomy) are some of the commonest in the specialty. The following need to be discussed and documented with the patient's full understanding:

- *Proposed method of incision:* e.g. Pfannensteil/midline/either if decision is genuinely uncertain and dependent on EUA for instance.
- *Primary purpose of procedure:* e.g. diagnostic/therapeutic/both.
- *Which, if any, organs will be removed:* including making the patient aware this may change depending upon intraoperative findings, e.g. total abdominal hysterectomy with ovarian conservation unless ovary(ies) abnormal at procedure.
- *Likely possibilities when the intra-abdominal pathology is genuinely unknown:* e.g. laparoscopy for pelvic pain of uncertain aetiology—diagnostic laparoscopy +/– adhesiolysis +/– diathermy to endometriosis.
- *Risks of all intra-abdominal procedures:* haemorrhage/infection (abdominal, skin, urinary)/injury to bowel, bladder, ureters, major blood vessels.
- *Risks of visceral injury increase in the presence of:* endometriosis, known adhesions, cancer or distorting pathology, multiple previous surgeries.
- *Larger procedures:* e.g. gynaeoncology debulking procedures, extra visceral risks, e.g. liver, spleen, may need discussion.
- *In the case of laparoscopy the small risk of conversion to laparotomy in the event of:* inadvertent visceral injury/intractable bleeding/operative inability to complete the procedure due to difficulty.
- *The small possibility of the need for blood transfusion:* in the event of unexpected bleeding.
- *If the patient refuses blood products:* then a preoperative meeting is mandatory with the surgeon, anaesthetist, and haematologist to establish what is and is not acceptable to the patient, sign advance directives, and re-evaluate risks.
- *The type of anaesthetic to be used:* individual anaesthetic risks should be explained by the anaesthetist.
- *Concurrent medical comorbidities:* need preoperative assessment and appropriate specialty input to establish operative risk.

Consent issues specific to laparoscopic sterilization

The following are mandatory for anyone requesting sterilization:

- Absolute certainty that their family is complete.
- The irreversible nature of sterilization.
- A recognized failure rate of 1:200.
- That male sterilization is a less risky procedure, done under LA, and has a failure rate of 1:2000 after two negative semen analyses.
- There has been a full consideration of all long-acting reversible contraceptives (LARCs), e.g. IUCD, Mirena®, implants.

⚠ Current recommendations are that sterilization should almost never be considered in patients <30yrs as later regret is common. A second opinion, at minimum, is good practice in these circumstances.

Further reading

RCOG. (2008). *Obtaining valid consent*. Clinical Governance Advice 6. ℘ http://www.rcog.org.uk/womens-health/clinical-guidance/obtaining-valid-consent

Consent for surgery that enters the uterine cavity

Procedures involving entry to the uterine cavity include hysteroscopy, evacuation, and TOP procedures.
- Primary purpose of procedure, e.g. diagnostic/therapeutic/both.
- What if anything will be removed, including making the patient aware this may change depending upon intraoperative findings, e.g. hysteroscopy +/– endometrial biopsy +/– resection of polyp +/– fibroid resection.
- Specifically consent for operative resection if this is a realistic possibility.
- Risks of all intrauterine procedures: haemorrhage/infection (endometritis)/small risk of uterine perforation with a small risk of injury to bowel, bladder, ureters, major blood vessels.
- Specifically for ERPC/TOP procedures the small risk of incomplete evacuation.
- Risks of intra-abdominal injury increase when operative resection and/or other energy sources are used.
- Small risk of the need for laparoscopy +/– laparotomy and repair in the event of uterine perforation.

Endometrial ablation procedures

In addition to the above issues the following are mandatory for anyone requesting endometrial ablation:
- Absolute certainty that their family is complete.
- The continued need for contraception post procedure.
- The possibility (procedure type dependent) of amenorrhoea.
- The possibility of the need for a second procedure in the next 5yrs.

Further reading

RCOG. (2008). *Obtaining valid consent*. Clinical Governance Advice 6. ♒ http://www.rcog.org.uk/womens-health/clinical-guidance/obtaining-valid-consent

Considerations for preoperative assessment in gynaecology

Preoperative assessment has all of the same general considerations as for all other surgical procedures—the majority of procedures are now done in day surgery. In terms of specific considerations they are procedure specific, but consider the following.

Specific gynaecological issues

- All women in the reproductive age are pregnant till proven otherwise—ensure that contraception and last normal menstrual period (LNMP) are clearly sought and documented in clinic and again immediately preoperatively (see 📖 Consent to treatment, p. 782).
- The above is especially true in those having surgery for fertility reasons—a preoperative pregnancy test is mandatory, but also *beware* unprotected sex in the cycle of the procedure—her pregnancy test may not be positive yet!
- If there is any doubt regarding possible pregnancy or the viability of a pregnancy prior to ERPC then do not continue until your doubts have been answered.
- NEVER assume a woman's future reproductive wishes—*always* ask them and document them.
- Do *not* operate on a pregnant women unless that is the indication for surgery (e.g. ERPC) or the benefits outweigh the risks.
- Do *not* forget anti-D administration for all Rh –ve women who have a uterine evacuation procedure or surgery for ectopic pregnancy.
- Where the uterine cavity is instrumented consider chlamydial prophylaxis to prevent ascending infection unless the patient has been screened recently and is –ve—the default position is to give it!
- Many of the women will *de facto* have risk factors for VTE, e.g. pregnancy, pelvic surgery, COCP use. *All* need a WHO VTE assessment.
- Woman having intraperitoneal surgery need consideration for bowel preparation if: multiple previous abdominal surgery, endometriosis, known adhesions, cancer.
- The need for specific preoperative investigations (e.g. ECG, CXR) is otherwise similar to general surgery, though nearly all will require an FBC and Group + Save at minimum.
- The majority of women will require ultrasound (or more rarely other imaging, e.g. CT/MRI) as part of their clinical pathway to provide information regarding their procedure—Ask yourself: 'Has this patient had an ultrasound?', and if not, 'does she need one?'

Clinical risk management: identifying and analysing risks

Clinical risk management is a mechanism for improving the quality of patient care. There are several steps in the process.

Identifying risk

What went wrong or what could go wrong

There are local and national sources used to identify risk issues outlined in the opposite box

Completing an incident reporting form

Most trusts have a dedicated reporting form to complete. These should be available in all clinical areas. All members of staff of all grades should be encouraged to complete forms when they are aware of risk incidents. A form should be completed for all actual adverse incidents affecting patients, as well as near misses.

Many units have a list of specific risk triggers that should prompt completion of a risk form. These might include an unplanned return to theatre, cord pH <7.10, or an operative blood loss of more than 800mL.

Serious incidents must be reported immediately to the local lead for clinical risk. All hospitals will have definitions for what constitutes such a serious untoward incident. When a serious incident has occurred, all staff concerned should prepare contemporaneous statements of their involvement whilst the incident is still fresh in their mind.

When writing incident reports and statements, only an account of the facts should be documented, *not* an opinion of what went wrong.

> ### Incident form information
> - Full patient details.
> - Date, time, and location of incident.
> - All staff involved (statements may be requested at a later date).
> - Brief factual report of the incident.

Risk analysis

Root cause analysis is a structured investigation that aims to identify the true cause of a problem and the actions necessary to eliminate it.

Adverse incidents rarely occur as a result of individual error alone. Factors contributing to the incident should be identified and an analysis report submitted.

Possible sources of risk identification

Local sources for identifying risk

- Incident report forms.
- Patient complaints.
- Audit results.

National sources for identifying risk

- NPSA alerts.
- Reports of national confidential enquiries.
- Care Quality Commission.

Possible contributory factors to a risk incident

- The patient.
- Individual staff.
- Communication.
- Team working (or not).
- Education and training of staff.
- Equipment and resources.
- Working conditions.

Risk analysis report

Will contain:

- Obvious outcomes that occurred.
- The chronology of events.
- The care management problems identified.
- A list of contributing factors.
- Recommended actions required.
- A timetable for implementation of recommendations.

Clinical risk management: risk reduction

Risk reduction

May be achieved by:
- Training.
- Introduction of guidelines.
- Increasing resources.

Risk elimination

May mean ceasing to provide a particular service.

Acceptance of risk

There is an acceptance that some risk cannot be reduced or eliminated. Hospitals attempt to keep litigation costs to a minimum by joining the Clinical Negligence Scheme for Trusts (CNST—see Box 24.1).

Dissemination of lessons learned

- *Local level:* sharing information with other units in the hospital.
- *National level:* through bodies such as the NPSA and Royal Colleges.
- Sharing information should include good practice points.

What risk management is not!

- 'Big brother.'
- A vehicle for individual blame or recrimination.
- An audit or research tool.
- A management policing policy (it is for everyone to learn from).
- Only designed to highlight bad care (good care should also be commended and fed back to staff, even if the outcome is poor or risk has occurred).
- A legal or negligence body.

Box 24.1 The Clinical Negligence Scheme for Trusts

- The CNST handles clinical negligence claims against member NHS bodies.
- Membership is voluntary, but currently all NHS and primary care trusts in England belong.
- The costs of the scheme are met by membership contributions:
  - the total projected claims cost are assessed in advance each year and contributions are determined for each trust (influenced by a range of factors including type of trust and specialties it provides)
  - discounts are available to trusts that achieve the relevant NHSLA risk management standards and to those with a good claims history.

When a claim is made against a member of the CNST, the body remains the legal defendant, but the NHSLA is responsible for handling the claim and associated costs.

Gynaecological imaging I

Gynaecological practice has changed enormously over last 20–30yrs principally due to improvements in pelvic imaging, particularly TVS.

Early pregnancy

USS is the imaging modality of choice for early pregnancy, allowing assessment of pregnancy location, viability, and gestational age. Table 16.1 summarizes the main diagnostic criteria used.

- In a normal intrauterine pregnancy, a gestational sac should be visible from 5wks gestation and fetal heart pulsations visible from 6wks using TVS.
- In the first trimester accurate dating is performed by measuring the CRL (optimum time is 8–12wks gestation).
- RCOG guidelines (2011) for the diagnosis of miscarriage. CRL ≥7mm with no FH and mean GS diameter ≥25mm.
- It should be possible to identify up to 90% of ectopic pregnancies on TVS.
- Other pathology may also be discovered, usually as an incidental finding, e.g. ovarian cysts.

Menstrual disorders

TVS can be used to reliably diagnose anatomical abnormalities such as:
- Endometrial polyps.
- Fibroids.
- Adenomyosis.

⚠ Other causes of bleeding disturbance, such as hormonal dysfunction, hormonal treatment, and infections, cannot be reliably established using imaging methods.
- TVS and saline infusion sonography allow assessment of endometrial pathology, such as polyps and submucous fibroids.
- USS and MRI have a similar ability to diagnose uterine fibroids, but MRI is superior to USS in determining the exact location, especially with a large uterus (>4 fibroids).

Postmenopausal bleeding

Approximately 10% of women with PMB will have gynaecological cancer, most of which is endometrial cancer.

A TVS examination with measurement of ET can discriminate between women at high and low risk.

Using a cut-off of an ET of 4mm:

- 96% of endometrial carcinomas can be identified using TVS.
- Endometrial cancer and hyperplasia can be suspected on TVS, but need a biopsy to confirm them histologically.
- If the ET is <4mm it is extremely unlikely that the woman has endometrial cancer—<1% (very high negative predictive value).
- Up to 55% of women with no disease will also have a positive result (much lower positive predictive value).
- Polyps may also be picked up as focal entities.
- Incidental ET measurements >4mm do not generally need further investigation in the absence of PMB.
- These ET measurements, in women before they are officially menopausal, cannot be used as their ET will vary depending upon cyclical activity.

Although the −ve predictive value is high for ET <4mm, in the presence of recurrent PMB the patient should have hysteroscopy.

Other methods for assessing the endometrium

- *Saline infusion sonography:*
    - infusion of saline into uterine cavity during scanning
    - allows assessment of focal endometrial lesions
    - agreement between saline infusion sonography and hysteroscopy is excellent.
- MRI may be indicated in the presence of fibroids if hysteroscopy is unhelpful.

Gynaecological imaging II

Pelvic pain

Acute pelvic pain
- USS is the diagnostic imaging method of choice.
- The following can reliably be diagnosed on TVS:
  - ovarian cysts
  - some sequelae of PID (including pyosalpinx and tubo-ovarian abscess)
  - hyrdosalpinges
  - fibroid degeneration.

▶ Colour Doppler may aid in adnexal torsion, but the findings are not specific enough and the diagnosis is usually made on clinical findings.

▶ Haemorrhagic ovarian cysts and ruptured ovarian cyst accidents have typical appearances on TVS.

Chronic pelvic pain
- Endometriosis may be diagnosed by the finding of endometriomas and occasionally by the visualization of endometriotic nodules elsewhere in the pelvis such as the rectovaginal septum, although these may be better visualized with MRI or rectal USS.
- Adenomyosis is associated with a thickening of the myometrium, uterine asymmetry, and with areas of both ↓ and ↑ echogenicity.
- The diagnostic accuracy of imaging to assess pelvic adhesions is uncertain.
- 'Soft markers' including immobile ovaries, site-specific tenderness, and loculated pelvic fluid may indicate pathology confirmed by laparoscopy.

Subfertility

USS is used in both the diagnosis and the management of infertility. It can be used to diagnose conditions such as polycystic ovarian disease and hydrosalpinx and to track follicular growth and rupture during normal and stimulated cycles during infertility treatment.
- Oocyte retrieval for assisted conception techniques is performed under USS guidance.
- Complications such OHSS can also be assessed by USS.
- HSG using radio-opaque dye and image intensification used to be the imaging method of choice to assess the uterine cavity and fallopian tubes:
  - has now been superseded by hysterosalpingo-contrast-sonography (HyCoSy) where a solution is infused into the uterine cavity whilst performing a TVS
  - combines a baseline TVS, assessment of the fallopian tubes and possibly even ovulation if the investigation is correctly timed.
- TVS is used to confirm viable or non-viable intrauterine pregnancy and indeed ectopic pregnancy as a result of IVF or other assisted reproduction techniques.

Gynaecological imaging III

Ovarian masses and gynaecological malignancy

- Experienced sonographers use pattern recognition to make a diagnosis.
- USS has been shown to be as good as or even superior to CT for the discrimination between different types of pelvic mass.
- When a pelvic mass is large and extending out of the pelvis a combined TVS and transabdominal scan (TAS) approach will ensure the whole mass is imaged.
- The following masses generally have characteristic sonographic appearances:
  - functional and luteal cysts
  - serous and mucinous cystadenomata
  - endometriomata
  - haemorrhagic cysts
  - teratomas (dermoids)
  - hydrosalpinges and para-ovarian cysts
  - tubo-ovarian abcess
  - 'typical' fibroids (when fibroids have undergone degeneration they can appear mixed solid/cystic and even have bizarre appearances—differentiation between fibroid and leiomyosarcoma cannot be made on TVS in these circumstances)
  - adhesional pockets of fluid.
- The following features are more suggestive of a malignant ovarian mass:
  - complex morphology—mixed solid/cystic appearance
  - large papillary cyst wall projections (>6mm)
  - thickened and irregular septations
  - ascites
  - evidence of peritoneal disease
  - highly vascularized solid elements or projections/septations.
- TVS or TAS can also be used to safely guide diagnostic ascitic taps or symptomatic drainage.
- MRI is superior to CT for discriminating between benign and malignant masses and may be better than USS due to a lower false positive rate.
- MRI can identify fat-containing fluid typical of dermoid cysts and blood typical of endometriomata due to their physical properties.
- Plain abdominal X-ray may occasionally give further information about pelvic mass:
  - fibroids may have become calcified
  - dermoid cysts may contain radio-opaque material (teeth or bone).
- MRI and CT are used in the imaging and staging and subsequent follow-up of gynaecological malignancies.
- A CXR is part of the routine assessment in cases of suspected malignancy (may show pleural effusions or metastases).

⚠ No single imaging modality can reliably distinguish between all benign and malignant masses even in the best hands.

Gynaecological imaging IV

Urogynaecology

- USS may be used to assess:
  - residual bladder volumes
  - the bladder neck in cases of incontinence.
- Urodynamic flow/pressure studies can be combined with the use of X-ray screening to gain additional information about the anatomy of the bladder and urethra (videocystourethography).
- Intravenous urography may be used to investigate continuous incontinence following childbirth, radiotherapy, or gynaecological surgery, which may be due to fistula formation between the ureters or bladder and the genital tract.
- 3D TVS is being used in some centres to aid in the diagnosis of pelvic floor dysfunction.

Other uses

- USS can be used to visualize intrauterine devices within the uterus:
  - lost IUDs may be located on plain abdominal X-ray
  - Mirenas® are radio-opaque.
- Ultrasound, HSG, and MRI can used to assess congenital abnormalities of the uterus.

Contrast studies of the renal tract (e.g. intravenous urography) should be considered when congenital malformations of the reproductive tract are diagnosed, as up to 40% are associated with abnormalities of the urinary tract.

Index

Common drugs: safety and usage in pregnancy and breast-feeding (Cont.)

Drug	Risk*	Conclude	Alternatives	Breast-feeding
Psychiatric medications				
Tricyclics	Largely safe	Use if high risk of relapse	Fluoxetine	Safe
SSRIs	Paroxetine teratogenic (3% risk) Others probably safe	Use if high risk of relapse (avoid paroxetine, fluoxetine best)	Fluoxetine	Safe
Lithium	Teratogenic (cardiac) (10% risk)	Use only if high risk of relapse	Difficult	Watch for toxicity
Neuroleptics	Possible very mild teratogenicity Largely unknown (avoid clozapine)	Usually continue because of risk of relapse	Difficult	Probably safe
Fundamentals: psychiatric disease is a major problem during/ after pregnancy so treatment may need to continue				
Antiepileptics				
Sodium valproate	Impaired childhood cognition Teratogenic (4–9% risk)	Minimize combinations	Carbamazepine N/A	Safe
Carbamazepine	Teratogenic (1–3% risk)	Consider change if <12 weeks	N/A	Safe
Lamotrigine	Teratogenic (1–5% risk)	Usually continue	N/A	Safe
		Usually continue		
Fundamentals: best sorted pre conceptually. Seizure control imperative, but minimize combinations and doses. High dose folic acid				
Other drugs				
Steroids (lung maturation: β– and dexamethasone)	Nil known with single course	Use if high risk for preterm delivery. Betamethasone best	N/A	N/A
Beta-agonists	Nil known at anti-asthmatic doses	Use if indicated, e.g. asthma	N/A	Safe
Ursodeoxycholic acid		Use if indicated, e.g. cholestasis	N/A	Not indicated

*Note background risk of congenital malformations 1–2%